Rare and Orphan Lung Diseases

Editors

ROBERT M. KOTLOFF
FRANCIS X. McCORMACK

CLINICS IN CHEST MEDICINE

www.chestmed.theclinics.com

September 2016 • Volume 37 • Number 3

ELSEVIER

1600 John F. Kennedy Boulevard • Suite 1800 • Philadelphia, Pennsylvania, 19103-2899

http://www.theclinics.com

CLINICS IN CHEST MEDICINE Volume 37, Number 3
September 2016 ISSN 0272-5231, ISBN-13: 978-0-323-46253-2

Editor: Patrick Manley
Developmental Editor: Casey Jackson

Clinics in Chest Medicine (ISSN 0272-5231) is published quarterly by Elsevier Inc., 360 Park Avenue South, New York, NY 10010-1710. Months of issue are March, June, September, and December. Periodicals postage paid at New York, NY and additional mailing offices. Subscription prices are $345.00 per year (domestic individuals), $621.00 per year (domestic institutions), $100.00 per year (domestic students/residents), $380.00 per year (Canadian individuals), $771.00 per year (Canadian institutions), $470.00 per year (international individuals), $771.00 per year (international institutions), and $230.00 per year (international and Canadian students/residents). International air speed delivery is included in all Clinics subscription prices. All prices are subject to change without notice. **POSTMASTER:** Send address changes to Clinics in Chest Medicine, Elsevier Health Sciences Division, Subscription Customer Service, 3251 Riverport Lane, Maryland Heights, MO 63043. **Customer Service: Telephone: 1-800-654-2452** (U.S. and Canada); **1-314-447-8871** (outside U.S. and Canada). **Fax: 1-314-447-8029. E-mail: journalscustomerservice-usa@elsevier.com (for print support); journalsonlinesupport-usa@elsevier.com (for online support).**

Reprints. For copies of 100 or more of articles in this publication, please contact the Commercial Reprints Department, Elsevier Inc., 360 Park Avenue South, New York, NY 10010-1710. Tel.: 212-633-3874; Fax: 212-633-3820; E-mail: reprints@elsevier.com.

Clinics in Chest Medicine is covered in *MEDLINE/PubMed (Index Medicus), Current Contents/Clinical Medicine, EMBASE/Excerpta Medica, Science Citation Index,* and *ISI/BIOMED.*

Contributors

EDITORS

ROBERT M. KOTLOFF, MD
Chair, Department of Pulmonary Medicine,
Cleveland Clinic; Professor of Medicine, Lerner
College of Medicine of Case Western Reserve
University, Cleveland, Ohio

FRANCIS X. McCORMACK, MD
Taylor Professor and Director, Division of
Pulmonary, Critical Care and Sleep Medicine,
Department of Internal Medicine, Cincinnati,
Ohio

AUTHORS

LAURIE L. CARR, MD
Assistant Professor of Medicine; Division of
Oncology, National Jewish Health, Denver,
Colorado

NEAL F. CHAISSON, MD
Staff Physician, Respiratory Institute,
Cleveland Clinic; Assistant Professor of
Medicine, Lerner College of Medicine of Case
Western Reserve University, Cleveland, Ohio

VINCENT COTTIN, MD, PhD
Department of Respiratory Diseases, Hospices
Civils de Lyon, Louis Pradel Hospital, National
Reference Center for Rare Pulmonary Diseases;
Professor of Respiratory Medicine, Univ Lyon,
Université Lyon I, INRA, UMR754, Lyon,
France

ERIN DeMARTINO, MD
Division of Pulmonary and Critical Care
Medicine, Mayo Clinic, Rochester,
Minnesota

GAIL H. DEUTSCH, MD
Associate Professor of Pathology; Seattle
Children's Hospital, University of Washington,
Seattle, Washington

MARK W. DODSON, MD, PhD
Fellow, Pulmonary Division, University of Utah,
Salt Lake City, Utah; Department of Medicine,
Intermountain Medical Center, Murray,
Utah

SOUHEIL EL-CHEMALY, MD, MPH
Assistant Professor, Division of Pulmonary and
Critical Care Medicine, Brigham and Women's
Hospital, Harvard Medical School, Boston,
Massachusetts

CHARLES GREGORY ELLIOTT, MD
Chairman, Department of Medicine,
Intermountain Medical Center, Murray, Utah;
Professor of Medicine, Pulmonary Division,
University of Utah, Salt Lake City, Utah

CAROL FARVER, MD
Director, Department of Anatomic Pathology,
Pathology and Laboratory Medicine Institute,
Cleveland Clinic; Professor of Pathology,
Cleveland Clinic Lerner College of Medicine of
Case Western Reserve University, Cleveland,
Ohio

ALEXANDRA F. FREEMAN, MD
Laboratory of Clinical Infectious Diseases,
NIAID, NHLBI, National Institutes of Health,
Bethesda, Maryland

RONALD S. GO, MD
Division of Hematology, Mayo Clinic,
Rochester, Minnesota

NISHANT GUPTA, MD
Division of Pulmonary, Critical Care and Sleep
Medicine, University of Cincinnati, Cincinnati,
Ohio

UMUR HATIPOĞLU, MD
Quality Improvement Officer, Respiratory
Institute, Cleveland Clinic Foundation,
Cleveland, Ohio

KRISTIN B. HIGHLAND, MD, MSCR, FCCP
Staff Physician, Department of Pulmonary
Medicine, Respiratory Institute, Cleveland
Clinic, Cleveland, Ohio

MAXIM ITKIN, MD, FSIR
Associate Professor of Radiology and
Pediatrics; Director of CHOP/HUP Center for
Lymphatic Imaging and Interventions,
Children's Hospital of Philadelphia, Penn
Medicine, Philadelphia, Pennsylvania

SIMON R. JOHNSON, BSc, MBBS, DM, FRCP
Division of Respiratory Medicine, National
Centre for Lymphangioleiomyomatosis,
University Hospitals NHS Trust, University of
Nottingham, Nottingham, United Kingdom

JEFFREY A. KERN, MD
Professor of Medicine; Division of Oncology,
National Jewish Health, Denver, Colorado

MICHAEL R. KNOWLES, MD
Department of Medicine, Marsico Lung
Institute/UNC CF Research Center, School of
Medicine, University of North Carolina at
Chapel Hill, Chapel Hill, North Carolina

ROBERT M. KOTLOFF, MD
Chair, Department of Pulmonary Medicine,
Cleveland Clinic; Professor of Medicine, Lerner
College of Medicine of Case Western Reserve
University, Cleveland, Ohio

MARGARET LEIGH, MD
Department of Pediatrics, Marsico Lung
Institute/UNC CF Research Center, School of
Medicine, University of North Carolina at
Chapel Hill, Chapel Hill, North Carolina

FRANCIS X. McCORMACK, MD
Taylor Professor and Director, Division of
Pulmonary, Critical Care and Sleep Medicine,
Department of Internal Medicine, Cincinnati,
Ohio

JOEL MOSS, MD, PhD
Deputy Chief, Cardiovascular and Pulmonary
Branch, National Heart, Lung, and Blood
Institute, National Institutes of Health,
Bethesda, Maryland

KENNETH N. OLIVIER, MD, MPH
Pulmonary Clinical Medicine Section,
Laboratory of Clinical Infectious Diseases,
NIAID, NHLBI, National Institutes of Health,
Bethesda, Maryland

GUSTAVO PACHECO-RODRIGUEZ, PhD
Staff Scientist, Cardiovascular and Pulmonary
Branch, National Heart, Lung, and Blood
Institute, National Institutes of Health,
Bethesda, Maryland

TANMAY S. PANCHABHAI, MD, FACP, FCCP
Staff Physician, Norton Thoracic Institute,
St. Joseph's Hospital and Medical Center;
Assistant Professor, Department of Medicine,
Creighton University School of Medicine,
Phoenix, Arizona

JOSEPH G. PARAMBIL, MD
Associate Professor of Medicine, Respiratory
Institute, Cleveland Clinic, Cleveland, Ohio

BRUCE K. RUBIN, MEngr, MD, MBA, FRCPC
The Jesse Ball DuPont Distinguished
Professor; Chair of Pediatrics; Physician in
Chief of the Children's Hospital of Richmond,
Virginia Commonwealth University, Richmond,
Virginia

JAY H. RYU, MD
Dr. David E. and Bette H. Dines Professor of
Pulmonary and Critical Care Medicine, Mayo
Clinic College of Medicine, Rochester,
Minnesota

ATSUSHI SAITO, MD, PhD
Department of Biochemistry and Department
of Respiratory Medicine and Allergology,
Sapporo Medical University, School of
Medicine, Sapporo, Japan

JAMES K. STOLLER, MD, MS
Professor and Chairman, Education Institute,
Cleveland Clinic; Jean Wall Bennett Professor
of Medicine, Cleveland Clinic Lerner College of
Medicine of Case Western Reserve University,
Cleveland, Ohio

BERNIE Y. SUNWOO, MBBS
Division of Pulmonary, Critical Care, Allergy
and Sleep Medicine, University of California,
San Francisco, California

TAKUJI SUZUKI, MD, PhD
Assistant Professor, Division of Pulmonary
Biology, Cincinnati Children's Hospital Medical
Center, Cincinnati, Ohio

ANGELO M. TAVEIRA-DASILVA, MD, PhD
Cardiovascular and Pulmonary Branch,
National Heart, Lung, and Blood Institute,
National Institutes of Health, Bethesda,
Maryland

BRUCE C. TRAPNELL, MD
Professor, Division of Pulmonary Biology,
Cincinnati Children's Hospital Medical Center,
Cincinnati, Ohio

ROBERT VASSALLO, MD
Division of Pulmonary and Critical Care
Medicine; Departments of Medicine,
Physiology and Biomedical Engineering,
Mayo Clinic, Rochester, Minnesota

EUNHEE S. YI, MD
Professor of Laboratory Medicine and
Pathology, Mayo Clinic College of Medicine,
Rochester, Minnesota

LISA R. YOUNG, MD
Associate Professor, Division of Pulmonary
Medicine and Allergy, Pulmonary, and
Critical Care, Departments of Pediatrics
and Medicine, Vanderbilt University
School of Medicine, Nashville,
Tennessee

MAIMOONA ZARIWALA, PhD
Department of Pathology and Laboratory
Medicine, Marsico Lung Institute/UNC CF
Research Center, School of Medicine,
University of North Carolina at Chapel Hill,
Chapel Hill, North Carolina

Contents

must be individualized. Pharmacologic treatment may include the use of chemotherapeutic agents. Smoking cessation is imperative in the management of pulmonary LCH.

Pulmonary alveolar proteinosis (PAP) is a rare syndrome characterized by the accumulation of surfactant in alveoli and terminal airways resulting in respiratory failure. PAP comprises part of a spectrum of disorders of surfactant homeostasis (clearance and production). The surfactant production disorders are caused by mutations in genes required for normal surfactant production. The PAP syndrome is identified based on history, radiologic, and bronchoalveolar lavage and/or histopathologic findings. The diagnosis of PAP-causing diseases in secondary PAP requires further studies. Whole-lung lavage is the current standard therapy and promising new pharmacologic therapies are in development.

Pulmonary alveolar microlithiasis (PAM) is a genetic lung disorder that is characterized by the accumulation of calcium phosphate deposits in the alveolar spaces of the lung. Mutations in the type II sodium phosphate cotransporter, NPT2b, have been reported in patients with PAM. PAM progresses gradually, often producing incremental dyspnea on exertion, desaturation in young adulthood, and respiratory insufficiency by late middle age. Treatment remains supportive, including supplemental oxygen therapy. For patients with end-stage disease, lung transplantation is available as a last resort. The recent development of a laboratory animal model has revealed several promising treatment approaches for future trials.

Primary ciliary dyskinesia (PCD) is a recessive genetically heterogeneous disorder of motile cilia with chronic otosinopulmonary disease and organ laterality defects in ~50% of cases. The prevalence of PCD is difficult to determine. Recent diagnostic advances through measurement of nasal nitric oxide and genetic testing has allowed rigorous diagnoses and determination of a robust clinical phenotype, which includes neonatal respiratory distress, daily nasal congestion, and wet cough starting early in life, along with organ laterality defects. There is early onset of lung disease in PCD with abnormal airflow mechanics and radiographic abnormalities detected in infancy and early childhood.

Lymphocytic interstitial pneumonia (LIP) is a rare lung disease on the spectrum of benign pulmonary lymphoproliferative disorders. LIP is frequently associated with connective tissue diseases or infections. Idiopathic LIP is rare; every attempt must be made to diagnose underlying conditions when LIP is diagnosed. Computed tomography of the chest in patients with LIP may reveal ground-glass opacities, centrilobular and subpleural nodules, and randomly distributed thin-walled cysts. Demonstrating polyclonality with immunohistochemistry is the key to differentiating

LIP from lymphoma. The 5-year mortality remains between 33% and 50% and is likely to vary based on the underlying disease process.

Birt-Hogg-Dubé Syndrome

Nishant Gupta, Bernie Y. Sunwoo, and Robert M. Kotloff

Birt-Hogg-Dubé syndrome (BHD) is a rare autosomal dominant disorder caused by mutations in the *Folliculin* gene and is characterized by the formation of fibrofolliculomas, early onset renal cancers, pulmonary cysts, and spontaneous pneumothoraces. The exact pathogenesis of tumor and lung cyst formation in BHD remains unclear. There is great phenotypic variability in the clinical features of BHD, and patients can present with any combination of skin, pulmonary, or renal findings. More than 80% of adult patients with BHD have pulmonary cysts on high-resolution computed tomography scan of the chest.

α_1-Antitrypsin Deficiency

Umur Hatipoğlu and James K. Stoller

α_1-Antitrypsin deficiency is an autosomal codominant condition that predisposes to emphysema and cirrhosis. The condition is common but grossly under-recognized. Identifying patients' α_1-antitrypsin deficiency has important management implications (ie, smoking cessation, genetic and occupational counseling, and specific treatment with the infusion of pooled human plasma α_1-antitrypsin). The weight of evidence suggests that augmentation therapy slows the progression of emphysema in individuals with severe α_1-antitrypsin deficiency.

Hermansky-Pudlak Syndrome

Souheil El-Chemaly and Lisa R. Young

Hermansky-Pudlak syndrome (HPS) is an autosomal recessive disorder that is associated with oculocutaneous albinism, bleeding diatheses, granulomatous colitis, and highly penetrant pulmonary fibrosis in some subtypes, including HPS-1, HPS-2, and HPS-4. HPS pulmonary fibrosis shows many of the clinical, radiologic, and histologic features found in idiopathic pulmonary fibrosis, but occurs at a younger age. Despite knowledge of the underlying genetic defects, there are currently no definitive therapeutic or preventive approaches for HPS pulmonary fibrosis other than lung transplant.

Hereditary Hemorrhagic Telangiectasia

Joseph G. Parambil

Hereditary hemorrhagic telangiectasia (HHT) is an underrecognized and under-diagnosed autosomal-dominant angiodysplasia that has an estimated prevalence of 1 in 5000 individuals, with variable clinical presentations even within family members with identical mutations. The most common manifestations are telangiectasias of the skin and nasal mucosa. However, HHT can often be complicated by the presence of arteriovenous malformations and telangiectasias in the lungs, brain, gastrointestinal tract, and liver that are often silent and can lead to life-threatening complications of stroke and hemorrhage. This article reviews HHT for the pulmonologist, who is not uncommonly the first practitioner to encounter these patients.

Diffuse Idiopathic Pulmonary Neuroendocrine Cell Hyperplasia and Neuroendocrine Hyperplasia of Infancy

Laurie L. Carr, Jeffrey A. Kern, and Gail H. Deutsch

Although incidental reactive pulmonary neuroendocrine cell hyperplasia (PNECH) is seen on biopsy specimens in adults with chronic lung disease, disorders characterized by marked PNECH are rare. Primary hyperplasia of neuroendocrine cells in the lung and obstructive lung disease related to remodeling or physiologic constriction of small airways define diffuse idiopathic neuroendocrine cell hyperplasia (DIPNECH) in the adult and neuroendocrine cell hyperplasia of infancy (NEHI) in children. DIPENCH and NEHI share a similar physiology, typical imaging appearance, and increased neuroendocrine cells on biopsy. However, there are important differences related to the underlying disease mechanisms leading to disparate outcomes.

Benign Metastasizing Leiomyoma

Gustavo Pacheco-Rodriguez, Angelo M. Taveira-DaSilva, and Joel Moss

Benign metastasizing leiomyoma (BML) is a rare and poorly characterized disease affecting primarily premenopausal women. Asymptomatic patients are often diagnosed incidentally by radiographs or other lung-imaging procedures performed for other indications, and the diagnosis is eventually confirmed by biopsy. Patients with BML are usually treated pharmacologically with antiestrogen therapies or surgically with oophorectomy or hysterectomy. Antiestrogen therapy is typically efficacious and, in general, most patients have a favorable prognosis. Asymptomatic patients with a confirmed diagnosis of BML, may be followed conservatively without treatment.

Index

PROGRAM OBJECTIVE
The goal of the *Clinics in Chest Medicine* is to provide practitioners with state-of-the-art information that is clinically useful, concise, well referenced, and comprehensive.

TARGET AUDIENCE
All practicing physicians and healthcare professionals who provide patient care utilizing findings from *Chest Medicine Clinics of North America*.

LEARNING OBJECTIVES
Upon completion of this activity, participants will be able to:
1. Review rare malignant and non-malignant disorders of the lung.
2. Discuss histiocytic and immunological lung diseases.
3. Recognize rare and orphan lung diseases such as Hermansky-Pudlak Syndrome, Birt-Hogg-Dubé Syndrome, and Primary Ciliary Dyskinesia, among others.

ACCREDITATION
The Elsevier Office of Continuing Medical Education (EOCME) is accredited by the Accreditation Council for Continuing Medical Education (ACCME) to provide continuing medical education for physicians.

The EOCME designates this enduring material for a maximum of 15 *AMA PRA Category 1 Credit*(s)™. Physicians should claim only the credit commensurate with the extent of their participation in the activity.

All other health care professionals requesting continuing education credit for this enduring material will be issued a certificate of participation.

DISCLOSURE OF CONFLICTS OF INTEREST
The EOCME assesses conflict of interest with its instructors, faculty, planners, and other individuals who are in a position to control the content of CME activities. All relevant conflicts of interest that are identified are thoroughly vetted by EOCME for fair balance, scientific objectivity, and patient care recommendations. EOCME is committed to providing its learners with CME activities that promote improvements or quality in healthcare and not a specific proprietary business or a commercial interest.

The planning committee, staff, authors and editors listed below have identified no financial relationships or relationships to products or devices they or their spouse/life partner have with commercial interest related to the content of this CME activity:
Laurie L. Carr, MD; Vincent Cottin, MD, PhD; Erin DeMartino, MD; Gail H. Deutsch, MD; Mark W. Dodson, MD, PhD; Souheil El-Chemaly, MD, MPH; Charles Gregory Elliot, MD; Rol Farver, MD; Anjali Fortna; Alexandra F. Freeman, MD; Ronald S. Go, MD; Nishant Gupta, MD; Umur Hatipoğlu, MD; Kristin B. Highland, MD, MSCR, FCCP; Maxim Itkin, MD, FSIR; Simon R. Johnson, BSc, MBBS, DM, FRCP; Michael R. Knowles, MD; Robert M. Kotloff, MD; Margaret Leigh, MD; Patrick Manley; Francis X. McCormack, MD; Joel Moss, MD, PhD; Palani Murugesan; Kenneth N. Olivier, MD, MPH; Gustavo Pacheco-Rodriguez, PhD; Tanmay S. Panchabhai, MD, FACP, FCCP; Joseph G. Parambil, MD; Jay H. Ryu, MD; Atsushi Saito, MD, PhD; Erin Scheckenbach; Bernie Y. Sunwoo, MBBS; Takuji Suzuki, MD, PhD; Angelo M. Taveira DaSilva, MD, PhD; Bruce C. Trapnell, MD; Robert Vassallo, MD; Eunhee S. Yi, MD; Lisa R. Young, MD; Maimoona Zariwala, PhD.

The planning committee, staff, authors and editors listed below have identified financial relationships or relationships to products or devices they or their spouse/life partner have with commercial interest related to the content of this CME activity:
Neal F. Chaisson, MD is a consultant/advisor for Actelion Pharmaceuticals US, Inc.
Jeffrey A. Kern, MD is a consultant/advisor for Strand Life Sciences Pvt Ltd and Uptake Medical.
Bruce K. Rubin, MEngr, MD, MBA, FRCPC has stock ownership in Koninklijke Philips N.V.; InspiRx, Boehringer Ingelheim GmbH; and Virginia Commonwealth University, has royalties/patents from Virginia Commonwealth University, and receives research support from Koninklijke Philips N.V.; InspiRx, and Boehringer Ingelheim GmbH.
James K. Stoller, MD, MS is a consultant/advisor for GRIFOLS USA, LLC; Baxalta Incorporated; Kamada; Arrowhead Pharmaceuticals, Inc; and CSL Behring, and has research support from CSL Behring.

UNAPPROVED/OFF-LABEL USE DISCLOSURE
The EOCME requires CME faculty to disclose to the participants:
1. When products or procedures being discussed are off-label, unlabelled, experimental, and/or investigational (not US Food and Drug Administration [FDA] approved); and
2. Any limitations on the information presented, such as data that are preliminary or that represent ongoing research, interim analyses, and/or unsupported opinions. Faculty may discuss information about pharmaceutical agents that is outside of FDA-approved labelling. This information is intended solely for CME and is not intended to promote off-label use of these medications. If you have any questions, contact the medical affairs department of the manufacturer for the most recent prescribing information.

TO ENROLL

To enroll in the *Chest Medicine Clinics* Continuing Medical Education program, call customer service at 1-800-654-2452 or sign up online at http://www.theclinics.com/home/cme. The CME program is available to subscribers for an additional annual fee of USD $225.

METHOD OF PARTICIPATION

In order to claim credit, participants must complete the following:

1. Complete enrolment as indicated above.
2. Read the activity.
3. Complete the CME Test and Evaluation. Participants must achieve a score of 70% on the test. All CME Tests and Evaluations must be completed online.

CME INQUIRIES/SPECIAL NEEDS

For all CME inquiries or special needs, please contact elsevierCME@elsevier.com.

CLINICS IN CHEST MEDICINE

THE CLINICS ARE AVAILABLE ONLINE!
Access your subscription at:
www.theclinics.com

Preface
Rare Lung Diseases: Occasionally the "Horse" Has Stripes

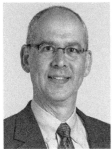

Robert M. Kotloff, MD   Francis X. McCormack, MD

Editors

When you hear hoofbeats, think of horses not zebras.

This oft-repeated adage, first offered by the sage diagnostician, Dr Theodore Woodward, cautions physicians to consider common rather than exotic entities when considering diagnostic possibilities. While a statistically sound principle, failure of the clinician to consider all possibilities runs the risk of incorrectly forcing a constellation of atypical features into a diagnosis of a common disorder. Those of us who specialize in rare pulmonary disorders witness these pitfalls in diagnosis, such as the patient with cystic lung disease labeled as emphysema, the patient with DIPNECH labeled as COPD, or the patient with benign metastasizing leiomyoma labeled as metastatic malignancy. Even a superficial familiarity with these unusual disorders might be sufficient to give a clinician pause before choosing the "horse" rather than the "zebra."

It is equally important to engage the scientific community in the study of rare pulmonary disorders as, in many cases, this provides the singular opportunity to approach disease pathogenesis from the vantage point of a primary molecular defect. Rapid progress is often possible, sometimes leading to discovery of new diseases, such as IgG4-related lung disease and pulmonary alveolar proteinosis due to GM-CSF receptor deficiencies, the genetic basis of old diseases such as EIF2AK4 in pulmonary veno-occlusive disease and pulmonary capillary hemangiomatosis, or novel treatments in record time, as with sirolimus in lymphangioleiomyomatosis or lymphatic interventions in plastic bronchitis.

In this issue, we review the genetic basis, cellular pathogenesis, and clinical presentation and management of uncommon pulmonary disorders, with a focus on the astounding progress made in the past decade. It is our hope that the reader will not only share in our fascination of the many unique features of these diseases but also appreciate the power of basic and translational research in providing insights into disease pathogenesis that ultimately can lead to development of effective therapeutics.

We would like to express our sincere gratitude to the authors who committed precious time to produce the scholarly works that comprise this issue. We would also like to thank Casey Jackson from Elsevier for orchestrating this effort and keeping everyone on task. Finally, we would like to

Clin Chest Med 37 (2016) xv–xvi
http://dx.doi.org/10.1016/j.ccm.2016.07.001
0272-5231/16/© 2016 Published by Elsevier Inc.

thank our wives, Debbie and Holly, who, despite our rare appearances at dinner and breakfast, support us unconditionally.

Robert M. Kotloff, MD
Cleveland Clinic
9500 Euclid Avenue, A90
Cleveland, OH 44195, USA

Francis X. McCormack, MD
MSB 6165
231 Albert Sabin Way
Cincinnati, OH 45267, USA

E-mail addresses:
kotlofr@ccf.org (R.M. Kotloff)
Frank.mccormack@uc.edu (F.X. McCormack)

Lymphangioleiomyomatosis

Simon R. Johnson, BSc, MBBS, DM, FRCP[a],*,
Angelo M. Taveira-DaSilva, MD, PhD[b], Joel Moss, MD, PhD[c]

KEYWORDS

- Cystic lung disease • Lymphatic disease • Angiomyolipoma • Pneumothorax • mTOR inhibitor

KEY POINTS

- Lymphangioleiomyomatosis (LAM) is a rare multisystem disease that almost exclusively affects women. It is categorized by lung cysts, lymphatic abnormalities, and angiomyolipomas.
- General management includes pulmonary rehabilitation, avoidance of estrogen-containing treatments, vaccinations against influenza and pneumococcus, and advice about complications and pregnancy if appropriate.
- Drug treatment may comprise bronchodilators if airflow obstruction is present and mammalian target of rapamycin (mTOR) inhibitors for those with progressive loss of lung function, chylous collections, or complex angiomyolipomas.
- Angiomyolipomas occur in half of those with sporadic LAM, almost all with tuberous sclerosis complex–LAM and should be screened for at diagnosis. Angiomyolipomas smaller than 3 cm can be followed by imaging with intervention considered for larger tumors.
- Those with advanced disease should be evaluated for the need for supplemental oxygen therapy, the presence of pulmonary hypertension, and for pulmonary transplantation if appropriate.

INTRODUCTION

Lymphangioleiomyomatosis (LAM) is a rare disease that affects between 5 to 9 million women.[1] Although men and children have been reported with LAM, this is highly unusual and LAM is one of the most sex-specific diseases described.[2–4] LAM affects the lungs, resulting in lung cysts, pneumothorax, and dyspnea. The lymphatics of the chest, abdomen, and pelvis are also affected, leading to lymphatic masses and chylous collections. Patients with LAM may also develop angiomyolipoma, a mixed mesenchymal tumor usually in the kidneys. LAM may occur sporadically, in the absence of other diseases but is common in adults with tuberous sclerosis complex (TSC). The natural history of LAM is highly variable but most women with LAM are at risk of pneumothorax, lose lung function at an accelerated rate, and develop progressive dyspnea, sometimes resulting in respiratory failure and death.

PATHOLOGIC EVALUATION
Histology

LAM lesions in the lungs are characterized by proliferation of neoplastic smooth muscle-like cells (LAM cells) in small clusters located on the edges of lung cysts and along blood vessels, lymphatics, and bronchioles.[5] LAM cell infiltrates cause airway obstruction, vascular wall thickening, disruption of lymphatic vessels, venous occlusion, and hemorrhage with hemosiderosis.[5–8] Nodular LAM lesions consist of spindle-shaped cells in the center and epithelioid cells at the periphery.[5] Enlargement of

Disclosure: The authors have nothing to disclose.
[a] Division of Respiratory Medicine, National Centre for Lymphangioleiomyomatosis, University Hospitals NHS Trust, University of Nottingham, Nottingham, NG7 2UH, UK; [b] Cardiovascular and Pulmonary Branch, National Institutes of Health, National Heart Lung and Blood Institute, Building 10, Room 6D05, Bethesda, MD 20814, USA; [c] Cardiovascular and Pulmonary Branch, National Institutes of Health, National Heart Lung and Blood Institute, Building 10, Room 6D03, Bethesda, MD 20814, USA
* Corresponding author.
E-mail address: simon.johnson@nottingham.ac.uk

Clin Chest Med 37 (2016) 389–403
http://dx.doi.org/10.1016/j.ccm.2016.04.002
0272-5231/16/$ – see front matter © 2016 Elsevier Inc. All rights reserved.

air spaces is associated with the proliferation of type II pneumocytes and destruction of elastin and collagen fibers in the walls of lung cysts.[5] Spindle and epithelioid LAM cells react with antibodies against smooth muscle antigens, for example, α-actin, vimentin, and desmin. The epithelioid cells also react with human melanin black (HMB)-45, an antibody that recognizes gp100, a premelanosomal protein.[5] Recently, non-neoplastic, actin-positive, fibroblast-like inflammatory cells have been identified in LAM nodules.[9,10] Lymphatic abnormalities are prominent in LAM, including cleft-like spaces in LAM nodules lined by lymphatic endothelial cells, which express vascular endothelial growth factor (VEGF)-3R and lymphangiogenic growth factors.[11,12] Extrapulmonary lymphangioleiomyomas are chyle-filled encapsulated masses of varying sizes, frequently located in the retroperitoneum, pelvis, and posterior mediastinum.[13] Lymphangioleiomyomas are lymphatics infiltrated by LAM cells arranged in fascicular, trabecular, and papillary patterns containing slit-like vascular channels.[5,6] Angiomyolipomas vary in size from a few millimeters to more than 20 cm in diameter[14,15] and are primarily located in the kidneys. Angiomyolipomas are characterized by proliferation of HMB-45 positive spindle cells, which express smooth muscle markers (LAM cells), poorly differentiated blood vessels, and adipocytes.[5,14]

Lymphangioleiomyomatosis Cell Biology

Several bioactive molecules with potential roles in disease progression are aberrantly expressed in LAM nodules. Estrogen and progesterone receptors are present in LAM cells and are thought to drive LAM cell proliferation and perhaps some of the sex specificity of LAM.[16,17] LAM cells express several chemokines and chemokine receptors potentially involved in LAM cell homing to the lung and lymphatics.[18,19] CD44v6, a transmembrane glycoprotein and adhesion molecule associated with metastatic behavior is also present.[20] Angiotensinogen, angiotensin II, renin, angiotensin-converting enzyme, and angiotensin I and II receptors are active in the microenvironment of LAM cells and serum, and may contribute to LAM cell proliferation and migration.[21,22] Erythropoietin receptors are present in LAM lung lesions[23] and an activated erythropoietin signaling pathway could lead to LAM cell proliferation.[23] LAM nodules express matrix metalloproteinase (MMP), MMP-2, MMP-9, MMP-1, MMP activators (MT1-MMP), and tissue inhibitors of metalloproteinases (TIMPs).[24–27] Serum MMP-9 is also elevated,[28] whereas serum levels of TIMP-3 are reduced.[29] MMPs have roles in remodeling, lymphangiogenesis, angiogenesis, cell migration, and metastasis.[24,25,30,31] Additionally, the serine proteases plasmin and plasminogen activator are elevated, whereas their inhibitor plasminogen activator inhibitor-1 is absent. Cathepsin K, a collagenase and elastase is also strongly expressed in LAM lesions.[32] These data suggest that a proteolytic environment may contribute to lung destruction in LAM.[25–29] It has been suggested that lung remodeling in LAM is a form of "frustrated" lymphangiogenesis that results in increased expression of MMP-2, MMP-9, and cathepsin-K mediated by VEGF-D and VEGF-C.[30–32]

Circulating Cells: Lymphangioleiomyomatosis as a Metastatic Neoplasm

The World Health Organization classified LAM as a low-grade malignant neoplasm. The National Cancer Institute lists it as a soft tissue neoplasm similar to leiomyomas and sarcomas.[33] Although LAM cells have a benign-appearing phenotype, they are able to metastasize and circulate in blood and lymph, appearing in chylous effusions and the urine of patients.[34–36] Furthermore, donor allografts can be invaded by the recipient's LAM cells.[37,38] The source of LAM cells is unknown but the potential primary sites include angiomyolipomas, uterine leiomyomas, and perivascular epithelioid cell tumors (**Fig. 1**).[12,31,39,40] LAM cells could enter the lumen of the lymphatic vessels and from there reach the systemic circulation and the lungs (see **Fig. 1**).

Tuberous Sclerosis Complex Genes and Mammalian Target of Rapamycin Activation

LAM cells in patients with TSC-LAM and sporadic LAM have mutations in the TSC genes, predominantly TSC-2.[41] The TSC1 and TSC2 genes[42,43] encode hamartin and tuberin proteins, respectively. Defective or deficient TSC1 or 2 activity causes accumulation of active Rheb-GTP and stimulation of mechanistic target of rapamycin (mTOR) complexes 1 and 2.[42,43] mTOR activation results in increased protein translation, proliferation, survival, and reduced autophagy.[42–46] These findings have led to the use of mTOR inhibitors in patients with LAM.

PRESENTATION AND DIAGNOSTIC STRATEGY
Presentation

Most LAM patients present with lung disease, predominantly dyspnea or pneumothorax. In the National Heart Lung and Blood Institute LAM registry approximately one-third of patients

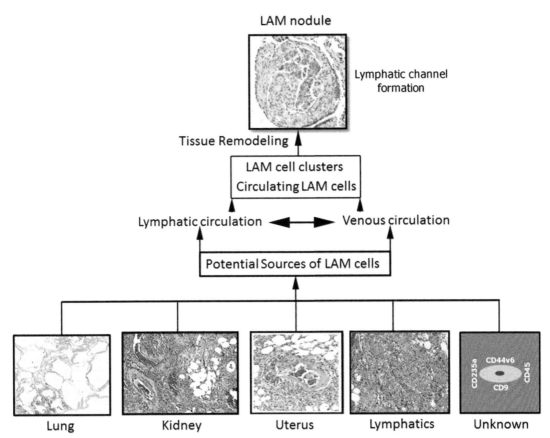

Fig. 1. The formation of the LAM nodule. The potential sources of LAM cells populating lung nodules could be neoplastic cells endogenous to the lung or from exogenous sources, including angiomyolipoma, uterus, or lymphatic system. Although the source of the LAM cells is unknown, disseminated LAM cells are found in blood, lymphatic lumen, chylous effusions, and urine. These cells of "unknown" origin have been mainly identified and characterized using density gradient and fluorescence-activated cell sorting (FACS) analysis with antibodies against cell surface antigens (CD44v6, CD9, CD45, CD235a). Other antigens (eg, erythropoietin receptor and syndecan 2) in cultured LAM cells have been identified. LAM cells may disseminate through the venous and lymphatic circulation or by interexchange between these routes. LAM cells or LAM cell clusters reaching the lung cause tissue remodeling and form the LAM lung nodule composed of spindle-shaped and epithelioid cells surrounded by hyperplastic type II pneumocytes. The LAM nodule is infiltrated with lymphatic channels, which are lined by cells reactive to D240 (podoplanin) antibodies and anti VEGFR-3 receptors.

presented with pneumothorax and one-third with dyspnea. One-quarter presented with other respiratory problems, including infections; hemoptysis; and, in patients with TSC identified by screening, the finding of lung cysts on computed tomography (CT) scan. The remaining 10% presented with extrapulmonary problems, including symptomatic angiomyolipoma (**Table 1**) and lymphangioleiomyomas.[47] Increasingly, patients are identified with early disease or without symptoms when undergoing CT scanning for unrelated problems. The chest radiograph is often normal in early disease but may reveal lung cysts, pneumothorax, or chylous effusions (**Fig. 2**). Most commonly, the possible diagnosis of LAM is first raised by the finding of lung cysts on a thoracic CT scan. The

findings of lung cysts are not specific for LAM, however, and emphysema, Birt-Hogg-Dubé (BHD) disease, Langerhans cell histiocytosis (LCH), Sjögren syndrome, lymphocytic interstitial pneumonitis (LIP), small airway disease with cystic change, type 1 neurofibromatosis, light chain deposition disease, and other diseases need to be considered in the differential.[48] Cysts in LAM tend to be round, very thin walled, and evenly distributed throughout all lung fields. They typically do not contain vessels or septations and do not occur in clusters (**Fig. 3**). Although these features may help distinguish LAM from other diseases, a definitive diagnosis cannot usually be made by thoracic CT alone.[49] Current diagnostic criteria from the European Respiratory Society require

Table 1
Demographic and clinical features of lymphangioleiomyomatosis patients followed at the National Heart, Lung, and Blood Institute

Demographics	All Patients	Sporadic LAM	TSC-LAM
Number of patients	554	460	94
Age of LAM diagnosis	40.4 ± 9.8	41.1 ± 9.4	36.4 ± 10.4[a]
Age, first symptom	36.4 ± 10	37.0 ± 9.9	33.2 ± 9.9[a]
Presenting Symptoms			
Dyspnea	353 (64%)	318 (69%)	35 (37%)
Pneumothorax	188 (34%)	150 (33%)	38 (40%)[b]
Hemoptysis	47 (9%)	44 (10%)	3 (3%)
Chylous effusions	43 (10%)	33 (7%)	10 (11%)
Abdominal, pelvic or back pain	67 (12%)	59 (13%)	8 (9%)
No respiratory symptoms	27 (5%)	8 (2%)	19 (19%)
Extrapulmonary Findings			
Lymphangioleiomyomas	189 (34%)	177 (38%)	12 (12.8%)[b]
Angiomyolipomas	280 (51%)	190 (41.3%)	90 (95.7%)[b]
Bilateral angiomyolipomas	141 (13.2%)	61 (13.2%)	80 (85.1%)[b]
Chylous effusions	106 (19%)	93 (20%)	13 (13.8%)

[a] *P*<.05. Significantly different from sporadic LAM.
[b] *P*<.01. Significantly different from sporadic LAM.

additional supportive features or a lung biopsy to make a definitive diagnosis of LAM.[50] Cases without these additional features and in the absence of a lung biopsy are classified as probable LAM if the chest CT is entirely consistent with LAM, or possible LAM when the chest CT is compatible but not entirely consistent with LAM (**Box 1**).[50]

Diagnostic Strategy

To make a clinically confident diagnosis in the least invasive manner when LAM is suspected, a stepwise approach is suggested (**Fig. 4**). A careful clinical examination should be made for cutaneous signs of TSC (facial angiofibromas, shagreen patch, periungual fibromas, retinal astrocytoma), BHD disease (facial acrochordons and trichodiscomas), and

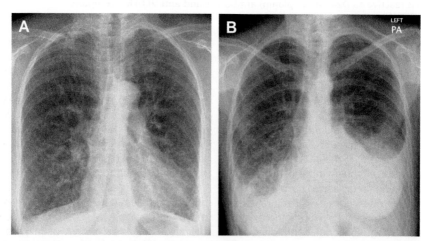

Fig. 2. Chest radiographs in LAM. (*A*) Characteristic radiograph findings of LAM with hyperexpanded lung fields and interstitial changes. (*B*) Patient with advanced LAM and bilateral chylous pleural effusions.

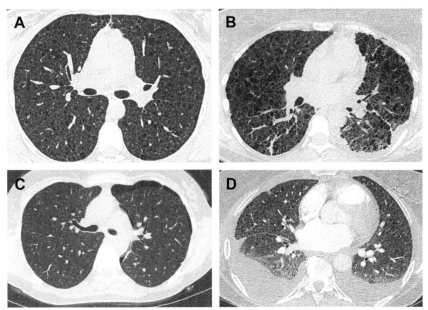

Fig. 3. Chest CT findings. (*A*) Characteristic appearances of LAM on CT with diffusely distributed round cysts and normal intervening lung parenchyma. (*B*) Patient with advanced disease and marked left sided pleural reaction following pleural surgery. (*C*) Patient with mild LAM and left sided pneumothorax. (*D*) Patient with LAM and bilateral chylous effusions.

connective tissue disease–related LIP (mechanic's hands and Raynaud phenomenon). A CT or MRI scan of the abdomen will identify angiomyolipoma in half of patients with LAM. Angiomyolipoma tend to have a characteristic radiological appearance as a heterogeneous lesion containing fat. A biopsy is not normally required, although renal masses without fat visible on CT may require biopsy to differentiate them from a renal carcinoma (**Fig. 5**). A further 25% to 30% of patients with LAM will have lymphatic abnormalities (lymphadenopathy, lymphangioleiomyomas, or chylous ascites) visible on the abdominal CT (**Fig. 6**). The presence of TSC or angiomyolipoma makes the diagnosis of LAM secure and, using this approach alone, a definite diagnosis can be made in two-thirds of women with LAM.[22]

Most women with LAM, particularly those with lymphatic abnormalities, have elevated levels of serum VEGF-D.[51] The finding of a serum VEGF-D level greater than 800 pg/mL can differentiate between LAM and other cystic lung diseases, including BHD, LIP, LCH, and emphysema, and reduce the need for a lung biopsy.[22,52,53]

In cases in which a diagnosis cannot be made noninvasively, a lung biopsy is usually required to make definite diagnosis. A definite diagnosis may not be required in a patient with few or no symptoms and a low risk of disease progression. In those with advanced disease and impaired lung function, a biopsy may carry a high risk and the risk and benefits of the procedure should be carefully considered. In general, however, a definitive diagnosis is required in patients being considered for long-term therapy with mTOR inhibitors. The most common diagnostic procedure is video-assisted thorascopic biopsy. A histologic diagnosis is often possible on morphologic grounds alone, although LAM cells may be sparse in early disease and immunostaining with α-smooth muscle actin, HMB-45, estrogen receptor, and progesterone receptor may be required to identify LAM cells.[5,54] Combining transbronchial biopsy with immunostaining is less invasive and is sufficient for diagnosis in 40% to 60% of cases.[55,56] Cryobiopsy and endobronchial ultrasound are new diagnostic techniques that may improve the yield of bronchoscopic approaches.[57]

MANAGEMENT AND DISEASE COURSE
Initial Assessment and Prognosis

When the diagnosis has been made, patients should undergo pulmonary function studies, including measurement of spirometry, lung volumes, and diffusion capacity. Exercise testing in the form of a 6-minute walk test or a cardiopulmonary exercise test should also be performed because gas exchange abnormalities during exercise are frequent in LAM (**Table 2**).[58,59] The clinical

---

Box 1
European Respiratory Society diagnostic criteria for lymphangioleiomyomatosis

Definite LAM

- Characteristic or compatible lung HRCT and lung biopsy fitting the pathologic criteria for LAM[a]
  Or

- Characteristic lung HRCT and any of the following

  ○ Angiomyolipoma (kidney)

  ○ Thoracic or abdominal chylous effusion

  ○ Lymphangioleiomyoma or lymph-node involved by LAM

  ○ TSC

Probable LAM

- Characteristic HRCT and compatible clinical history
  Or

- Compatible HRCT and any of the following

  ○ Angiomyolipoma (kidney)

  ○ Thoracic or abdominal chylous effusion

Possible LAM

- Characteristic or compatible HRCT

  ○ Pathologic samples from patients with suspected LAM should be examined by a pathologist experienced in LAM.

  ○ LAM should be considered when there is a variable predominance of cysts, multifocal, nodular proliferating immature smooth muscle, and perivascular epithelioid cells.

  ○ Immunohistochemistry for α-smooth muscle actin and HMB-45 should be performed especially if morphologic features do not allow a secure diagnosis to be made. Estrogen and progesterone receptor staining may be an adjunct to diagnosis.

[a] Pathologic criteria for diagnosis of LAM.

Johnson SR, Cordier JF, Lazor R, et al. European Respiratory Society guidelines for the diagnosis and management of lymphangioleiomyomatosis. Eur Respir J 2010;35:14–26.

---

manifestations and the rate of progression of lung disease is highly variable between individuals. Mean loss of lung function varies from 70 to 140 mL/y for loss of forced expiratory volume in 1 second (FEV_1).[60–64] Ten years from presentation, approximately 50% of patients will have Medical Research Council grade 3 dyspnea and have to stop walking on flat ground at a normal pace, whereas approximately 10% will have grade 5 dyspnea and be too breathless to leave the house.[65] Although no one factor can predict prognosis, a combination of clinical features, lung function, and VEGF-D levels provide a means to grade disease severity, to predict rate of decline and response to therapy, and to advise patients regarding prognosis (**Table 3**).[66]

General Principles of Management

Patients should be told that LAM, in most of those affected, is a chronic disease with an estimated median transplant-free survival from the time of diagnosis of 23 years.[67] Therefore, as much as possible, patients with the disease should lead a normal life with a healthy lifestyle. They should be encouraged to lose excess weight, engage in physical activities, and exercise regularly. The 2 major limiting factors in carrying out activities of daily living are dyspnea on exertion and fatigue.[68] Anecdotal reports suggest that pulmonary rehabilitation is beneficial. Levels of exercise should be limited only by the severity of lung disease. Use of supplemental oxygen during exercise can be best assessed by enrollment in a rehabilitation program. Sports involving physical contact and martial arts should be avoided because of the potential for trauma-induced bleeding in patients who have larger angiomyolipomas. Because of potential risks of estrogens in the pathogenesis of LAM, patients should be advised against using estrogen-containing contraceptives.[69–71] Patients should receive vaccination against influenza and

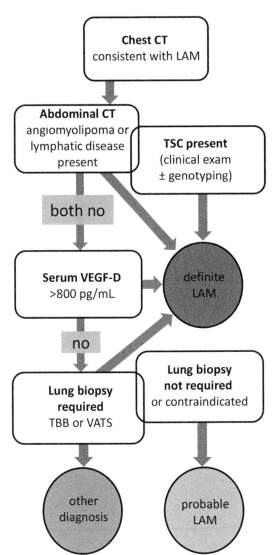

Fig. 4. Diagnostic strategy for patients with suspected LAM. A full clinical examination should be conducted for signs of TSC and other cystic lung diseases, including cutaneous stigmata of BHD syndrome and connective tissue disease. An abdominal CT scan should be performed. If TSC, an angiomyolipoma, or lymphatic disease is found, or if serum VEGF-D is greater than 800 pg/mL, no further tests are required to make the diagnosis. If these criteria are not met, then either a transbronchial or video-assisted thoracic surgery (VATS) biopsy is required to make a definite diagnosis. If the CT is characteristic but neither clinical criteria nor pathologic analysis are definitive, the diagnosis of probable LAM is made.

pneumococcal pneumonia, and should be advised of the risk of pneumothorax and, if appropriate, angiomyolipoma bleeding. Patient groups are an excellent source of patient-specific support and on-line communities are accessible to those with all levels of disability.

Pregnancy and Contraception

Pneumothorax, chylous effusions, worsening of respiratory symptoms, hemorrhage of angiomyolipomas, and premature births are over-represented during pregnancy in women with LAM.[72–74] Pregnancy should be discouraged in patients with severe disease or those in whom lung function is declining rapidly. Patients with mild disease who wish to become pregnant should be informed about the potential risks. With close medical and obstetric supervision, some women with LAM have tolerated pregnancy without apparent short-term or long-term sequela. Estrogen-based contraceptives are contraindicated in LAM. For women who wish to avoid pregnancy, progesterone-based oral contraceptives or low-dose, drug-eluting, intrauterine or cervical devices are recommended.

Tuberous Sclerosis–Related Clinical Problems

Screening women with TSC for LAM using CT scanning has revealed that approximately 20% of women at 18 years and up to 80% at 40 years have lung cysts consistent with LAM. Lung cysts are also seen in approximately 10% of men with TSC, although these men and many women with TSC-LAM remain asymptomatic.[3] Although most patients with TSC-LAM have clinical problems distinct from LAM, such as seizures, cognitive impairment, or behavioral disorders, women with TSC may have LAM as their most significant clinical manifestation.[75] LAM is a major cause of death in adult women with TSC.[75,76] These patients commonly also have multiple angiomyolipomas and other renal manifestations, including adult polycystic kidney disease associated with the TSC-2 contiguous gene syndrome.[77] Cerebral involvement may cause epilepsy, learning difficulties, autism, and obsessive-compulsive disorder, and there may be skin lesions, including facial angiofibromas, which may require treatment for cosmetic reasons.

Bronchodilators

Approximately 25% to 30% of LAM patients have a significant bronchodilator response either to β-adrenergic or anticholinergic agents.[74,78] In those with airflow obstruction who respond to bronchodilators, use of short-acting bronchodilators is recommended during exacerbations associated with upper respiratory infections, before exercise, or every 6 hours as recommended for other obstructive lung diseases. Treatment with long-acting β-adrenergic or anticholinergic agents

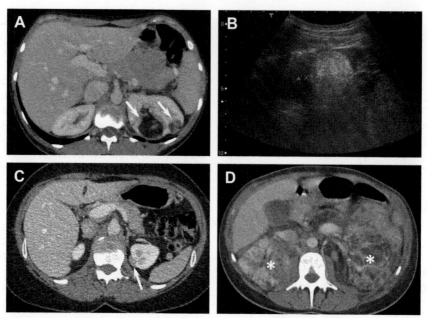

Fig. 5. CT appearances of angiomyolipoma. (*A*) Classic appearances of renal angiomyolipoma showing 2 hetero-geneous fat-containing tumors in the left kidney (*arrows*). (*B*) Characteristic echogenic ultrasound appearance of the same 4 cm angiomyolipoma shown in (*A*). (*C*) Small fat-poor angiomyolipoma at medial border of the left kidney (*arrow*). (*D*) Bilateral complex angiomyolipomas massively enlarging both kidneys in a patient with TSC (*asterisks*).

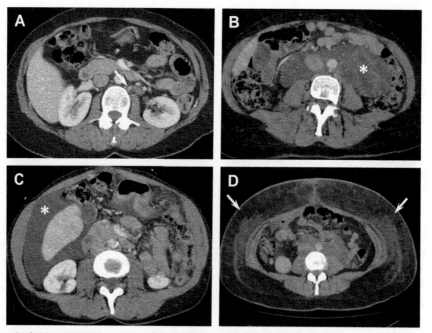

Fig. 6. Abdominal CT appearances. (*A*) Subtle retroperitoneal lymphatic disease (*arrow*). (*B*) Large complex abdominal lymphangioleiomyomas in a patient with no abdominal symptoms and only mild lung disease (*asterisk*). (*C*) Abdominal CT showing chylous ascites (*asterisk*). (*D*) CT showing chylous infiltration of the subcu-taneous fat in a patient with TSC and advanced LAM (*arrows*).

Table 2
Pulmonary function abnormalities in lymphangioleiomyomatosis

	All Patients	Sporadic LAM	TSC-LAM
Number of patients	554	460	94
Reduced FEV_1 and FEV_1/FVC	48%	51%	33%
Reduced DL_{CO}	58%	61%	40%
Reduced FEV_1 and DL_{CO}	40%	42%	27%
No air flow obstruction or diffusion impairment	29%	27%	43%

Abbreviations: DL_{CO}, diffusing capacity of lung for carbon monoxide; FEV_1, forced expiratory volume in 1 second; FVC, forced vital capacity.

may be considered in patients who consistently respond to short-acting bronchodilators.

Mammalian Target of Rapamycin Activation Inhibitors

The identification of somatic mutations in TSC-2 in LAM nodules,[41] the subsequent identification that the TSC-2 protein inhibits mTOR,[79] and the existence of a licensed inhibitor targeting mTOR lead to rapid translation of mTOR inhibitors to patients with LAM. Initial studies demonstrated that mTOR inhibition was associated with reduction in the volume of LAM and TSC associated angiomyolipomas.[80,81] A randomized placebo controlled trial of sirolimus (rapamycin) in patients with moderate LAM showed a significant reduction in loss of lung function from a reduction in FEV_1 of 134 mL/y in the placebo group to plus 19 mL/y in the treatment group. There were also improvements in forced vital capacity, quality of life, and functional performance. After discontinuation of sirolimus, loss of lung function resumed.[63] In an open-label study of 26 weeks of

everolimus treatment, similar improvements were seen in FEV_1 and also in the 6-minute walk distance.[82] Sirolimus has also shown efficacy in patients with lymphatic disease. In a case series and several case reports, there were improvements in lymphangioleiomyoma volume and thoracic and abdominal chylous effusions.[83] Presumably due to an effect on lymphatic remodeling, the full benefit took up to 12 months to achieve in some subjects. In those with TSC, which shares a common genetic basis with LAM, sirolimus also reduced the volume of subependymal giant cell astrocytomas[84] and improved the size and appearance of facial angiofibromas.[85]

Currently, sirolimus is approved by the US Food and Drug Administration (FDA) and the Japanese Pharmaceutical and Medical Devices Agency for LAM. Everolimus is approved by the FDA and European Medicines Agency for treatment of angiomyolipoma in TSC. Because the effect of mTOR inhibitors in LAM is suppressive, with lung function decline and angiomyolipoma growth recurring after cessation of therapy, treatment is usually

Table 3
Prognostic indicators in patients with lymphangioleiomyomatosis

Prognostic Factor	Association	Setting
Elevated serum VEGF-D	Increased loss of FEV_1	Prospective study[66]
Postmenopausal	Reduced loss of FEV_1	Retrospective studies[60,62]
Presentation with pneumothorax	Reduced loss of lung function	Retrospective studies[106]
Low K_{CO} at presentation	Increased loss of FEV_1	Retrospective study[107]
Positive bronchodilator response	Increased loss of FEV_1	Prospective cohort[78]
Higher LAM histology score	Worse survival	Prospective cohort[6]
Elevated serum osteopontin	Increased loss of FEV_1 and DL_{CO}	Prospective cohort[20]
Genotype in TSC-LAM	More severe LAM in TSC-2 vs TSC-1	Retrospective cohort[108]

Abbreviation: K_{CO}, carbon monoxide transfer coefficient.

indefinite. Because the LAM phenotype is variable and not all patients have progressive disease, mTOR inhibitors should be reserved for those with progressive loss of lung function, symptomatic chylous complications, or problematic angiomyolipomas. In initial studies, treatment was titrated to a serum trough level of 5 to 15 ng/mL, although similar efficacy and fewer side effects have been reported using serum levels of 3 to 5 ng/ml.[63,86] Side effects are common and include aphthous ulcers, diarrhea, edema, rashes, and nausea. Sirolimus pneumonitis seems less common in those treated for LAM than for other indications, such as renal transplant or cancer[87]; however, it was recently reported in 5% of subjects in a trial of long-term sirolimus in Japan.[86] Longer term treatment of up to 8 years seems safe and efficacious with side effects tending to reduce with duration of treatment.[88]

Pneumothorax

Pneumothorax occurs at some point in the disease in approximately 70% of women with LAM, often requires surgical treatment, and frequently recurs.[89,90] Conservative treatment, including aspiration and chest tube drainage, is associated with a greater than 60% recurrence rate in studies; whereas surgical treatments, including pleurodesis, abrasion, and pleurectomy, are associated with much lower recurrence rates.[89,90] Pneumothorax is a source of significant morbidity for patients and for these reasons the European Respiratory Society LAM guidelines and the LAM Foundation Pleural Disease Consensus Group recommended chemical pleurodesis and surgical intervention, respectively, at first pneumothorax for women with LAM.[50,90]

Chylous Complications

Lymphatic occlusion can result in chylous leaks from the thoracic duct, causing pleural effusions, or from the abdominal lymphatics, causing ascites. Enlargement of lymphatic tissue is commonly visible on CT scan, including thickening of the thoracic duct, retroperitoneal, abdominal, and pelvic lymphadenopathy in approximately 30% of patients. Larger cystic lymphatic collections, called lymphangioleiomyomas, are present in the abdomen or pelvis in 30% of sporadic LAM patients and 10% of TSC LAM patients[13,91] (see **Fig. 6**). Although lymphadenopathy tends to be asymptomatic, lymphangioleiomyomas may cause pressure symptoms on the bowel and bladder or bloating and abdominal distention that is worse in the later parts of the day, and often wrongly attributed to irritable bowel syndrome.

Chylous collections tend to be associated with more advanced disease, with pleural effusions causing dyspnea and ascites causing abdominal swelling. Rarely, chylous stasis at other sites can lead to chyloptysis, lymphedema, pericardial effusions, and chyluria.[53] If chylous effusions are causing significant dyspnea, paracentesis may provide the diagnosis and result in transient symptomatic improvement. Previously pleural surgery, including pleurodesis, pleurectomy, and thoracic duct ligation, has been used to control chylous pleural effusion, albeit with mixed results.[92] Surgical resection of abdominal or pelvic lymphatic masses may result in prolonged chylous leakage and should generally be avoided. In expert centers, imaging of lymphatic abnormalities and minimally invasive lymphatic embolization has been successful in isolated cases.[93] Recent series have shown that use of mTOR inhibitors for symptomatic abdominal and thoracic chylous complications can be highly effective, reducing the need for repeated abdominal or thoracic taps, and reducing the size of abdominal masses.[83,86]

Angiomyolipomas

Although angiomyolipomas have been reported at multiple sites, most of these tumors occur in the kidneys and occasionally the liver. Angiomyolipoma occur in about 50% of patients with sporadic LAM and most of those with TSC-LAM.[94,95] Tumors vary in size from millimeters to many centimeters and may be present unilaterally or bilaterally. Multiple, bilateral, large tumors are more frequent in TSC-LAM than sporadic LAM[95] (see **Fig. 5**). Most angiomyolipomas are asymptomatic; however, larger lesions are prone to spontaneous bleeding and may present with hematuria or symptoms of retroperitoneal hemorrhage. Potential loss of renal function as a consequence of diffuse infiltration or acute hemorrhage mandates that these tumors should be detected early in the disease course and that all women with LAM should have cross-sectional imaging at diagnosis.[50] Management is aimed at preventing renal hemorrhage. Because only large tumors are associated with bleeding, smaller lesions can be safely observed with serial imaging every 1 to 2 years.[94,96] Risk factors for angiomyolipoma hemorrhage include increasing tumor size and the presence of aneurysmal blood vessels.[97] Hemorrhage is extremely rare in tumors less than 3 cm but increases significantly in those greater than 4 cm. Larger tumors should be imaged with MRI scanning to delineate their vascular supply with a view to intervention, including selective embolization of tumor vasculature or nephron-sparing surgery. Recently, mTOR inhibitors have been shown to reduce the size of angiomyolipomas.[80,98,99] Although no studies have been specifically powered to determine the effect of mTOR inhibition on angiomyolipomas-related hemorrhage, the recent tuberous sclerosis guidelines suggest that mTOR inhibitor therapy, rather than other treatment modalities, is first-line treatment of patients with angiomyolipomas in tuberous sclerosis that are enlarging and are greater than 3 cm.[100]

Meningioma

Meningioma occurs in up to 2% of patients with LAM, a figure that far exceeds that expected in an age-matched general population.[101] Although frequently asymptomatic, meningiomas may present with symptoms of a space-occupying lesion or epilepsy.[101] LAM patients with cerebral symptoms should have brain imaging to exclude meningioma.

Advanced Disease

LAM patients with progressive lung disease may develop respiratory failure and related complications, including susceptibility to respiratory infections, hypoxemia, and pulmonary hypertension. Respiratory infections should be treated aggressively with attention paid to colonization by resistant organisms. Hypoxemia on exertion is common, even in those with early disease,[59] and patients with advanced disease may require oxygen at rest, with sleep, and with ambulation. Pulmonary hypertension can result from chronic hypoxia as well as from LAM cell infiltration of the pulmonary vasculature.[102] Pulmonary hypertension should be screened for in patients with advanced disease and those with hypoxemia and dyspnea disproportionate to their lung function impairment.

Pulmonary transplantation can be considered in LAM patients with advanced disease. The outcome for those with LAM is at least as good for those with other pulmonary indications. LAM-specific comorbidities, particularly chylous accumulations and angiomyolipomas, should be optimally treated to prevent post-transplant complications.[50,103] Previous pleural surgery is associated with longer operative times and increased perioperative hemorrhage but is not associated with increased post-transplant mortality and is regarded as a relative contraindication.[104,105]

SUMMARY

LAM is a rare multisystem disease that predominantly affects women. The disease is categorized by lung cysts, lymphatic abnormalities, and angiomyolipomas. Patients develop airflow obstruction and abnormalities of gas exchange that progress at a variable rate and may be complicated by pneumothorax, chylous collections of the thorax and abdomen, and angiomyolipoma hemorrhage. The diagnosis of LAM is made by a combination chest CT scan, the presence of angiomyolipoma, lymphatic abnormalities, and, if required, serum VEGF-D, lung biopsy, and testing for TSC. Baseline assessment should comprise abdominal imaging, full pulmonary function testing, exercise testing, and exclusion of tuberous sclerosis. General management includes pulmonary rehabilitation, avoidance of estrogen-containing treatments, vaccinations against influenza and pneumococcus, and advice about complications and pregnancy if appropriate. Drug treatment should include bronchodilators when airflow obstruction is present and mTOR inhibitors for those with progressive loss of lung function, chylous collections, or large angiomyolipomas. Pneumothorax is common and should be treated early and definitively to prevent recurrence. Patients with angiomyolipomas should be screened for LAM at diagnosis because these occur in half of patients with sporadic LAM and almost all with TSC-LAM. Those with tumors less than 3 cm can be followed by serial imaging and intervention should be considered for larger tumors. LAM patients with advanced disease should be evaluated for the need for supplemental oxygen therapy, the presence of pulmonary hypertension, and for pulmonary transplantation, if appropriate.

REFERENCES

1. Harknett EC, Chang WYC, Byrnes S, et al. Regional and National variability suggests underestimation of prevalence of lymphangioleiomyomatosis. Q J Med 2011;104:971–9.
2. Aubry MC, Myers JL, Ryu JH, et al. Pulmonary lymphangioleiomyomatosis in a man. Am J Respir Crit Care Med 2000;162:749–52.
3. Adriaensen ME, Schaefer-Prokop CM, Duyndam DAC, et al. Radiological evidence of lymphangioleiomyomatosis in female and male patients with tuberous sclerosis complex. Clin Radiol 2011;66:625–8.
4. Schiavina M, Di Scioscio V, Contini P, et al. Pulmonary lymphangioleiomyomatosis in a karyotypically normal man without tuberous sclerosis complex. Am J Respir Crit Care Med 2007;176:96–8.
5. Ferrans VJ, Yu ZX, Nelson WK, et al. Lymphangioleiomyomatosis (LAM): a review of clinical and

morphological features. J Nippon Med Sch 2000; 67:311–29.

6. Matsui K, Beasley MB, Nelson WK, et al. Prognostic significance of pulmonary lymphangioleiomyomatosis histologic score. Am J Surg Pathol 2001;25:479–84.

7. Corrin B, Liebow AA, Friedman PJ. Pulmonary lymphangioleiomyomatosis. Am J Pathol 1975;79: 348–82.

8. Carrington CB, Cugell DW, Gaensler EA, et al. Lymphangioleiomyomatosis. Physiologic-pathologic-radiologic correlations. Am Rev Respir Dis 1977; 116:977–95.

9. Clements D, Dongre A, Krymskyaya V, et al. Wild type mesenchymal cells contribute to the lung pathology of lymphangioleiomyomatosis. PLoS One 2015;10(5):e0126025.

10. Atochina-Vasserman EN, Guo C-J, Abramova E, et al. Surfactant dysfunction and lung inflammation in the female mouse model of lymphangioleiomyomatosis. Am J Respir Cell Mol Biol 2014;53:96–104.

11. Kumasaka T, Seyama K, Mitani K, et al. Lymphangiogenesis in lymphangioleiomyomatosis: its implication in the progression of lymphangioleiomyomatosis. Am J Surg Pathol 2004;28:1007–16.

12. Mitani K, Kumasaka T, Takemura H, et al. Cytologic, immunocytochemical and ultrastructural characterization of lymphangioleiomyomatosis cell clusters in chylous effusions of patients with lymphangioleiomyomatosis. Acta Cytol 2009;53:402–9.

13. Avila NA, Dwyer AJ, Rabel A, et al. Sporadic lymphangioleiomyomatosis and tuberous sclerosis complex with lymphangioleiomyomatosis: comparison of CT features. Radiology 2006;242: 277–85.

14. Matsui K, Tatsuguchi A, Valencia J, et al. Extrapulmonary lymphangioleiomyomatosis (LAM): clinico-pathologic features in 22 cases [Review] [21 refs]. Hum Pathol 2000;31:1242–8.

15. Avila NA, Kelly JA, Chu SC, et al. Lymphangioleiomyomatosis: abdominopelvic CT and US findings. Radiology 2000;216:147–53.

16. Matsui K, Takeda K, Yu ZX, et al. Downregulation of estrogen and progesterone receptors in the abnormal smooth muscle cells in pulmonary lymphangioleiomyomatosis following therapy. An immunohistochemical study. Am J Respir Crit Care Med 2000;161:1002–9.

17. Gu X, Yu JJ, Ilter D, et al. Integration of mTOR and estrogen–ERK2 signaling in lymphangioleiomyomatosis pathogenesis. Proc Natl Acad Sci U S A 2013;110:14960–5.

18. Pacheco-Rodriguez G, Kumaki F, Steagall WK, et al. Chemokine-enhanced chemotaxis of lymphangioleiomyomatosis cells with mutations in the tumor suppressor TSC2 gene. J Immunol 2009; 182:1270–7.

19. Clements D, Markwick LJ, Puri N, et al. Role of the CXCR4/CXCL12 Axis in lymphangioleiomyomatosis and angiomyolipoma. J Immunol 2010;185: 1812–21.

20. Pacheco-Rodriguez G, Steagall WK, Crooks DM, et al. TSC2 loss in lymphangioleiomyomatosis cells correlated with expression of CD44v6, a molecular determinant of metastasis. Cancer Res 2007;67: 10573–81.

21. Valencia JC, Pacheco-Rodriguez G, Carmona AK, et al. Tissue-specific renin-angiotensin system in pulmonary lymphangioleiomyomatosis. Am J Respir Cell Mol Biol 2006;35:40–7.

22. Chang W, Cane JL, Blakey J, et al. Clinical utility of diagnostic guidelines and putative biomarkers in lymphangioleiomyomatosis. Respir Res 2012;13:34.

23. Ikeda Y, Taveira-DaSilva AM, Pacheco-Rodriguez G, et al. Erythropoietin-driven proliferation of cells with mutations in the tumor suppressor gene TSC2. Am J Physiol Lung Cell Mol Physiol 2011;300:L64–72.

24. Hayashi T, Fleming MV, Stetler-Stevenson WG, et al. Immunohistochemical study of matrix metalloproteinases (MMPs) and their tissue inhibitors (TIMPs) in pulmonary lymphangioleiomyomatosis (LAM). Hum Pathol 1997;28:1071–8.

25. Fukuda Y, Ishizaki M, Kudoh S, et al. Localization of matrix metalloproteinases-1, -2, and -9 and tissue inhibitor of metalloproteinase-2 in interstitial lung diseases. Lab Invest 1998;78:687–98.

26. Matsui K, Takeda K, Yu ZX, et al. Role for activation of matrix metalloproteinases in the pathogenesis of pulmonary lymphangioleiomyomatosis. Arch Pathol Lab Med 2000;124:267–75.

27. Zhe X, Yang Y, Jakkaraju S, et al. Tissue inhibitor of metalloproteinase-3 downregulation in lymphangioleiomyomatosis: potential consequence of abnormal serum response factor expression. Am J Respir Cell Mol Biol 2003;28:504–11.

28. Odajima N, Betsuyaku T, Nasuhara Y, et al. Matrix metalloproteinases in blood from patients with LAM. Respir Med 2009;103:124–9.

29. Papakonstantinou E, Dionyssopoulos A, Aletras AJ, et al. Expression of matrix metalloproteinases and their endogenous tissue inhibitors in skin lesions from patients with tuberous sclerosis. J Am Acad Dermatol 2004;51:526–33.

30. Gupta R, Kitaichi M, Inoue Y, et al. Lymphatic manifestations of lymphangioleiomyomatosis. Lymphology 2014;47:106–17.

31. Henske EP, McCormack FX. Lymphangioleiomyomatosis - a wolf in sheep's clothing. J Clin Invest 2012;122:3807–16.

32. Chilosi M, Pea M, Martignoni G, et al. Cathepsin-k expression in pulmonary lymphangioleiomyomatosis. Mod Pathol 2009;22:161–6.

33. Travis WD, Brambilla E, Nicholson AG, et al. The 2015 World Health Organization Classification of

lung tumors: impact of genetic, clinical and radiologic advances since the 2004 classification. J Thorac Oncol 2015;10(9):1243–60.

34. Crooks DM, Pacheco-Rodriguez G, DeCastro RM, et al. Molecular and genetic analysis of disseminated neoplastic cells in lymphangioleiomyomatosis. Proc Natl Acad Sci U S A 2004;101(50): 17462–7.

35. Cai X, Pacheco-Rodriguez G, Fan Q-Y, et al. Phenotypic characterization of disseminated cells with TSC2 loss of heterozygosity in patients with lymphangioleiomyomatosis. Am J Respir Crit Care Med 2010;182:1410–8.

36. Steagall WK, Zhang L, Cai X, et al. Genetic heterogeneity of circulating cells from patients with lymphangioleiomyomatosis with and without lung transplantation. Am J Respir Crit Care Med 2015; 191:854–6.

37. Bittmann I, Rolf B, Amann G, et al. Recurrence of lymphangioleiomyomatosis after single lung transplantation: new insights into pathogenesis. Hum Pathol 2003;34:95–8.

38. Karbowniczek M, Astrinidis A, Balsara BR, et al. Recurrent lymphangiomyomatosis after transplantation: genetic analyses reveal a metastatic mechanism. Am J Respir Crit Care Med 2003; 167:976–82.

39. Grzegorek I, Zuba-Surma E, Chabowski M, et al. Characterization of cells cultured from chylous effusion from a patient with sporadic lymphangioleiomyomatosis. Anticancer Res 2015;35:3341–51.

40. Hayashi T, Kumasaka T, Mitani K, et al. Prevalence of uterine and adnexal involvement in pulmonary lymphangioleiomyomatosis: a clinicopathologic study of 10 patients. Am J Surg Pathol 2011; 35(12):1776–85.

41. Carsillo T, Astrinidis A, Henske EP. Mutations in the tuberous sclerosis complex gene TSC2 are a cause of sporadic pulmonary lymphangioleiomyomatosis. Proc Natl Acad Sci U S A 2000;97: 6085–90.

42. Zoncu R, Efeyan A, Sabatini DM. mTOR: from growth signal integration to cancer, diabetes and ageing. Nat Rev Mol Cell Biol 2011;12:21–35.

43. Rosner M, Hanneder M, Siegel N, et al. The tuberous sclerosis gene products hamartin and tuberin are multifunctional proteins with a wide spectrum of interacting partners. Mutat Res 2008;658: 234–46.

44. Dos DS, Ali SM, Kim D-H, et al. Rictor, a Novel Binding Partner of mTOR, defines a rapamycin-insensitive and raptor-independent pathway that regulates the cytoskeleton. Curr Biol 2004;14: 1296–302.

45. Huang J, Manning Brendan D. A complex interplay between Akt, TSC2 and the two mTOR complexes. Biochem Soc Trans 2009;37:217–22.

46. Goncharova EA, Goncharov DA, Li H, et al. mTORC2 is required for proliferation and survival of TSC2-Null cells. Mol Cell Biol 2011;31:2484–98.

47. Ryu JH, Moss J, Beck GJ, et al. The NHLBI lymphangioleiomyomatosis registry: characteristics of 230 patients at enrollment. Am J Respir Crit Care Med 2006;173:105–11.

48. Cordier JF, Johnson S. Multiple cystic lung disease. Orphan Lung Diseases. European Respiratory Monograph 2011. p. 46–83.

49. Gupta N, Meraj R, Tanase D, et al. Accuracy of chest high-resolution computed tomography in diagnosing diffuse cystic lung diseases. Eur Respir J 2015;46:1196–9.

50. Johnson SR, Cordier JF, Lazor R, et al. European Respiratory Society guidelines for the diagnosis and management of lymphangioleiomyomatosis. Eur Respir J 2010;35:14–26.

51. Seyama K, Kumasaka T, Souma S, et al. Vascular endothelial growth factor-D is increased in serum of patients with lymphangioleiomyomatosis. Lymphatic Res Biol 2006;4:143–52.

52. Young LR, VanDyke R, Gulleman PM, et al. Serum vascular endothelial growth factor-D prospectively distinguishes lymphangioleiomyomatosis from other diseases. Chest 2010;138:674–81.

53. Glasgow CG, Taveira-Dasilva AM, Darling TN, et al. Lymphatic involvement in lymphangioleiomyomatosis. Ann N Y Acad Sci 2008;1131:206–14.

54. Zhe X, Schuger L. Combined smooth muscle and melanocytic differentiation in lymphangioleiomyomatosis. J Histochem Cytochem 2004;52:1537–42.

55. Meraj R, Wikenheiser-Brokamp K, Young L, et al. Utility of transbronchial biopsy in the diagnosis of lymphangioleiomyomatosis. Front Med 2012;6: 395–405.

56. Kai-Feng X, Han C, Hongrui L, et al. Transbronchial lung biopsy in Lymphangioleiomyomatosis (LAM): diagnostic value and safety. A35. I've got a feeling we're going to solve this one: insights into lymphangioleiomyomatosis. American Thoracic Society; 2015. p. A1399.

57. Fruchter O, Fridel L, El Raouf BA, et al. Histological diagnosis of interstitial lung diseases by cryo-transbronchial biopsy. Respirology 2014;19:683–8.

58. Crausman RS, Jennings CA, Mortenson RL, et al. Lymphangioleiomyomatosis: the pathophysiology of diminished exercise capacity. Am J Respir Crit Care Med 1996;153:1368–76.

59. Taveira-DaSilva AM, Stylianou MP, Hedin CJ, et al. Maximal oxygen uptake and severity of disease in lymphangioleiomyomatosis. Am J Respir Crit Care Med 2003;168:1427–31.

60. Johnson SR, Tattersfield AE. Decline in lung function in lymphangioleiomyomatosis: relation to menopause and progesterone treatment. Am J Respir Crit Care Med 1999;160:628–33.

61. Urban T, Lazor R, Lacronique J, et al. Pulmonary lymphangioleiomyomatosis. A study of 69 patients. Groupe d'Etudes et de Recherche sur les Maladies "Orphelines" Pulmonaires (GERM"O"P). Medicine (Baltimore) 1999;78:321–37.

62. Taveira-DaSilva AM, Stylianou MP, Hedin CJ, et al. Decline in lung function in patients with lymphangioleiomyomatosis treated with or without progesterone. Chest 2004;126:1867–74.

63. McCormack FX, Inoue Y, Moss J, et al. Efficacy and safety of sirolimus in lymphangioleiomyomatosis. N Engl J Med 2011;364:1595–606.

64. Chang WYC, Cane JL, Kumaran M, et al. A 2-year randomised placebo-controlled trial of doxycycline for lymphangioleiomyomatosis. Eur Respir J 2014; 43:1114–23.

65. Johnson SR, Whale CI, Hubbard RB, et al. Survival and disease progression in UK patients with lymphangioleiomyomatosis. Thorax 2004;59:800–3.

66. Young LR, Lee H-S, Inoue Y, et al. Serum VEGF-D concentration as a biomarker of lymphangioleiomyomatosis severity and treatment response: a prospective analysis of the Multicenter International Lymphangioleiomyomatosis Efficacy of Sirolimus (MILES) trial. Lancet Respir Med 2013;1(6):445–52.

67. Oprescu N, McCormack FX, Byrnes S, et al. Clinical predictors of mortality and cause of death in lymphangioleiomyomatosis: a population-based registry. Lung 2013;191:35–42.

68. Belkin A, Albright K, Fier K, et al. "Getting stuck with LAM": patients perspectives on living with Lymphangioleiomyomatosis. Health Qual Life Outcomes 2014;12:1–6.

69. Ohori NP, Yousem SA, Sonmez-Alpan E, et al. Estrogen and progesterone receptors in lymphangioleiomyomatosis, epithelioid hemangioendothelioma, and sclerosing hemangioma of the lung. Am J Clin Pathol 1991;96:529–35.

70. Brunelli A, Catalini G, Fianchini A. Pregnancy exacerbating unsuspected mediastinal lymphangioleiomyomatosis and chylothorax. Int J Gynaecol Obstet 1996;52:289–90.

71. Yano S. Exacerbation of pulmonary lymphangioleiomyomatosis by exogenous oestrogen used for infertility treatment. Thorax 2002;57:1085–6.

72. Fujimoto M, Ohara N, Sasaki H, et al. Pregnancy complicated with pulmonary lymphangioleiomyomatosis: case report. Clin Exp Obstet Gynecol 2005;32:199–200.

73. Iruloh C, Keriakos R, Smith DJ, et al. Renal angiomyolipoma and lymphangioleiomyomatosis in pregnancy. J Obstet Gynaecol 2013;33:542–6.

74. Taveira-DaSilva AM, Steagall WK, Rabel A, et al. Reversible airflow obstruction in lymphangioleiomyomatosis. Chest 2009;136:1596–603.

75. Seibert D, Hong C-H, Takeuchi F, et al. Recognition of tuberous sclerosis in adult women: delayed presentation with life-threatening consequences. Ann Intern Med 2011;154:806–13.

76. Shepherd CW, Gomez MR, Lie JT, et al. Causes of death in patients with tuberous sclerosis. Mayo Clin Proc 1991;66:792–6.

77. Harris PC. The TSC2/PKD1 contiguous gene syndrome. Contrib Nephrol 1997;122:76–82.

78. Taveira-DaSilva AM, Hedin C, Stylianou MP, et al. Reversible airflow obstruction, proliferation of abnormal smooth muscle cells, and impairment of gas exchange as predictors of outcome in Lymphangioleiomyomatosis. Am J Respir Crit Care Med 2001;164:1072–6.

79. Goncharova EA, Goncharov DA, Eszterhas A, et al. Tuberin regulates p70 S6 kinase activation and ribosomal protein S6 phosphorylation. A role for the TSC2 tumor suppressor gene in pulmonary lymphangioleiomyomatosis (LAM). J Biol Chem 2002;277:30958–67.

80. Bissler JJ, McCormack FX, Young LR, et al. Sirolimus for angiomyolipoma in tuberous sclerosis complex or lymphangioleiomyomatosis. N Engl J Med 2008;358:140–51.

81. Davies DM, Johnson SR, Tattersfield AE, et al. Sirolimus therapy in tuberous sclerosis or sporadic lymphangioleiomyomatosis. N Engl J Med 2008; 358:200–3.

82. Goldberg HJ, Harari S, Cottin V, et al. Everolimus for the treatment of lymphangioleiomyomatosis: a phase II study. Eur Respir J 2015;46:783–94.

83. Taveira-DaSilva AM, Hathaway O, Stylianou M, et al. Changes in lung function and chylous effusions in patients with lymphangioleiomyomatosis treated with sirolimus. Ann Intern Med 2011;154: 797–805.

84. Krueger DA, Care MM, Holland K, et al. Everolimus for subependymal giant-cell astrocytomas in tuberous sclerosis. N Engl J Med 2010;363:1801–11.

85. Hofbauer GFL, Marcollo-Pini A, Corsenca A, et al. The mTOR inhibitor rapamycin significantly improves facial angiofibroma lesions in a patient with tuberous sclerosis. Br J Dermatol 2008;159:473–5.

86. Ando K, Kurihara M, Kataoka H, et al. The efficacy and safety of low-dose sirolimus for treatment of lymphangioleiomyomatosis. Respir Investig 2013; 51(3):175–83.

87. Somers MJ, Paul E. Safety considerations of mammalian target of rapamycin inhibitors in tuberous sclerosis complex and renal transplantation. J Clin Pharmacol 2015;55:368–76.

88. Yao J, Taveira-DaSilva AM, Jones AM, et al. Sustained effects of sirolimus on lung function and cystic lung lesions in lymphangioleiomyomatosis. Am J Respir Crit Care Med 2014;190(11):1273–82.

89. Johnson SR, Tattersfield AE. Clinical experience of lymphangioleiomyomatosis in the UK. Thorax 2000; 55:1052–7.

90. Almoosa KF, Ryu JH, Mendez J, et al. Management of pneumothorax in lymphangioleiomyomatosis: effects on recurrence and lung transplantation complications. Chest 2006;129:1274–81.

91. Chu SC, Horiba K, Usuki J, et al. Comprehensive evaluation of 35 patients with lymphangioleiomyomatosis. Chest 1999;115:1041–52.

92. Ryu JH, Doerr CH, Fisher SD, et al. Chylothorax in lymphangioleiomyomatosis. Chest 2003;123: 623–7.

93. Chen E, Itkin M. Thoracic duct embolization for chylous leaks. Semin Intervent Radiol 2011;28: 63–74.

94. Yeoh Z, Navaratnam V, Bhatt R, et al. Natural history of angiomyolipoma in lymphangioleiomyomatosis: implications for screening and surveillance. Orphanet J Rare Dis 2014;9:151.

95. Rakowski SK, Winterkorn EB, Paul E, et al. Renal manifestations of tuberous sclerosis complex: incidence, prognosis, and predictive factors. Kidney Int 2006;70:1777–82.

96. Sooriakumaran P, Gibbs P, Coughlin G, et al. Angiomyolipomata: challenges, solutions, and future prospects based on over 100 cases treated. BJU Int 2010;105:101–6.

97. Lane BR, Aydin H, Danforth TL, et al. Clinical correlates of renal angiomyolipoma subtypes in 209 patients: classic, fat poor, tuberous sclerosis associated and epithelioid. J Urol 2008;180: 836–43.

98. Bissler JJ, Kingswood JC, Radzikowska E, et al. Everolimus for angiomyolipoma associated with tuberous sclerosis complex or sporadic lymphangioleiomyomatosis (EXIST-2): a multicentre, randomised, double-blind, placebo-controlled trial. Lancet 2013;381:817–24.

99. Davies DM, de Vries PJ, Johnson SR, et al. Sirolimus therapy for Angiomyolipoma in tuberous sclerosis and sporadic lymphangioleiomyomatosis: a phase 2 trial. Clin Cancer Res 2011;17:4071–81.

100. Krueger DA, Northrup H. Tuberous sclerosis complex surveillance and management: recommendations of the 2012 International Tuberous Sclerosis Complex Consensus Conference. Pediatr Neurol 2013;49:255–65.

101. Moss J, DeCastro R, Patronas NJ, et al. Meningiomas in lymphangioleiomyomatosis. JAMA 2001; 286:1879–81.

102. Cottin V, Harari S, Humbert M, et al. Pulmonary hypertension in lymphangioleiomyomatosis: characteristics in 20 patients. Eur Respir J 2012;40: 630–40.

103. McCormack FX. Lymphangioleiomyomatosis: a clinical update. Chest 2008;133:507–16.

104. Boehler A, Speich R, Russi EW, et al. Lung transplantation for lymphangioleiomyomatosis. N Engl J Med 1996;335:1275–80.

105. Benden C, Rea F, Behr J, et al. Lung transplantation for lymphangioleiomyomatosis: the European experience. J Heart Lung Transplant 2008;28(1): 1–7.

106. Cohen MM, Pollock-BarZiv S, Johnson SR. Emerging clinical picture of lymphangioleiomyomatosis. Thorax 2005;60:875–9.

107. Lazor R, Valeyre D, Lacronique J, et al. Low initial KCO predicts rapid FEV1 decline in pulmonary lymphangioleiomyomatosis. Respir Med 2004;98: 536–41.

108. Muzykewicz DA, Sharma A, Muse V, et al. TSC1 and TSC2 mutations in patients with lymphangioleiomyomatosis and tuberous sclerosis complex. J Med Genet 2009;46(7):465–8.

Plastic Bronchitis

Bruce K. Rubin, MEngr, MD, MBA, FRCPC

KEYWORDS

- Mucus • Mucin • Secretory hyperresponsiveness • Cast bronchitis • Fontan physiology
- Congenital heart disease • Pulmonary lymphatics

KEY POINTS

- Plastic bronchitis associated with congenital heart disease or with lymphatic anomalies is caused by aberrant pulmonary lymphatic vessels and drainage. This true form of plastic bronchitis can usually be treated by selective lymphatic vessel ablation.
- Plastic bronchitis is probably more common than reported. This speculation is based on the observation that many clinicians are unfamiliar with the disease and may fail to recognize milder forms of the syndrome.
- Plastic bronchitis with cohesive branching airway casts should not be confused with the more common, but smaller and more etiologically distinct, casts that are associated with mucus plugging.
- For nonlymphatic plastic bronchitis associated with eosinophils and Charcot-Leyden crystals within casts, the most effective therapy seems to be cast removal followed by high-dose or pulse corticosteroids.

INTRODUCTION

Plastic bronchitis (PB) is an uncommon pulmonary disease characterized by production of cohesive and branching casts filling the airways (**Fig. 1**). This disease has been recognized for thousands of years and was first described by Galen in patients who he thought were expectorating pulmonary veins. PB has had many other names through the years, including fibrinous bronchitis and cast bronchitis.

PATIENT EVALUATION OVERVIEW

The diagnosis of PB is confirmed by a history of expectoration of branching airways casts, or by removing branching casts at the time bronchoscopy. Life-threatening respiratory distress can occur because of obstruction of airways with casts in children with congenital heart disease or as a consequence of lymphatic engorgement following surgical correction of congenital heart disease.[1] The casts of PB often contain an abundance of mucin but unlike mucin polymers in normal mucus, which are linearly linked, there is significant cross-linking between adjacent mucin strands (**Fig. 2**). Most casts have only small amounts of fibrin.[2]

True PB associated with expectoration of branching casts has not been reported in patients with cystic fibrosis or bronchiectasis. Although there are large amounts of polymeric DNA and F-actin in cystic fibrosis, this rarely, if ever, supports the formation of the complex branching casts that are diagnostic of PB.[3] Furthermore, polymeric DNA and F-actin are not abundant in PB casts, so aerosol dornase alfa is typically ineffective as therapy (discussed later). PB must also be differentiated from the mucous plugging that is associated with fungal inflammation of the airway in allergic bronchopulmonary aspergillosis.

Disclosure: Dr Rubin is a Board member of the Plastic Bronchitis Foundation, he directs the International Plastic Bronchitis Registry and Specimen Repository, and his lab is partially funded by the American Respiratory Care Foundation to study this condition.
The Children's Hospital of Richmond at Virginia Commonwealth University, 1000 East Broad Street, Richmond, VA 23298, USA
E-mail address: brubin@vcu.edu

Clin Chest Med 37 (2016) 405–408
http://dx.doi.org/10.1016/j.ccm.2016.04.003
0272-5231/16/$ – see front matter © 2016 Elsevier Inc. All rights reserved.

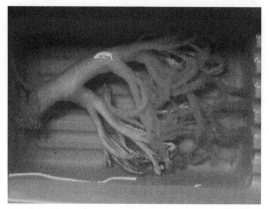

Fig. 1. Typical expectorated branching cast from a child with plastic bronchitis caused by congenital heart disease.

It is not clear whether true PB can be part of the asthma spectrum in patients with severe asthma and secretory hyperresponsiveness.[2]

The author examined PB casts from more than 50 adults and children with a variety of associated conditions. All showed the presence of inflammatory cell infiltrates that predominantly comprised lymphocytes and, at times, eosinophils. Inflammatory cells are more commonly seen in association with asthma and allergy and other non–cardiac-associated conditions.[4]

PB is underdiagnosed and may be first discovered at autopsy. Patients with milder

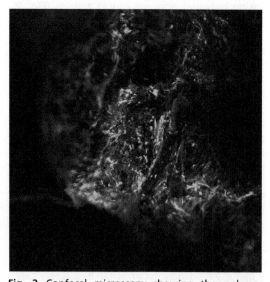

Fig. 2. Confocal microscopy showing the polymer structure of a plastic bronchitis cast. Polymeric mucin is pseudocolored red by Texas Red–UEA (Ulex europaeus agglutinin I) lectin, intracellular (nuclear) DNA is green (Yoyo-1), and fibrin polymers are blue (by immunohistochemistry).

forms of cardiogenic PB may undergo spontaneous recovery as cardiac function improves.

DISEASE ASSOCIATIONS

PB in children is usually associated with congenital heart disease and especially those with single-ventricle, Fontan physiology (**Box 1**).[5] The occurrence, severity, and the frequency of exacerbations of PB vary markedly among patients with congenital heart disease, sometimes first appearing years after surgery. Some patients have subclinical disease with the expectoration of small casts or resolution of casts between exacerbations. PB has been associated with lymphatic abnormalities both in patients with congenital heart disease and in patients with primary abnormalities of lymphatic flow. MRI mapping of thoracic lymphatics has conclusively shown that all of these patients have aberrant pulmonary lymphatics and, in patients with congenital heart disease, these vessels have a distinctive appearance.[6] Ablation of these abnormal lymph vessels using direct injection of tissue glue is almost uniformly effective in reducing, and often eliminating, cast formation.[7]

A PB-like condition can be triggered by the inhalation of toxic gases, such as sulfur mustard. In experimental animals that have inhaled sulfur mustard there is extensive plugging of the airway with fibrin-rich casts that are histologically different from PB. In these animal models, casts can be effectively treated with inhaled heparin[8] or tissue plasminogen activator (tPA).[9]

Box 1
Conditions associated with plastic bronchitis

Proven conditions

Congenital heart disease with Fontan physiology

Pulmonary lymphatic anomalies

Influenza A pulmonary infection

Possible conditions

Toxic inhalation

Sickle cell acute chest syndrome

Hypersecretory and near-fatal asthma (eosinophilic casts)

Unlikely and unproven conditions

Cystic fibrosis

Chronic obstructive pulmonary disease

Bronchiectasis

Bacterial pneumonia

PB is not associated with pulmonary bacterial infection and in general antibiotics are not recommended as part of therapy. However, PB has been associated with influenza A infection in children and similar cast formation has been described in birds that have been experimentally infected with avian influenza.[10,11]

It is controversial whether severe asthma and airway plugging should be considered true PB. Fatal asthma secretions are extremely cohesive and, when extracted from the airway, appear to form branching casts. In that respect, they more closely resemble PB than mucous plugging. These casts contain eosinophils and their degradation products (Charcot-Leyden crystals).[4]

PHARMACOLOGIC TREATMENT OPTIONS

Because PB is an uncommon condition, most reports of effective therapy are based on subjective criteria detailed in case reports or small case series (**Box 2**). Further, most patients in

these small studies have received many different medications, making it difficult to ascertain which of these therapies, if any, are effective. Evaluation of data from the Plastic Bronchitis Registry (http://rubinlab.pediatrics.vcu.edu/research/plastic-bronchitis/) suggests that there is no benefit to the use of asthma medications like beta agonists or inhaled corticosteroids in most cases of PB. There is also no apparent therapeutic benefit from using inhaled dornase alfa (Pulmozyme), expectorants such as guaifenesin or hypertonic saline, or mucolytics such as N-acetylcysteine. These medications should only be used with caution because some can induce mucus secretion or increase airway inflammation.

There have been case reports that the inhalation of tPA can improve PB through fibrin depolymerization.[12] tPA is irritating to the airway, and can result in hemoptysis or dyspnea after inhalation. It is also extremely expensive. In patients with PB and severe airway obstruction who are not stable enough to undergo bronchoscopy, a trial of aerosol tPA can be considered at a dose of 0.7 to 1.0 mg/kg every 4 hours. Inhaled heparin has also been reported to be effective in patients with PB.[13] Heparin has no effect on fibrin-containing casts but it has antiinflammatory properties that can decrease mucin secretion, prevent Tissue Factor activation of the fibrin pathway, and attenuate vascular leak. Heparin is less irritating to the airway than tPA and is far less expensive.

Isolated reports suggest that inhaled anticholinergics may reduce cast formation. Despite concern that inhaled anticholinergics may thicken secretions, this has not been substantiated in other diseases, such as asthma or chronic obstructive pulmonary disease.[14] Low-dose macrolides can decrease mucin production by inhibiting activation of extracellular regulated kinase 1 and 2[15] and attenuating the severity of PB.[16]

NONPHARMACOLOGIC AND SURGICAL TREATMENT OPTIONS

In patients with lymphatic abnormalities, the most effective therapy for PB is MRI-guided selective lymphatic embolization.[7] Improving cardiac output has been reported to reduce the severity of PB, but surgical attempts to optimize Fontan physiology by fenestration of the atrial septum or taking down the shunt are generally unsuccessful. Cardiac transplant in patients with heart failure has also been reported to improve PB.[17]

Airway clearance using standard pulmonary toilet techniques seems to be among the safest and most effective of therapies. Routine, daily use of a high-frequency chest compression vest

---

Box 2
Recommendations for therapy

Good evidence

Selective embolization or gluing of aberrant lymphatics

Thoracic duct ligation

Airway clearance, including physical therapy devices like high-frequency chest compression vest

Aerosolized heparin

Cardiac transplant

Improving cardiac function

Anecdotal or case report evidence

Hyperosmolar saline

Low-dose oral macrolides (clarithromycin or azithromycin)

Oral or inhaled corticosteroids (only for eosinophilic casts)

Aerosol tissue plasminogen activator

No evidence and potentially harmful

Beta agonist aerosol

Dornase alfa (Pulmozyme)

Mucolytics such as N-acetylcysteine

Expectorants such as guaifenesin

Nonmacrolide antibiotics

Modifications of Fontan (fenestration or takedown)

for those with an effective cough, or a Cough Assist (Philips Respironics) device for those with impaired cough, may help prevent cast reaccumulation. The author also recommend an exercise regimen and good nutrition, which may consist of protein repletion in children with protein-losing enteropathy, or weight loss in obese adults with PB.

EVALUATION OF OUTCOMES AND LONG-TERM RECOMMENDATIONS

The primary considerations when treating PB are facilitating the clearance of casts that have formed in the airways, and preventing future casting and airway obstruction. Cast clearance by bronchoscopy allows inhaled medications to gain access to the distal conducting airways and promote airway clearance and reduce inflammation and bronchospasm. In addition, extensive cast removal may make surgical and radiologic interventions easier for patients to tolerate.

THE FUTURE

Through the US National Institutes of Health, Office of Rare Diseases, an International Plastic Bronchitis Registry has been established to collect data on patients with PB throughout the world (ClinicalTrials.gov identifier NCT01663948). This database will help clinicians to generate hypotheses that can be tested clinically, including the use of genomic or inflammasome screening for potential causes for this debilitating disease. Through the Office of Rare Diseases, a tissue repository of expectorated bronchial casts has also been established and will make these samples available to investigators interested in studying PB (https://ncats.nih.gov/grdr/partners).

REFERENCES

1. Soyer T, Yalcin Ş, Emiralioğlu N, et al. Use of serial rigid bronchoscopy in the treatment of plastic bronchitis in children. J Pediatr Surg 2016 [Epub ahead of print].
2. Rubin BK, Priftis KN, Schmidt HJ, et al. Secretory hyperresponsiveness and pulmonary mucus hypersecretion. Chest 2014;146(2):496–507.
3. Kater A, Henke MO, Rubin BK. The role of DNA and actin polymers on the polymer structure and rheology of cystic fibrosis sputum and depolymerization by gelsolin or thymosin Beta 4. Ann N Y Acad Sci 2007;1112:140–53.
4. Madsen P, Shah SA, Rubin BK. Plastic bronchitis: new insights and a classification scheme. Paediatr Respir Rev 2005;6:292–300.
5. Goldberg DJ, Dodds K, Rychik J. Rare problems associated with the Fontan circulation. Cardiol Young 2010;20:113–9.
6. Dori Y, Keller MS, Fogel MA, et al. MRI of lymphatic abnormalities after functional single-ventricle palliation surgery. AJR Am J Roentgenol 2014;203(2):426–31.
7. Dori Y, Keller MS, Rychik J, et al. Successful treatment of plastic bronchitis by selective lymphatic embolization in a Fontan patient. Pediatrics 2014;134(2):e590–5.
8. Houin PR, Veress LA, Rancourt RC, et al. Intratracheal heparin improves plastic bronchitis due to sulfur mustard analog. Pediatr Pulmonol 2015;50(2):118–26.
9. Veress LA, Anderson DR, Hendry-Hofer TB, et al. Airway tissue plasminogen activator prevents acute mortality due to lethal sulfur mustard inhalation. Toxicol Sci 2015;143(1):178–84.
10. Deng J, Zheng Y, Li C, et al. Plastic bronchitis in three children associated with 2009 influenza A(H1N1) virus infection. Chest 2010;138:1486–8.
11. Zhang J, Kang X. Plastic bronchitis associated with influenza virus infection in children: a report on 14 cases. Int J Pediatr Otorhinolaryngol 2015;79(4):481–6.
12. Heath L, Ling S, Racz J, et al. Prospective, longitudinal study of plastic bronchitis cast pathology and responsiveness to tissue plasminogen activator. Pediatr Cardiol 2011;32:1182–9.
13. Eason DE, Cox K, Moskowitz WB. Aerosolized heparin in the treatment of Fontan related plastic bronchitis. Cardiol Young 2014;24(1):140–2.
14. Bateman ED, Rennard S, Barnes PJ, et al. Alternative mechanisms for tiotropium. Pulm Pharmacol Ther 2009;22:533–42.
15. Kanoh S, Rubin BK. Macrolides as immunomodulatory medications. Mechanisms of action and clinical applications. Clin Microbiol Rev 2010;23:590–615.
16. Schultz KD, Oermann CM. Treatment of cast bronchitis with low-dose oral azithromycin. Pediatr Pulmonol 2003;35:135–43.
17. Laubisch JE, Green DM, Mogayzel PJ, et al. Treatment of plastic bronchitis by orthotopic heart transplantation. Pediatr Cardiol 2011;32:1193–5.

Nonmalignant Adult Thoracic Lymphatic Disorders

Maxim Itkin, MD, FSIR[a],*, Francis X. McCormack, MD[b]

KEYWORDS

- Lymphangioma • Lymphangiomatosis • Lymphangiectasia • Generalize lymphatic anomaly (GLA)
- Gorham-Stout disease (GSD) • Kaposiform lymphangiomatosis (KL) • Pulmonary lymphangiectasia
- Yellow nail syndrome

KEY POINTS

- The thoracic lymphatic disorders typically present with symptoms of cough, shortness of breath, chyloptysis, or expectoration of branching casts.
- Typical pulmonary manifestations of the thoracic lymphatic disorders include chylous effusions, peribronchiolar interstitial infiltrates, and mediastinal masses.
- The emergence of sophisticated imaging techniques that characterize abnormal lymphatic flow promises to improve the classification and therapeutic approaches to the thoracic lymphatic disorders.

INTRODUCTION

Primary lymphatic anomalies comprise a bewildering array of congenital and acquired conditions that can affect every organ system containing lymphatic channels, generally considered to be all tissues except brain and bone marrow. Lymphatic anomalies usually come to medical attention during childhood or early adulthood, but can also present later in life. For the purpose of this article, the discussion focuses on the lymphatic disorders that involve thoracic structures, either primarily or as part of a more global lymphatic disease process, and which preferentially affect older children and adults.

The pulmonary lymphatics are a network of vessels that function to transport cells and fluids from the periphery of the lung to the central lymphatic conduits, in order to regulate tissue pressure and facilitate regional immune responses. The peripheral lymphatic vessels converge on the larger conduits coursing on the surface of major airways in the hila and mediastinum and ultimately drain into the right lymphatic duct and thoracic duct (TD). The right lymphatic duct inserts into the subclavian vein in the neck and drains the right upper lobe. The TD inserts into the left innominate vein at the junction with the internal jugular vein and drains the left lung, right middle and lower lobes of the right lung, as well as all structures below the diaphragm (Fig. 1). A broad discussion of lymphatic anatomy is beyond the scope of this article, but it is important to note that intestinal lymph (chyle) that contains chylomicrons (dietary fats) enters the TD at the level of cisterna chyli in the upper abdomen and is transported to the venous system in the neck. The primary route thorough which chylous fluid reaches the pleural space or other thoracic structures in subjects with chylous effusions, therefore, is either through (1) reflux from an obstructed or pressure-overloaded

Disclosures: None.
[a] Interventional Radiology, Hospital of the University of Pennsylvania, Penn Medicine, 1 Silverstein, 3400 Spruce Street, Philadelphia, PA 19104, USA; [b] Division of Pulmonary, Critical Care and Sleep Medicine, University of Cincinnati, MSB 6165, 231 Albert Sabin Way, Cincinnati, OH 45267-0564, USA
* Corresponding author.
E-mail address: itkinmax@uphs.upenn.edu

Clin Chest Med 37 (2016) 409–420
http://dx.doi.org/10.1016/j.ccm.2016.04.004
0272-5231/16/$ – see front matter © 2016 Elsevier Inc. All rights reserved.

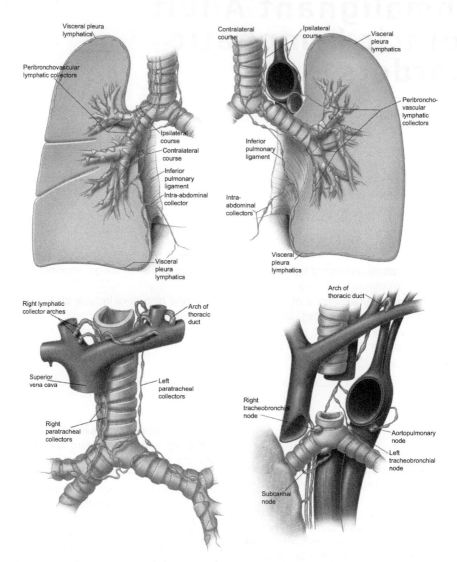

Fig. 1. Schematic representation of pulmonary lymphatic anatomy. (*Adapted from* Riquet M. Bronchial arteries and lymphatics of the lung. Thorac Surg Clin 2007;17:619–38; with permission.)

TD into the pulmonary lymphatic stream, or (2) through a pathologic connection between chylous lymphatics and the pleural space, airways, or lung parenchyma, as can occur following surgery or trauma or as part of a pathologic process. Other thoracic chylous complications that can result from these 2 processes include chylous congestion in the lung parenchyma,[1] plastic bronchitis (PB; expectoration of branching casts),[2] chylopericardium, and chyloptysis.

The thoracic lymphatic disorders (TLD) comprise a group of diseases that are variably associated with mediastinal or pulmonary masses, interstitial infiltrates, airway disorders including chyloptysis, PB, pleural effusions that are often chylous, and repeated pulmonary infections and bronchiectasis (eg, yellow nail syndrome, YNS).

Extrapulmonary manifestations of the TLDs can include lymphatic leaks in various distributions (eg, chylous ascites), protein-losing enteropathy, recurrent fevers and prostration, lymphatic obstruction resulting in lymphedema of extremities, coagulopathy, and bony lesions. The TLDs often present in protean manner and can be congenital or acquired, localized or systemic. Attempts to classify these disorders have generally been based on defining commonalities of a limited number of cases or the consensus of experts.[3–6] Most of the published classification systems use inconsistent terminology and lack clear diagnostic, clinical, laboratory, or imaging standards. The TLDs are often grouped based on symptoms, age of presentation, histologic appearance, associated illnesses, or secondary imaging findings rather than on unifying pathologic processes.

Common terms that have been used to describe primary lymphatic disorders include lymphangioma, lymphangiectasia, lymphangiomatosis, primary lymphedema,[7] pulmonary lymphangiectasia (PL),[8–10] intrathoracic lymphangiomatosis,[11] thoracic lymphangiomatosis,[12] diffuse pulmonary lymphangiomatosis,[13] and mediastinal lymphangiomatosis.[14] The mode of clinical presentation is often added to modify these disease classifications, using terms idiopathic, congenital, neonatal, or acquired to describe chylothorax, chylous ascites, or chylopericardium.[15–18]

In particular, the terms lymphangioma and lymphangiectasia have been used interchangeably to describe a heterogeneous group of disorders associated with excess lymphatic tissue. Although both conditions are very similar histologically,[6,19] by definition lymphangiomas are sequestered from the main lymphatic system, and lymphangiectasias are connected to it. The primary means to differentiate between these 2 disorders clinically is with imaging capable of revealing lymphatic flow. Revealing lymphatic flow was formerly accomplished with pedal lymphangiogram and lymphoscintigraphy,[20,21] which have been reported to demonstrate pathologic lymphatic flow ("lymphatic reflux") in lymphangiectasia despite its limitations in anatomic definition.[22–24] Over the last few decades, however, these procedures have been less frequently performed and the expertise required to execute them has been lost to many radiology departments. Intranodal lymphangiogram (IL)[25] and dynamic contrast-enhanced magnetic resonance lymphangiogram (DCMRL)[26,27] are new imaging techniques that can better define lymphatic anatomy and lymphatic flow. These approaches have opened new vistas in the understanding the importance of lymphatic flow in primary lymphatic disorders[26,27] and will likely lead to more rational approaches to classification.

The International Society for the Study of Vascular Anomalies (ISSVA) approved new guidelines for classification of the lymphatic disorders at the 20th ISSVA Workshop in Melbourne, Australia in 2014. Disorders of the pulmonary lymphatic system include macrocystic, microcystic, and mixed lymphatic malformations, generalized lymphatic anomalies (GLA, also previously known as diffuse lymphangiomatosis), lymphatic malformations in Gorham-Stout disease (GSD), channel-type lymphatic malformations, and primary lymphedema. Not mentioned in the ISSVA classification are disorders associated with combinations of lymphatic and other tissue anomalies, including lymphangioleiomyomatosis (LAM), or YNS. The disorders we have chosen to discuss below are a subset of TLDs that might conceivably present with pulmonary infiltrates, thoracic masses, or chylous leaks in an adult pulmonary clinic, including lymphangioma (a term that has now been replaced with microcystic or macrocystic lymphatic malformation), diffuse pulmonary lymphangiomatosis (DPL; a term that is obsolete but without an accepted replacement, here called primary pulmonary lymphatic anomaly [PPLA]), GLA with pulmonary involvement, a new subtype of GLA called Kaposiform lymphangiomatosis (KLA), lymphatic malformation in GSD, PB, and YNS. Disorders that are exclusively found in neonates primarily, are malignant, or which do not typically involve thorax, such as congenital chylothorax, primary lymphedema, Kaposi sarcoma, or lymphangiosarcoma, are not discussed in this article. An overriding theme in this review is the importance of lymphatic imaging in classifying and treating these disorders.

THORACIC LYMPHANGIOMAS (MICROCYSTIC AND MACROCYSTIC LYMPHATIC MALFORMATIONS)

Lymphangiomas are focal proliferations of well-differentiated lymphatic tissue that present as multicystic or sponge-like accumulations.[19,28] In many cases, they represent embryologic remnants of lymphatic tissues. Acquired or secondary lymphangiomas can occur at the site of radiation, trauma, or infection. Cystic lymphangiomas (also known as cystic hygromas or cystic hydromas) can occur anywhere but are most common in the armpit and the neck. In the thorax, they manifest as masses in the mediastinum,[29,30] pleura,[31,32] or intrapulmonary[33] distributions (**Fig. 2**). Mediastinal lymphangiomas are equally distributed between the anterior, posterior, and medial mediastinal compartments and often envelop and displace mediastinal vessels. Thoracic lymphangiomas are usually detected as nodules or cystic masses on chest radiographs. MRI is the most useful diagnostic modality, because it accurately predicts intraoperative findings, and heavy T2 weighting brightly elucidates tumor boundaries. Histologically, lymphangiomas are composed of an increased number dilated lymphatic channels and are filled with proteinaceous fluid. Although most lymphangiomas occur in the first 2 years of life, 40% of 151 lymphangiomas reviewed in consultation by the Air Force Institute of Pathology were from patients who were older than 16 years of age.[34] Clinically, intrathoracic lymphangiomas

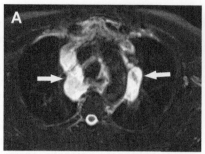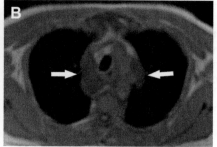

Fig. 2. MRI features of patient with mediastinal lymphangioma (*arrows*). (*A*) Axial T2-weighted MRI shows high signal pretracheal and paratracheal masses. The high signal is due to high water content in lymphangiomas. (*B*) The signal on T1-weighted image is similar to smooth muscle.

can present as incidental findings or associated with symptoms of organ compression, such as cough, dyspnea, stridor, or Horner syndrome. Because they are often isolated from the main lymphatic system, intrathoracic lymphangiomas are typically not associated with chylous pleural effusions. Surgical resection of mediastinal lymphangiomas has been successfully performed to relieve compression on adjacent organs.[35,36] Recently, a high prevalence of PIK3CA mutations have been reported in patients with lymphatic malformations and malformative syndromes.[37]

LYMPHANGIOLEIOMYOMATOSIS

LAM, also known as lymphangiomyomatosis, is a rare cystic lung disease that occurs most commonly in women.[38] Recent research from multiple laboratories has revealed that LAM is a progressive, low-grade metastasizing neoplasm associated with smooth muscle-like cell infiltration of the lung interstitium and cystic remodeling of the pulmonary parenchyma.[39,40] Cystic changes consistent with LAM occur in both men and women with tuberous sclerosis complex,[41] associated with germ-line mutations in either TSC1 or TSC2.[42] Sporadic LAM occurs in patients who do not have TSC, has been reported only in women, and is driven by somatic mutations in TSC2.[43,44] Although the source of LAM cells that infiltrate the lung is unknown, available evidence suggests that the disease spreads primarily through lymphatic channels.[45,46] Lymph node involvement is greatest in low abdominal and pelvic locations and decreases in a gradient-like fashion to the thoracic mediastinum, suggestive of an origin in the pelvis.[47] The uterus is a prime candidate for the source of LAM cells, a notion that is supported by the estrogen and progesterone receptor positivity of the neoplastic cells and multiple case reports of uterine involvement in LAM.[48–51]

Lymphatic manifestations of LAM include TD wall invasion, mediastinal lymphangioleiomyoma formation, and chylous fluid collections in the peritoneal, pleural, and pericardial spaces. Abnormal communications between lymphatic channels and hollow viscera can result in protein-losing enteropathy, chyluria, chyloptysis, chylocolporrhea (chylometrorrhea), chyle leak from the umbilicus, chylous pulmonary congestion, and lower extremity lymphedema. LAM lesions express lymphangiogenic growth factors, vascular endothelial growth factor (VEGF)-C and VEGF-D,[45] growth factor receptors, VEGFR-2 and VEGFR-3 (Flt-4), and markers LYVE-1 and podoplanin, and are laced with chaotic lymphatic channels.[52] Serum VEGF-D is elevated in 70% of patients with LAM and is a clinically useful diagnostic and prognostic biomarker.[53–56] Molecular targeted therapy with sirolimus is antilymphangiogenic and is effective at stabilizing lung function and for the lymphatic and chylous complications of LAM,[51,57] although little is known about the optimal dose and duration of the drug. Other approaches to control chylous pleural effusions include pleurodesis, TD embolization, and TD ligation. Patients with problematic or refractory chylous fluid collections and leaks should undergo imaging with IL[25] or DCMRL[26,27] to identify the source of the leak (**Fig. 3**). As an example of the importance of understanding underlying pathologic lymphatic anatomy and flow before intervening, chylous pleural effusions requiring repeated taps may be revealed by IL or DCMRL to arise from lymphatic leakage into the abdomen rather than into the chest. Because in those cases the thoracic effusion arises from chylous ascites that is drawn into the chest by negative pleural pressures generated during respiration, TD ligation would be contraindicated. In this situation, embolization, pleurodesis, or sirolimus treatment would be preferred approaches.

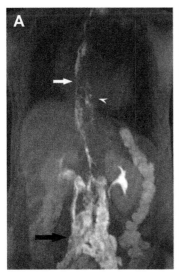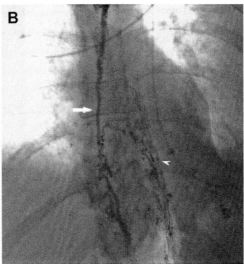

Fig. 3. (*A*) DCMRL imaging of a patient with LAM, demonstrating large retroperitoneal masses (*black arrow*), prominent TD (*white arrow*), and abnormal branching of the lymphatic vessels from TD, resulting in development of chylothorax (*arrowhead*). (*B*) Corresponding fluoroscopy image of the TD of the same patient, following injection of contrast material through the microcatheter positioned in the proximal part of TD. Injection confirms mild dilation of the TD (*white arrow*) and abnormal branching of the lymphatic vessels from the TD, resulting in development of chylothorax (*arrowhead*).

PRIMARY PULMONARY LYMPHATIC ANOMALY

In rare cases, especially in children, primary lymphatic anomalies may be entirely restricted to the thoracic cavity. These disorders have been reported in the literature as DPL,[13,19] pulmonary lymphangiectasis,[58] intrathoracic lymphangiomatosis,[11] thoracic lymphangiomatosis,[59] and diffuse pulmonary angiomatosis.[60] Tazelaar and colleagues[13] originally proposed the term "diffuse pulmonary lymphangiomatosis," but the most recent ISSVA guidelines support the use of the suffix "-oma" only in cases where the lymphatic abnormality is known to be neoplastic. Indeed, most lymphatic disorders discussed here are likely due to persistence or duplication of well-differentiated lymphatics rather than clonal tumor growth. Tazelaar also proposed that DPL be distinguished from PL, which he thought should be restricted to the very rare congenital or secondary cause cases where pulmonary lymphatics are dilated but not increased in number. In the new classification of vascular malformations, the ISSVA avoids using the term lymphangiomatosis and describes 2 distinct lymphatic malformation conditions[4]: GLA, and GSD. Because the ISSVA group does not appear to have directly addressed the nomenclature for the organ-restricted disorder formerly known as DPL, the term PPLA is used here. On gross examination, the lung parenchyma in cases of PPLA does not reveal any discrete nodules or masses. At low power, the lung may reveal spongiform expansion of interlobular septa, but no true cysts. Histologically, PPLA is associated with extensively anastomosing, variably sized, endothelial cell-lined spaces distributed along lymphatic routes throughout the lung. According to Tazelaar and colleagues,[13] compared with PL, there is a prominence of collagen and spindle-shaped cells surrounding endothelial lined channels. Compared with LAM, although hemosiderin-laden macrophages can be prominent in either, the surrounding lung parenchyma is usually normal in PPLA. Chest radiographs and computed tomography (CT) scans reveal alveolar and interstitial infiltrates, and pulmonary function tests often reveal a restrictive abnormality.[61] PPLA can be confused with LAM because of the presence of vimentin and desmin–positive spindle cell smooth muscle infiltrates and chylous accumulations, but PPLA is generally not associated with cystic change in the pulmonary parenchyma or with positivity for HMB-45. There are no known treatments for PPLA, but if proven to be a true lymphangiectasia, it is possible that the disorder could be treated by interruption of caudal lymphatic flow, such as TD ligation or TD embolization.

GENERALIZED LYMPHATIC ANOMALY WITH PULMONARY INVOLVEMENT

GLA may affect the skin, superficial soft tissue, abdominal and thoracic viscera, and bone.[62] GLA has been described in all ages, from birth to age 80. Thoracic involvement is common and often includes mediastinal lymphangioma, chylothorax, chylopericardium, chyloptysis, or PB, and interstitial changes that are often most prominent along bronchovascular bundles. Extrapulmonary features can include chylous ascites, protein-losing enteropathy, peripheral lymphedema, lymphopenia, hemihypertrophy, and disseminated intravascular coagulopathy. Bony involvement is common in GLA. When present, GLA tends to spare the cortex and to follow a more stable course than GSD.[63] Single or multiple lymphangiomyomas can be found within the mediastinum, diffusely infiltrating mediastinal fat, or adherent to the pleura or chest wall. Lymphangiography reveals multiple lesions of the TD, dilated lymphatic channels, and lymphangiomas throughout the bones and lungs. Bilateral interstitial infiltrates or pericardial and pleural effusions are often present on the chest radiograph. Pulmonary function tests may reveal a restrictive pattern, but mixed patterns are also found. CT scans of the thorax reveal diffuse thickening of intralobular septa and bronchovascular bundles with extensive involvement of mediastinal fat and perihilar regions. Histopathology demonstrates anastomosing endothelial-lined spaces along pulmonary lymphatic routes. Heavy T2-weighted MRI may reveal lymphatic anomalies in the thorax and abdomen, and IL[25] or DCMRL[26,27] can be used to define abnormal lymphatic low. A recent phase II trial demonstrated that sirolimus resulted in at least partial responses in 100% of patients with GLA.[64]

GORHAM-STOUT DISEASE

GSD, also called vanishing bone disease, is associated with abdominal and thoracic visceral lymphatic involvement, effusions, and destructive bony disease (**Fig. 4**).[65] In contrast to GLA, GSD involves the bone cortex and can result in progressive osteolysis.[63] Tissue samples are positive for lymphatic endothelial cell markers, suggesting that GSD is primarily a disease of disordered lymphangiogenesis.[66] Current treatments for GSD are primarily symptomatic and supportive and include control of mass effect using sclerotherapy,[67] and conservative and surgical treatment of chylous leaks. In a recent phase II trial of sirolimus treatment, 3 of 3 patients with GSD had partial responses.[64]

KAPOSIFORM LYMPHANGIOMATOSIS

KLA is a newly characterized entity that was initially described as a subtype of GLA but is now

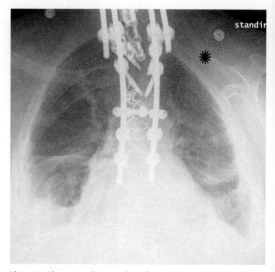

Fig. 4. Chest radiograph of an 11-year-old patient with GSD. Note the absence of the left clavicle (*black star*) due to osteolysis.

pathologically differentiated from that disorder by the presence of clusters or sheets of spindle-shaped lymphatic endothelial cells infiltrating malformed lymphatic channels.[68] It is important to distinguish KLA from PPLA or GLA because it tends to follow a more aggressive course, at least in children. Characteristic hematological abnormalities that occur in KLA can be helpful in that regard, including elevated fibrin split products and D-dimer, low fibrinogen and platelet count. Hemorrhagic complications also occur, including bloody effusions and expectorations. As with GLA, dilated, malformed lymphatic channels are lined by a single layer of endothelial cells in KLA. However, in KLA, foci of pattern-less clusters of intralymphatic or perilymphatic podoplanin, PROX1, and LYVE-1-positive spindled cells are found associated with platelet microthrombi, extravasated red blood cells, hemosiderin, and fibrosis without significant atypia or mitoses. It is not known whether spindled cells are clonal/neoplastic or reactive. Although the disease typically presents in early childhood, later onset has also been reported.[69] The most common manifestations of KLA are respiratory symptoms, including cough, shortness of breath and hemoptysis (50%), hemostatic abnormalities (50%), enlarging, palpable masses (35%),[68] mediastinal masses, interstitial infiltrates (**Fig. 5**), and effusions, which can be chylous or hemorrhagic. Dilated, blood-filled lymphatic channels may be visualized on the pleural surface during video-assisted thoracoscopic surgery. Hemorrhagic lesions have also been seen on peritoneal and pericardial surfaces. Progressive interstitial lung disease and chylous

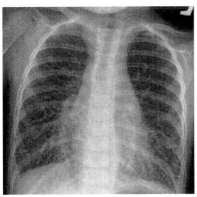
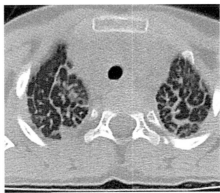

Fig. 5. Chest radiograph and chest CT of a patient with KLA shows increased interstitial markings.

pleural effusions can lead to respiratory failure. Vincristine and sirolimus treatment have been reported in KLA.[70,71] In a recent phase II sirolimus trial, 5 of 7 patients with KLA had a partial response and 1 had stable disease.[64]

CHYLOPTYSIS AND PLASTIC BRONCHITIS

PB describes a heterogenous group of allergic, immunologic, infectious, cardiac, neoplastic, and lymphatic disorders that are associated with expectoration of bronchial casts.[72] PB as it has been defined is not a single disease with a unifying mechanism that explains cast formation in all conditions. Indeed, it is not clear that PB is always associated with bronchitis, defined as disruption, dysfunction, or inflammation of bronchial mucosa.

In most cases of true PB, the bronchial system may be serving as no more than a mold for congealing bronchial contents. This finding is certainly true in the most common form of PB, which follows cardiac surgery for congenital heart disease, especially the Fontan procedure. In these cases, abnormal pulmonary lymphatic flow (**Fig. 6**) results in leakage of proteinaceous and lipid-rich fluids into the bronchial tree.[73] Recently, heavy T2-weighted MRI has revealed that occult lymphatic anomalies that represent developmental remnants or subclinical GLA are present in adults who present with expectoration of large multiantennary, branching casts.[2] IL[25] and DCMRL[26,27] have been used to more precisely image the leaks, and in the small number of patients who have been treated to date, embolization of the TD has

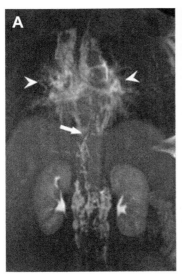
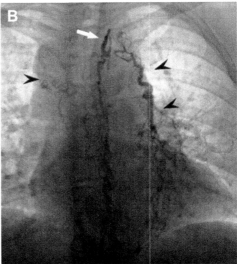

Fig. 6. (A) DCMRL in patient with idiopathic PB demonstrating small TD (*white arrow*) and abnormal pulmonary lymphatic perfusion in the mediastinum and lung hila (*white arrowheads*). (B) Corresponding fluoroscopy image of the TD of the same patient, following injection of contrast material through the microcatheter positioned in the proximal part of TD, demonstrating occlusion of the distal part of the TD (*white arrow*) and retrograde flow of the contrast in the mediastinal lymphatic ducts (*black arrowheads*).

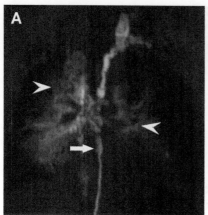 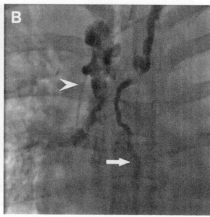

Fig. 7. (A) DCMRL in a patient with pulmonary lymphangiectasia demonstrating dilated TD (*white arrow*) and abnormal pulmonary lymphatic perfusion in the lung hilum (*white arrowheads*). (B) Corresponding fluoroscopy image of the TD of the same patient, following injection of contrast material through the microcatheter positioned in proximal part of TD, confirms the dilation of the TD (*white arrow*) and retrograde flow of the contrast in the mediastinal lymphatic ducts (*white arrowhead*).

been highly successful in controlling cast formation (Maxim Itkin, Francis X. McCormack, Yoav Dori, unpublished data, 2016). The authors submit that lymphatic causes should be considered in all patients who present with expectoration of complex, multiantennary branching casts. Heavy T2-weighted MRI, and, as appropriate, IL and/or DCMRL may be useful for identifying pathogenic lymphatic tissue and lymphatic flow. Cannulation of the TD followed by embolization should be considered in those patients who are shown to have leakage of lymphatic fluid into the airway.[27] Therapeutic interventions with medium-chain triglyceride-enriched low-fat diets, intratracheal heparin, inhaled tissue plasminogen activator, and steroids have also been reported and have met with variable success.[74–77]

PULMONARY LYMPHANGIECTASIA

PL describes pathologic dilation of lymphatic vessels in the lungs. Both primary and secondary forms have been described. The former primarily occurs in neonates due to failure of pulmonary interstitial tissues to regress and is typically fatal, and the secondary forms are usually due to processes that impair lymphatic flow or increase lymph production. The ISSVA defined isolated lymphangiectasia as a lymphatic conductive disorder,[4] highlighting that the ectatic lymphatic vessels are connected to the main lymphatic system. As a result, a common presentation of thoracic lymphangiectasia is chylous effusion. The cause of lymphangiectasia is unknown, but may be due to congenital occlusion of parts of the central lymphatic system, such as the TD, absence of

the lymphatic valves, or lymphatic fluid overproduction that results in overdistention and overgrowth of the lymphatic vessels.[78]

The clinical presentation of PL includes respiratory symptoms of wheezing, chronic cough or chest pain, bilateral interstitial infiltrates, restrictive pulmonary physiology, and pericardial and pleural effusions.[13]

The diagnosis of PL is based on dilated lymphatic vessels in perivascular and peribronchial distributions on pathologic analysis, patchy ground glass opacification and thickening of the interlobular septa on CT,[61] or reflux of contrast into the lung parenchyma on lymphangiogram.[79]

Occlusion and narrowing of the upper part of the TD with retrograde pulmonary lymphatic flow occurs in patients with idiopathic chylopericardium and chylothorax on DCMRL and IL (**Fig. 7**). For that reason, the authors recommend DCMRL and IL as the first imaging modalities for a patient presenting with idiopathic chylothorax/chylopericardium with and without lung disease.

Treatments that have been attempted for PL include thoracentesis, dietary modification, pleurodesis, octreotide, and interruption of cranial thoracic lymphatic flow (TD embolization, TD ligation).[80] Prognosis is usually good in cases where chylothorax and chylopericardium can be controlled.

THE YELLOW NAIL SYNDROME

Of all the TLDs, the YNS is one of the most likely to present in adulthood, at a median age of 40 to 50 years.[81,82] The YNS was first described by

White and Samman in 1964,[83] now defined as the triad of yellow dystrophic fingernails (86%), pleural effusion (36%), and idiopathic lymphedema (80%). Only 20% to 30% of cases have all 3 manifestations, and the presence of any 2 is generally considered to be diagnostic. More than 60% of patients develop sinopulmonary manifestations other than pleural effusion, which can include chronic cough, repeated infection, rhinosinusitis, recurrent pneumonia, bronchiectasis, and sinusitis. Whether YNS represents a genetic or acquired disorder remains controversial.[84,85] Wells described an extended family with 8 affected members.[86] The proband developed lower extremity lymphedema as well as edema in the vocal cords, genitalia, hands, and face. Although cases of YNS have occurred in patients with connective tissue disease, neoplasms, immunodeficiencies, and endocrine disorders, it is unclear if these disorders play a direct role in disease pathogenesis or simply represent chance associations. In the largest retrospective study of YNS to date, 9 of 150 patients were found to have a family history of lymphedema or YNS.[81] Two reports of infants born with hydrops and chylothorax to mothers with YNS suggest a heritable cause in some cases.[87,88] Mutations in the FOXC2 gene have been described in patients with the lymphedema-distichiasis (LD) syndrome, some of whom also have yellow nails, leading Finegold and colleagues[89] to conclude that there is phenotypic overlap between LD and YNS. A subsequent analysis of 4 families with YNS revealed no evidence of FOXC2 mutations, however.[90] It is important to note that although nail changes and yellowing occur in other forms of lymphedema, the nail manifestations of YNS are quite distinctive and include marked thickening, very slow growth, excessive side-to-side curvature, loss of lunulae and cuticles, and detachment from the nail bed (onycholysis).[91] It is interesting that the nail changes in YNS can spontaneously regress. The male:female ratio of affected patients is 1.2/1. Pulmonary effusions are bilateral in 68% of cases and are most commonly lymphocytic exudates.[81] Chylothorax is documented in a minority of cases in retrospective series (~20%), but it is unclear if the diagnosis was rigorously pursued in all cases. Pleural effusions routinely reoccur despite repeated taps, but pleurodesis is effective in more than 80% of cases. Pericardial effusions have also been described, and in some cases, have required pericardiectomy. Nail matrix biopsies reveal ectatic endothelial lined channels and dense stromal fibrosis, and pleural biopsies demonstrate dilated lymphatics associated with lymphocytic pleuritis and moderate fibrosis.

Lymphangiograms and lymphoscintigraphy often reveal hypoplasia of lymphatics. There is no effective treatment for YNS, but octreotide therapy has been attempted in some cases.[92,93]

SUMMARY AND FUTURE DIRECTIONS

There has been an explosion in molecular understanding of lymphatic development in the last 2 decades, yielding powerful new markers to probe disease pathogenesis in the TLD.[94] More detailed histopathologic and immunohistochemical characterization using these tools is defining subsets of GLA that exhibit more aggressive behavior. Improved imaging of the lymphatic system (eg, DCMRL) promises to rapidly enhance the understanding of the pathogenesis of TLD. Genetic analyses are revealing the genetic basis of lymphatic malformation and primary lymphedema disorders. Recent trials of the antilymphangiogenic drug sirolimus have revealed stabilizing effects on lung function, reversal of chylous effusions, shrinkage of lymphatic masses, and promising benefits in many of the complex vascular anomalies described here. Lymphatic biomarkers that are useful diagnostically and correlate with disease progression have been reported. Recent technical advances have resulted in novel approaches to controlling lymphatic leaks. Powerful new approaches to molecular and genetic characterization promise to shed new light on disease pathogenesis and uncover novel therapeutic targets.

REFERENCES

1. Moua T, Olson EJ, St Jean HC, et al. Resolution of chylous pulmonary congestion and respiratory failure in LAM with sirolimus therapy. Am J Respir Crit Care Med 2012;186(4):389–90.
2. Mouhadi El S, Taillé C, Cazes A, et al. Plastic bronchitis related to idiopathic thoracic lymphangiectasia. Noncontrast magnetic resonance lymphography. Am J Respir Crit Care Med 2015;192(5):632–3.
3. Noonan JA, Walters LR, Reeves JT. Congenital pulmonary lymphangiectasis. Am J Dis Child 1970; 120(4):314–9.
4. Wassef M, Blei F, Adams D, et al. Vascular anomalies classification: recommendations from the International Society for the Study of Vascular Anomalies. Pediatrics 2015;136(1):e203–14.
5. Esther CR, Barker PM. Pulmonary lymphangiectasia: diagnosis and clinical course. Pediatr Pulmonol 2004;38(4):308–13.
6. Hilliard RI, McKendry JB, Phillips MJ. Congenital abnormalities of the lymphatic system: a new clinical classification. Pediatrics 1990;86(6):988–94.

7. Smeltzer DM, Stickler GB, Schirger A. Primary lymphedema in children and adolescents: a follow-up study and review. Pediatrics 1985;76(2):206–18.

8. Felman AH, Rhatigan RM, Pierson KK. Pulmonary lymphangiectasia. Observation in 17 patients and proposed classification. Am J Roentgenol Radium Ther Nucl Med 1972;116(3):548–58.

9. Lloyd ES, Press HC. Congenital pulmonary lymphangiectasis. South Med J 1979;72(9):1205–6.

10. Kirchner J, Jacobi V, Schneider M, et al. Primary congenital pulmonary lymphangiectasia–a case report. Wien Klin Wochenschr 1997;109(23): 922–4.

11. Swank DW, Hepper NG, Folkert KE, et al. Intrathoracic lymphangiomatosis mimicking lymphangioleiomyomatosis in a young woman. Mayo Clin Proc 1989;64(10):1264–8.

12. Margraf LR. Thoracic lymphangiomatosis. Pediatr Pathol Lab Med 1996;16(1):155–60.

13. Tazelaar HD, Kerr D, Yousem SA, et al. Diffuse pulmonary lymphangiomatosis. Hum Pathol 1993; 24(12):1313–22.

14. Caballero Y, Pérez D, Cano JR. Diffuse pulmonary lymphangiomatosis with mediastinal affectation. Arch Bronconeumol 2011;47(9):474–5.

15. Bulbul A, Okan F, Nuhoglu A. Idiopathic congenital chylothorax presented with severe hydrops and treated with octreotide in term newborn. J Matern Fetal Neonatal Med 2009;22(12):1197–200.

16. Bialkowski A, Poets CF, Franz AR, Erhebungseinheit für seltene pädiatrische Erkrankungen in Deutschland Study Group. Congenital chylothorax: a prospective nationwide epidemiological study in Germany. Arch Dis Child Fetal Neonatal Ed 2015; 100(2):F169–72.

17. de Winter RJ, Bresser P, Römer JW, et al. Idiopathic chylopericardium with bilateral pulmonary reflux of chyle. Am Heart J 1994;127(4 Pt 1):936–9.

18. Miyoshi K, Nakagawa T, Kokado Y, et al. Primary chylopericardium with pulmonary lymphedema. Thorac Cardiovasc Surg 2008;56(5):306–8.

19. Faul JL, Berry GJ, Colby TV, et al. Thoracic lymphangiomas, lymphangiectasis, lymphangiomatosis, and lymphatic dysplasia syndrome. Am J Respir Crit Care Med 2000;161(3 Pt 1):1037–46.

20. Beveridge N, Allen L, Rogers K. Lymphoscintigraphy in the diagnosis of lymphangiomatosis. Clin Nucl Med 2010;35(8):579–82.

21. Kinmonth J. Management of some abnormalities of the chylous return. Proc R Soc Med 1972;65(8): 721–2.

22. Bellini C, Villa G, Sambuceti G, et al. Lymphoscintigraphy patterns in newborns and children with congenital lymphatic dysplasia. Lymphology 2014; 47(1):28–39.

23. Kinmonth J, Taylor G. Chylous reflux. Br Med J 1964; 1(5382):529–32.

24. Freundlich IM. The role of lymphangiography in chylothorax. A report of six nontraumatic cases. Am J Roentgenol Radium Ther Nucl Med 1975;125(3): 617–27.

25. Nadolski GJ, Itkin M. Feasibility of ultrasound-guided intranodal lymphangiogram for thoracic duct embolization. J Vasc Interv Radiol 2012;23(5): 613–6.

26. Dori Y, Zviman MM, Itkin M. Dynamic contrast-enhanced MR lymphangiography: feasibility study in swine. Radiology 2014;273(2):410–6.

27. Dori Y, Keller MS, Rychik J, et al. Successful treatment of plastic bronchitis by selective lymphatic embolization in a Fontan patient. Pediatrics 2014; 134(2):e590–5.

28. Elluru RG, Balakrishnan K, Padua HM. Lymphatic malformations: diagnosis and management. Semin Pediatr Surg 2014;23(4):178–85.

29. Oshikiri T, Morikawa T, Jinushi E, et al. Five cases of the lymphangioma of the mediastinum in adult. Ann Thorac Cardiovasc Surg 2001;7(2):103–5.

30. Charruau L, Parrens M, Jougon J, et al. Mediastinal lymphangioma in adults: CT and MR imaging features. Eur Radiol 2000;10(8):1310–4.

31. Benninghoff MG, Todd WU, Bascom R. Incidental pleural-based pulmonary lymphangioma. J Am Osteopath Assoc 2008;108(9):525–8.

32. Wilson C, Askin FB, Heitmiller RF. Solitary pulmonary lymphangioma. Ann Thorac Surg 2001;71(4): 1337–8.

33. Shaffer K, Rosado-de-Christenson ML, Patz EF, et al. Thoracic lymphangioma in adults: CT and MR imaging features. AJR Am J Roentgenol 1994;162(2): 283–9.

34. Kransdorf MJ. Benign soft-tissue tumors in a large referral population: distribution of specific diagnoses by age, sex, and location. AJR Am J Roentgenol 1995;164(2):395–402.

35. Pike MG, Wood AJ, Corrin B, et al. Intrathoracic extramediastinal cystic hygroma. Arch Dis Child 1984; 59(1):75–7.

36. Miyake H, Shiga M, Takaki H, et al. Mediastinal lymphangiomas in adults: CT findings. J Thorac Imaging 1996;11(1):83–5.

37. Luks VL, Kamitaki N, Vivero MP, et al. Lymphatic and other vascular malformative/overgrowth disorders are caused by somatic mutations in PIK3CA. J Pediatr 2015;166(4):1048–54.e1–5.

38. Seyama K, Kumasaka T, Kurihara M, et al. Lymphangioleiomyomatosis: a disease involving the lymphatic system. Lymphat Res Biol 2010;8(1): 21–31.

39. Henske EP, McCormack FX. Lymphangioleiomyomatosis—a wolf in sheep's clothing. J Clin Invest 2012;122(11):3807–16.

40. McCormack FX, Travis WD, Colby TV, et al. Lymphangioleiomyomatosis: calling it what it is: a

low-grade, destructive, metastasizing neoplasm. Am J Respir Crit Care Med 2012;186(12):1210–2.

41. Muzykewicz DA, Sharma A, Muse V, et al. TSC1 and TSC2 mutations in patients with lymphangioleiomyomatosis and tuberous sclerosis complex. J Med Genet 2009;46(7):465–8.

42. Dabora SL, Jozwiak S, Franz DN, et al. Mutational analysis in a cohort of 224 tuberous sclerosis patients Indicates increased severity of TSC2, compared with TSC1, disease in multiple organs. Am J Hum Genet 2001;68(1):64–80.

43. Carsillo T, Astrinidis A, Henske EP. Mutations in the tuberous sclerosis complex gene TSC2 are a cause of sporadic pulmonary lymphangioleiomyomatosis. Proc Natl Acad Sci U S A 2000;97(11): 6085–90.

44. Astrinidis A, Khare L, Carsillo T, et al. Mutational analysis of the tuberous sclerosis gene TSC2 in patients with pulmonary lymphangioleiomyomatosis. J Med Genet 2000;37(1):55–7.

45. Kumasaka T, Seyama K, Mitani K, et al. Lymphangiogenesis in lymphangioleiomyomatosis: its implication in the progression of lymphangioleiomyomatosis. Am J Surg Pathol 2004;28(8):1007–16.

46. Kumasaka T, Seyama K, Mitani K, et al. Lymphangiogenesis-mediated shedding of LAM cell clusters as a mechanism for dissemination in lymphangioleiomyomatosis. Am J Surg Pathol 2005;29(10): 1356–66.

47. Tobino K, Johkoh T, Fujimoto K, et al. Computed tomographic features of lymphangioleiomyomatosis: evaluation in 138 patients. Eur J Radiol 2015;84(3): 534–41.

48. Gao L, Yue MM, Davis J, et al. In pulmonary lymphangioleiomyomatosis expression of progesterone receptor is frequently higher than that of estrogen receptor. Virchows Arch 2014;464(4):495–503.

49. Longacre TA, Hendrickson MR, Kapp DS, et al. Lymphangioleiomyomatosis of the uterus simulating high-stage endometrial stromal sarcoma. Gynecol Oncol 1996;63(3):404–10.

50. Hayashi T, Kumasaka T, Mitani K, et al. Prevalence of uterine and adnexal involvement in pulmonary lymphangioleiomyomatosis: a clinicopathologic study of 10 patients. Am J Surg Pathol 2011;35(12): 1776–85.

51. Taveira-DaSilva AM, Hathaway O, Stylianou M, et al. Changes in lung function and chylous effusions in patients with lymphangioleiomyomatosis treated with sirolimus. Ann Intern Med 2011;154(12): 797–805. W–292–3.

52. Davis JM, Hyjek E, Husain AN, et al. Lymphatic endothelial differentiation in pulmonary lymphangioleiomyomatosis cells. J Histochem Cytochem 2013; 61(8):580–90.

53. Young LR, Vandyke R, Gulleman PM, et al. Serum vascular endothelial growth factor-D prospectively distinguishes lymphangioleiomyomatosis from other diseases. Chest 2010;138(3):674–81.

54. Young LR, Inoue Y, McCormack FX. Diagnostic potential of serum VEGF-D for lymphangioleiomyomatosis. N Engl J Med 2008;358(2):199–200.

55. Young LR, Lee H-S, Inoue Y, et al. Serum VEGF-D concentration as a biomarker of lymphangioleiomyomatosis severity and treatment response: a prospective analysis of the Multicenter International Lymphangioleiomyomatosis Efficacy of Sirolimus (MILES) trial. Lancet Respir Med 2013;1(6): 445–52.

56. Seyama K, Kumasaka T, Souma S, et al. Vascular endothelial growth factor-D is increased in serum of patients with lymphangioleiomyomatosis. Lymphat Res Biol 2006;4(3):143–52.

57. McCormack FX, Inoue Y, Moss J, et al. Efficacy and safety of sirolimus in lymphangioleiomyomatosis. N Engl J Med 2011;364(17):1595–606.

58. Toyoshima M, Suzuki S, Kono M, et al. Mildly progressive pulmonary lymphangiectasis diagnosed in a young adult. Am J Respir Crit Care Med 2014; 189(7):860–2.

59. Liu NF, Yan ZX, Wu XF. Classification of lymphatic-system malformations in primary lymphoedema based on MR lymphangiography. Eur J Vasc Endovasc Surg 2012;44(3):345–9.

60. Canny GJ, Cutz E, MacLusky IB, et al. Diffuse pulmonary angiomatosis. Thorax 1991;46(11):851–3.

61. Swensen SJ, Hartman TE, Mayo JR, et al. Diffuse pulmonary lymphangiomatosis: CT findings. J Comput Assist Tomogr 1995;19(3):348–52.

62. Ozeki M, Fujino A, Matsuoka K, et al. Clinical features and prognosis of generalized lymphatic anomaly, Kaposiform lymphangiomatosis, and Gorham-Stout disease. Pediatr Blood Cancer 2016; 63(5):832–8.

63. Lala S, Mulliken JB, Alomari AI, et al. Gorham-Stout disease and generalized lymphatic anomaly–clinical, radiologic, and histologic differentiation. Skeletal Radiol 2013;42(7):917–24.

64. Adams DM, Trenor CC, Hammill AM, et al. Efficacy and safety of sirolimus in the treatment of complicated vascular anomalies. Pediatrics 2016;137(2):1–10.

65. Trenor CC, Chaudry G. Complex lymphatic anomalies. Semin Pediatr Surg 2014;23(4):186–90.

66. Radhakrishnan K, Rockson SG. Gorham's disease: an osseous disease of lymphangiogenesis? Ann N Y Acad Sci 2008;1131(1):203–5.

67. Molitch HI, Unger EC, Witte CL, et al. Percutaneous sclerotherapy of lymphangiomas. Radiology 1995; 194(2):343–7.

68. Croteau SE, Kozakewich HPW, Perez-Atayde AR, et al. Kaposiform lymphangiomatosis: a distinct aggressive lymphatic anomaly. J Pediatr 2014; 164(2):383–8.

69. Safi F, Gupta A, Adams D, et al. Kaposiform lymphangiomatosis, a newly characterized vascular anomaly presenting with hemoptysis in an adult woman. Ann Am Thorac Soc 2014;11(1):92–5.

70. Fernandes VM, Fargo JH, Saini S, et al. Kaposiform lymphangiomatosis: unifying features of a heterogeneous disorder. Pediatr Blood Cancer 2014;62(5):901–4.

71. Wang Z, Li K, Yao W, et al. Successful treatment of kaposiform lymphangiomatosis with sirolimus. Pediatr Blood Cancer 2015;62(7):1291–3.

72. Eberlein MH, Drummond MB, Haponik EF. Plastic bronchitis: a management challenge. Am J Med Sci 2008;335(2):163–9.

73. Dori Y, Keller MS, Rome JJ, et al. Percutaneous lymphatic embolization of abnormal pulmonary lymphatic flow as treatment of plastic bronchitis in patients with congenital heart disease. Circulation 2016;133(12):1160–70.

74. Avitabile CM, Goldberg DJ, Dodds K, et al. A multifaceted approach to the management of plastic bronchitis after cavopulmonary palliation. Ann Thorac Surg 2014;98(2):634–40.

75. Parikh K, WITTE MH, Samson R, et al. Successful treatment of plastic bronchitis with low fat diet and subsequent thoracic duct ligation in child with fontan physiology. Lymphology 2012;45(2):47–52.

76. Turgut T, In E, Ozercan IH, et al. A case of plastic bronchitis. Arch Iran Med 2014;17(8):589–90.

77. Houin PR, Veress LA, Rancourt RC, et al. Intratracheal heparin improves plastic bronchitis due to sulfur mustard analog. Pediatr Pulmonol 2015;50(2):118–26.

78. Gray M, Kovatis KZ, Stuart T, et al. Treatment of congenital pulmonary lymphangiectasia using ethiodized oil lymphangiography. J Perinatol 2014;34(9):720–2.

79. Toltzis RJ, Rosenthal A, Fellows K, et al. Chylous reflux syndrome involving the pericardium and lung. Chest 1978;74(4):457–8.

80. Nadolski GJ, Itkin M. Thoracic duct embolization (TDE) for non-traumatic chylous effusion: experience in 34 patients. Chest 2013;143(1):158–63.

81. Valdes L, Huggins JT, Gude F, et al. Characteristics of patients with yellow nail syndrome and pleural effusion. Respirology 2014;19(7):985–92.

82. Maldonado F, Ryu JH. Yellow nail syndrome. Curr Opin Pulm Med 2009;15(4):371–5.

83. Samman PD, White WF. The "yellow nail" syndrome. Br J Dermatol 1964;76:153–7.

84. Razi E. Familial yellow nail syndrome. Dermatol Online J 2006;12(2):15.

85. Lambert EM, Dziura J, Kauls L, et al. Yellow nail syndrome in three siblings: a randomized double-blind trial of topical vitamin E. Pediatr Dermatol 2006;23(4):390–5.

86. Wells GC. Yellow nail syndrome: with familiar primary hypoplasia of lymphatics, manifest late in life. Proc R Soc Med 1966;59(5):447.

87. Slee J, Nelson J, Dickinson J, et al. Yellow nail syndrome presenting as non-immune hydrops: second case report. Am J Med Genet 2000;93(1):1–4.

88. Govaert P, Leroy JG, Pauwels R, et al. Perinatal manifestations of maternal yellow nail syndrome. Pediatrics 1992;89(6 Pt 1):1016–8.

89. Finegold DN, Kimak MA, Lawrence EC, et al. Truncating mutations in FOXC2 cause multiple lymphedema syndromes. Hum Mol Genet 2001;10(11):1185–9.

90. Rezaie T, Ghoroghchian R, Bell R, et al. Primary non-syndromic lymphoedema (Meige disease) is not caused by mutations in FOXC2. Eur J Hum Genet 2008;16(3):300–4.

91. Hoque SR, Mansour S, Mortimer PS. Yellow nail syndrome: not a genetic disorder? Eleven new cases and a review of the literature. Br J Dermatol 2007;156(6):1230–4.

92. Makrilakis K, Pavlatos S, Giannikopoulos G, et al. Successful octreotide treatment of chylous pleural effusion and lymphedema in the yellow nail syndrome. Ann Intern Med 2004;141(3):246–7.

93. Widjaja A, Gratz KF, Ockenga J, et al. Octreotide for therapy of chylous ascites in yellow nail syndrome. Gastroenterology 1999;116(4):1017–8.

94. Alitalo K. The lymphatic vasculature in disease. Nat Med 2011;17(11):1371–80.

Langerhans Cell Histiocytosis and Other Histiocytic Diseases of the Lung

Erin DeMartino, MD[a], Ronald S. Go, MD[b],
Robert Vassallo, MD[a,c,d],*

KEYWORDS

- Histiocyte • Langerhans cell • Macrophage • Cigarette smoking • Lung • Interstitial • BRAF

KEY POINTS

- Several of the primary histiocytic disorders may affect the lung in varying ways: among the histiocytic disorders occurring in adult patients, Langerhans cell histiocytosis is the most commonly encountered and usually is associated with cigarette smoking.
- The histiocytic disorders are rare, and all manifest variable clinical courses that may range from benign disease with spontaneous regression to life-threatening aggressive disorders associated with high morbidity and mortality.
- Definitive diagnosis of these rare clinical entities requires histopathologic confirmation.
- Activating mutations associated with specific cell regulatory pathways have been described in Langerhans cell histiocytosis and Erdheim-Chester disease and provide information about the natural biology of these diseases as well as potential for specific targeted treatment using inhibitors of these pathways.
- Management includes specific treatment of the underlying histiocytic disorder, avoidance of exacerbating factors like cigarette smoking or second-hand smoke exposure, management of complications (such as pneumothorax or pulmonary hypertension), and lung transplantation in selected instances.

INTRODUCTION

The histiocytic syndromes are a diverse collection of diseases caused by proliferative abnormalities in the macrophage and dendritic cell lineage, but resulting in strikingly varied clinical behavior. Although some syndromes are life-threatening, others follow an indolent course and require minimal therapeutic intervention. The Langerhans cell histiocytoses (LCH) are a subclassification of these syndromes caused by infiltration of specialized dendritic cells (Langerhans cells) into the lung as a single disease site, or multiple organs.[1] These infiltrating cells trigger an inflammatory cascade and varying degrees of organ dysfunction.[2,3] Other, less common, histiocytic syndromes that can involve the lung include Erdheim-Chester disease (ECD) and Rosai-Dorfman disease (RDD). Key aspects of these histiocytic entities are summarized in **Table 1**. Pulmonary LCH (PLCH) is reviewed in detail in the current review, because it is the predominant

Disclosure Statement: The authors have nothing to disclose.
R. Vassallo is supported by a Flight Attendant Medical Research Institute grant (FAMRI CIA_123022).
[a] Division of Pulmonary and Critical Care Medicine, Mayo Clinic, 200 First Street SW, Rochester, MN 55905, USA; [b] Division of Hematology, Mayo Clinic, 200 First Street SW, Rochester, MN 55905, USA; [c] Department of Medicine, Mayo Clinic, 200 First Street SW, Rochester, MN 55905, USA; [d] Department of Physiology and Biomedical Engineering, Mayo Clinic, 200 First Street SW, Rochester, MN 55905, USA
* Corresponding author. Division of Pulmonary and Critical Care Medicine, Mayo Clinic, 200 First Street SW, Rochester, MN 55905.
E-mail address: vassallo.robert@mayo.edu

Clin Chest Med 37 (2016) 421–430
http://dx.doi.org/10.1016/j.ccm.2016.04.005
0272-5231/16/$ – see front matter © 2016 Elsevier Inc. All rights reserved.

Table 1
Summary of certain contrasting features between pulmonary Langerhans cell histiocytosis, Erdheim-Chester disease, and Rosai-Dorfman disease

	Pulmonary LCH	Erdheim-Chester Disease	Rosai-Dorfman Disease
Association with cigarette smoking	Yes	No	No
Key histopathologic findings	Bronchiolocentric lesions with Langerhans cells, eosinophils, and other inflammatory cells forming loosely formed nodular lesions	Tissue infiltration by foamy histiocytes with interspersed inflammatory cells and multinucleate giant cells in a background of variable fibrosis	Tissue infiltration by histiocytic cells with mixed inflammatory infiltrates. Emperipolesis (histiocytic cells engulfing leukocytes) is a cardinal feature
Immunostaining profile of lung biopsy	S-100+, CD1a+, Langerin+ Factor XIIIa−	CD68+, CD163+, Factor XIIIa+ CD1a−, S-100−, Langerin−	S100+, CD14+, CD68+, and CD11c+ CD1a−, Langerin−, Factor XIIIa−
Birbeck granules on electron microscopy	Present	Absent	Absent
Detection of BRAF-V600E mutation	Approximately 30% of cases	At least 50%	Usually negative
Predominant chest CT findings	Cysts and lung nodules distributed mainly in the mid and upper lung fields with sparing of the lung base.	Mediastinal infiltration, pleural thickening/effusion, interlobular septal thickening, centrilobular nodular opacities, ground-glass opacities, and lung cysts	Mediastinal and hilar adenopathy most common feature. Cystic change, parenchymal infiltrates, and airway disease are less common

histiocytic disorder encountered by pulmonary specialists, while key features of ECD and RDD will also be outlined.

EPIDEMIOLOGY AND DEMOGRAPHICS

Although considered an uncommon disease, the exact prevalence and incidence of LCH are unknown. One study described greater than 500 patients with lung diseases who underwent surgical lung biopsy; PLCH was identified in 3.4% of cases.[3] PLCH can affect all ethnic groups and all ages, although most often patients are diagnosed between the ages of 20 and 40 years.[4,5] Heritable genetic factors do not appear to play a prominent role in pathogenesis.[6] Isolated PLCH is primarily a disease of young adult smokers, with greater than 90% of patients endorsing a smoking history in several series.[4,7,8] In multisystem LCH, the smoking connection is less clear. Although multisystem LCH is 3 times more prevalent in the pediatric population than adults, isolated PLCH is exceedingly rare in children.[9,10] Case reports of PLCH recurrence in adolescents who smoke with childhood multisystem LCH in remission support the

hypothesis that tobacco smoke exposure plays a critical role in the pathogenesis of PLCH.[11]

PATHOLOGY AND PATHOPHYSIOLOGY

In cases of advanced PLCH, gross pathologic inspection may reveal cysts on the pleural surface and palpable nodules of various sizes.[12] Although most nodules are between 1 and 5 mm in size, they can grow to sizes of up to 15 mm. In late disease, nodules are replaced by advanced bullous and cystic lesions, often in association with hyperinflation and late-stage fibrosis with honeycombing.[13] PLCH affects the bronchiolar, interstitial, alveolar, and vascular compartments of the lung to variable degrees in different patients. Although traditionally considered an interstitial lung disease, it is arguably more appropriate to consider PLCH as an inflammatory bronchiolitis with loosely formed nodules of dendritic cells aggregating around small airways,[8,12,14] resulting in varying degrees of interstitial inflammation, alveolar macrophage infiltration,[13] and proliferative vasculopathy of both arteries and veins.[8,15,16]

Loosely formed cellular nodules cluster adjacent to the small airways and are scattered throughout the lung parenchyma in early disease.[13] The composition of these early lesions includes abundant Langerhans' cells and varying numbers of lymphocytes, macrophages, monocytes, plasma cells, and eosinophils.[13] Extensive eosinophilic infiltration is commonly encountered, hence the former descriptor "eosinophilic granulomas."[12] Pathologic findings evolve from symmetric stellate lesions with adjacent pigmented alveolar macrophage accumulation in early disease (so-called pseudo-desquamative pneumonia)[8,12,16] to destruction of bronchiolar and alveolar structures in advanced disease, typically with diminished cellularity.[12]

Ultrastructurally, Langerhans' cells have distinctive, elongated nuclei and pale cytoplasm. Langerhans' cells are definitively identified by the presence on electron microscopy of Birbeck granules, pathognomonic rod-shaped intracellular inclusions, or by immunohistochemical staining for CD1a surface antigen.[17] S-100 staining can detect the presence of Langerhans' cells, but macrophages may also react with S-100. The mere presence of Langerhans' cells is not sufficient to establish the diagnosis of LCH, because this cell population can be present in lung cancer and idiopathic fibrosis.[18,19] Irregular, stellate-shaped cystic lesions result from destruction of bronchiolar walls by peribronchiolar inflammation, with progressive dilation and fibrotic envelopment of small airway lumina.[13,15]

Langerhans' cells, epithelial-associated antigen-presenting dendritic cells regulating innate and acquired immune responses of the skin, gastrointestinal and airway mucosa, are central to the pathogenesis of PLCH.[20–22] Langerhans' cells sample epithelial lining fluid for "danger" signals by projecting periscopelike extensions between epithelial cells.[23,24] If an antigen breaches the epithelial barrier, it encounters a web of Langerhans' cell dendritic projections. Following antigen exposure, toll-like receptor, and CD40 receptor activation, the Langerhans' cell undergoes maturation, upregulating cell surface receptors, migrating to regional lymphoid tissue and facilitating costimulation of T and B cells.[24] By surveying and processing a vast array of inhaled antigens and pathogens, Langerhans' cells play a crucial role in modulating the regional immune response. Langerhans' cells in healthy individuals must intricately balance tolerance to harmless antigens and induction of immunity to pathogens. Although the mechanism of this sensitive balance is incompletely understood, cytokines, chemokines, and other signaling by local macrophages clearly influence Langerhans' cell functions.

Despite a clear epidemiologic link between cigarette smoke exposure and PLCH, the role of smoking in disease pathogenesis is incompletely understood. In murine models, exposure to tobacco smoke stimulates expansion of the lung dendritic cell population.[25] In one study, mice chronically exposed to cigarette smoke developed loosely formed granulomas,[25] but this observation has not been reproduced, and an animal model does not exist. Although tobacco smoke exposure appears important in PLCH pathogenesis, the relatively low frequency of the disease implies that other factors, including environmental exposures, viruses, or genetic modifiers, may also predispose to the disease.

Clonal expansion is a hallmark of neoplastic processes. Demonstration of clonal patterns in lesional tissues of adults and children with extrapulmonary LCH has led to categorization of this process as a neoplasm, yet clonal expansion has not been detected in all PLCH lesions.[26,27] The different derivations of Langerhans' cell populations in the lesional tissue of patients with systemic LCH versus PLCH suggest distinct mechanisms of disease. BRAF-V600E mutations have been reported in patients with both isolated pulmonary and multisystemic LCH, although the frequency of activating BRAF mutations is higher in the latter.[28,29] Badalian-Very and colleagues[29] found that 57% of archived nonpulmonary LCH specimens contained an activating mutation in the BRAF pathway, whereas Roden and colleagues[28] reported BRAF-V600E expression in 28% of patients with PLCH. Although clonal Langerhans' cells are not universally observed in PLCH, this may be explained by a low mutant allele frequency in the cells as well as the potential effect of cigarette smoke exposure, causing a mixture of clonal and nonclonally expanded Langerhans' cell populations.[28,29] A recent study showed that the BRAF-V600E mutation in predominantly pediatric patients with so-called high-risk LCH (LCH associated with involvement of the spleen, liver, bone marrow, lung, and skeleton; usually more difficult and resistant to treatment) may be identified in circulating somatic cells, whereas the BRAF-V600E mutation in low-risk LCH patients (disease involving skin, bones, lymph nodes, or pituitary gland, which is usually associated with better prognosis) is likely to only be identified in lesional tissue.[30] These recent observations support a causative role for BRAF-V600E mutations in the pathogenesis of both pediatric and adult LCH (including PLCH) and suggest that at least a proportion of cases are consistent with classification of the disease as a myeloid neoplasm with varied biological expression. Activating mutations involving the mitogen-activated protein kinase pathway (MAPK) have also been described in systemic LCH.[31] Recent studies using whole exome and transcriptome sequencing of tissue samples from multisystem LCH and ECD subjects have identified recurrent kinase fusions involving BRAF, ALK (anaplastic lymphoma kinase), and NTRK1 (neurotrophic tyrosine kinase), as well as recurrent, activating mutations of MAPK and other cellular proliferative pathways.[32] The overall frequency of occurrence of MAPK and other activating mutations in PLCH is not well defined.

CLINICAL FEATURES AND DIAGNOSTIC EVALUATION

Approximately one-third of PLCH patients are asymptomatic when diagnosed.[4] The remaining two-thirds of subjects present with subacute onset of cough, dyspnea on exertion, and fatigue, although in 10% to 20% of patients spontaneous pneumothorax may lead to an acute presentation.[4,33,34] Extrapulmonary organ involvement occurs in 10% to 15% of patients, predominantly affecting skin, lymph nodes, hypothalamus, and bone, especially the skull and axial skeleton.[4] Asking patients about skin rashes, polyuria, and bony pain can elicit these symptoms and may direct further testing, such as skin biopsy or skeletal survey. Chest physical examination may be normal or demonstrate evidence of obstructive lung disease. No useful biochemical or serum diagnostic tests exist. Screening for hypothalamic dysfunction by measuring serum sodium and serum and urine osmolality may be informative in patients with polyuria.

IMAGING AND PULMONARY FUNCTION TESTING

Chest radiography is frequently abnormal, although findings are nonspecific. Early disease is characterized by bilateral nodular and reticulonodular changes, whereas advanced disease may exhibit a prominent cystic appearance.[35] Contiguous cysts measuring up to 20 mm may assume the appearance of advanced emphysema. High-resolution computed tomography scan (HRCT) of the chest should be obtained in any patient suspected of having PLCH. Not only does it provide useful information about disease distribution but also the characteristic appearance of lesions can obviate surgical biopsy (**Fig. 1**). Small nodules spanning several millimeters to 2 cm in diameter are often found, including some with central cavitation in early stages.[36–38] In later disease stages, nodules are less common and bizarrely shaped, and moderately thin-walled cysts predominate. The "classical" HRCT pattern of PLCH includes both nodular and cystic changes with apical and midlung predominance, sparing the bases and costophrenic angles (see **Fig. 1**). In the appropriate clinical context, these radiographic findings can be sufficiently persuasive that a lung biopsy can be avoided. In the setting of constitutional symptoms or bone pain suggestive of systemic disease, PET may be useful. A PET scan can identify sites of multisystem LCH involvement, can elucidate concurrent disease processes (such as lymphoma), and has been described as a biomarker to assess response to therapy.[39]

One-fifth of PLCH patients have normal spirometry, diffusing capacity, and lung volumes at the time of diagnosis.[4] When abnormal, the most common finding in pulmonary function is a reduced diffusing capacity to carbon monoxide (DLCO), occurring in approximately two-thirds of patients.[4,40] Spirometry may demonstrate obstruction, restriction, or a mixed airflow defect.[4] Lung volumes may be normal, reduced, or increased due to hyperinflation and coexistent emphysema. The diversity of pulmonary function abnormalities may be influenced by the stage at which testing is performed, with early restriction eclipsed by later obstruction.[4] Exercise physiology is typically impaired in PLCH patients, including those with relatively normal baseline pulmonary function testing.[40] Crausman and colleagues[40] correlated measures of pulmonary vascular function with overall exercise performance, suggesting that pulmonary vascular dysfunction is the primary insult in early disease.[40] In advanced disease, pulmonary vascular dysfunction and ventilatory limitation both contribute to impaired exercise capacity.

APPROACH TO THE DIAGNOSIS OF PULMONARY LANGERHANS CELL HISTIOCYTOSIS

The role of bronchoscopy in diagnosing PLCH is relatively limited. Bronchoalveolar lavage (BAL) cellular composition may demonstrate an increase in CD1a-positive cells, with 5% or greater considered highly supportive of the diagnosis; however, patients with biopsy-proven disease may have only 2% to 4% CD1a-positive cells on BAL, suggesting the test is not very sensitive.[41] Transbronchoscopic lung biopsy may provide evidence for alternative diagnoses, but has a relatively low diagnostic yield for PLCH.[21] The diagnostic yield

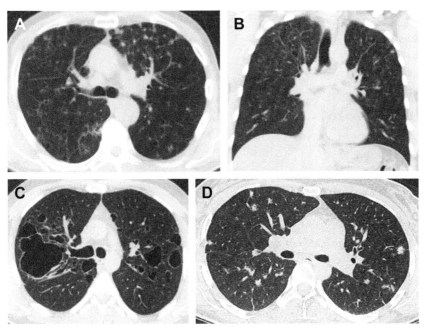

Fig. 1. Chest CT image findings in PLCH. (*A*) 60-year-old smoker with biopsy-proven PLCH. The combination of cystic lesions and nodular abnormalities is highly suggestive of PLCH. (*B*) Coronal section from a 46-year-old woman with biopsy-proven PLCH. The representative image shows a combination of cystic change, emphysema, and occasional small nodules in an upper lobe distribution with sparing of the lower lung fields. (*C*) A 34-year-old man with advanced biopsy-proven PLCH. The representative image shows extensive cystic change in both lung fields. (*D*) A 35-year-old woman who was asymptomatic at presentation. Chest radiography demonstrated bilateral pulmonary nodules. Biopsy of the nodules showed PLCH. The representative image shows bilateral nodules of varying size in the midlung region.

appears improved with cryo-transbronchial biopsy.[42] Surgical lung biopsy may be necessary if definitive diagnosis must be established. If skin or bone biopsy is consistent with LCH in a patient with classic HRCT findings, lung biopsy is not pursued.

PLCH should be suspected in patients with a smoking history and diffuse lung infiltrates and/or cysts, spontaneous pneumothorax, obstructive defect on spirometry, skin rash, or diabetes insipidus in a patient with lung infiltrates, or "emphysema" in young adulthood. All patients in whom PLCH is suspected should undergo pulmonary function testing and HRCT. Interrogation of the hypothalamic-pituitary axis may be useful in patients with nocturia or polyuria. In the correct clinical context, a classical HRCT pattern may be sufficient to establish a provisional diagnosis, although histologic examination of lung tissue is the gold standard for definite diagnosis.

MANAGEMENT

No therapy has prospectively demonstrated a reduction in the mortality of PLCH. Smoking cessation stabilizes or improves symptoms in a substantial proportion of patients (**Fig. 2**), and abstinence from smoking is recommended for all patients.[10,43–46] Unfortunately, PLCH advances in some patients despite smoking cessation.[44]

Although corticosteroids are often prescribed for PLCH management, their use is not supported by prospective or randomized trials. Retrospective studies and case reports correlate symptom improvement with steroid initiation, although these findings are often confounded by other interventions such as smoking cessation.[4,9,47–49] Because of the substantial side-effect profile and limited evidence of efficacy, these authors rarely prescribe corticosteroids in patients with evidence of progressive disease. If a trial of corticosteroids is pursued, it should be ideally reserved for patients who demonstrate progression of disease (decline in pulmonary function parameters, particularly forced expiratory volume in the first second of expiration [FEV_1] or DLCO) despite smoking cessation.

Chemotherapeutic agents have been used in patients with progressive disease or multisystem involvement.[50–53] Although few efficacy data are available, in several case reports and small series, cladribine has been reported to induce

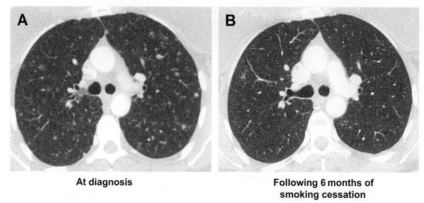

At diagnosis

Following 6 months of smoking cessation

Fig. 2. A 40-year-old woman with surgical lung biopsy-proven PLCH. (*A*) Characteristic chest CT imaging features with diffuse nodular and small cystic lesions. (*B*) Follow-up representative chest CT image demonstrating marked improvement in the parenchymal abnormalities noted at the time of presentation.

radiographic improvement or partial clinical remission of both isolated pulmonary and systemic LCH.[50–56] Further study of longitudinal toxicity from this treatment is warranted. With recent recognition of BRAF mutations in PLCH, therapies with specific BRAF inhibitors show promise.[57] Treatment should be managed by a center with expertise in PLCH.

Pneumothorax and cor pulmonale are managed in a standard fashion in this population, although pleurodesis or pleurectomy should be avoided in potential lung transplant candidates. Pulmonary hypertension is another important complication to recognize. The prevalence of pulmonary hypertension and the mechanisms by which it develops in PLCH are still not fully defined. A suggested approach is to obtain screening 2-dimensional echocardiography at diagnosis and as clinically indicated, particularly in patients who are markedly dyspneic or whose DLCO declines over time.[58] If echocardiography suggests features consistent with pulmonary hypertension, right heart catheterization should be considered.[58] In carefully selected instances, patients may experience significant symptomatic improvement with vasodilator therapies approved for the treatment of pulmonary arterial hypertension.[59,60] Lung transplantation should be considered in patients whose lung function or symptoms decline rapidly despite abstinence from smoking and a trial of immunosuppression. PLCH may recur in the transplanted lung if the recipient resumes smoking.[61]

If PLCH is diagnosed early and smoking cessation is achieved before development of serious lung impairment, the prognosis is often good. The effects of immunosuppression and abstinence from smoking on disease course or mortality are not clearly delineated. Several factors are correlated with a worse clinical outcome, including a

decline in the FEV_1 or DLCO over longitudinal follow-up.[4,44] Literature on pregnancy in PLCH is sparse, but several case reports describe stability of pulmonary function and healthy pregnancy outcomes,[62] and even spontaneous complete remission of cutaneous and nodal involvement.[63]

Case reports and series describe a wide range of neoplasms in association with childhood and adult LCH, including lymphoma, myelodysplastic syndrome, multiple myeloma, myeloproliferative neoplasms, lung adenocarcinomas, and other solid organ tumors.[4,20,64,65]

ERDHEIM-CHESTER DISEASE

ECD is a non-Langerhans histiocytic disorder that may rarely affect the lung or thoracic cavity. Although the incidence is not known with certainty, ECD is rare, and pulmonary manifestations from ECD are distinctly uncommon. The pathogenesis is poorly understood, but ECD is associated with activating BRAF mutations in greater than 50% of cases.[66] Unlike LCH, there is no association with cigarette smoking. Clinically, most patients present with bony involvement (bone pain), whereas a proportion of patients is asymptomatic despite having bone involvement (usually detected by radiography performed for other indications).[67,68] Neurologic manifestations, diabetes insipidus, and constitutional symptoms are also commonly encountered at the time of presentation.[67] Up to 25% of patients will have pulmonary findings that may manifest on chest computed tomographic (CT) scan as mediastinal involvement, pleural effusions, pulmonary opacities, or lung cysts (**Fig. 3**).[69] Histopathology is required for definite diagnosis and typically will show histiocytic infiltrates in a lymphangitic pattern associated with varying degrees of fibrosis and

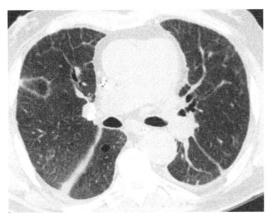

Fig. 3. A representative chest CT image from a 70-year-old man with biopsy-proven ECD. Interlobular septal thickening, pleural thickening, and fluid in the fissure (*right side*), nonspecific areas of reticulation and a single lung cyst can be appreciated in the right lower lobe.

lymphoplasmacytic infiltrates.[70] Immunophenotyping of ECD cells reveals positive expression for CD68 (macrophage marker) and CD163. Markers of Langerhans cells including CD1a or S100 are negative on immunostaining.[70] Management should be individualized and directed by centers with relevant expertise. Patients with minimal disease burden or minimal symptoms may be observed without specific therapy. Pharmacologic treatment should be considered in symptomatic patients or those with evidence of organ dysfunction. There is no standard treatment approach, and interferon-α, chemotherapy agents, corticosteroids, and radiation therapy have all been used with varying reported success.[71] BRAF inhibitor therapy has been successfully used in patients known to carry the BRAF-V600E mutation who fail to respond to other treatments.[57,72]

ROSAI-DORMAN DISEASE (SINUS HISTIOCYTOSIS WITH MASSIVE LYMPHADENOPATHY)

RDD is a histiocytic disorder of unknown cause characterized primarily by lymphadenopathy. In one series, 9 of 21 patients with RDD had intrathoracic manifestations.[73] Of these 9 patients, mediastinal lymphadenopathy was observed in 5: the remaining patients had evidence of cystic change, interstitial lung disease, or airway disease on imaging.[73] Although LCH is a dendritic cell disorder, RDD is a macrophage lineage disorder that most commonly presents in young adults and is not linked to cigarette smoking. The histopathologic features in RDD are distinct from other histiocytic disorders. A typical light

microscopy feature of RDD is emperipolesis, a term used to describe histiocytic engulfment of erythrocytes, lymphocytes, and plasma cells.[74] Immunohistochemistry demonstrates positive histiocytic staining for the S100 protein, CD14, CD68 (macrophage markers), and CD11c (early dendritic cell marker).[74] Langerhans cell markers like CD1a or Langerin are negative.[75] The differential diagnoses include chronic infections, low-grade lymphomas, immunoglobulin G4 disease, ECD, and LCH.[75] The prognosis in most patients appears to be relatively good, although longitudinal studies are lacking. Treatment of RDD is not well established, but cladribine has been successfully used in anecdotal cases.[76,77]

SUMMARY

The thoracic cavity and its contents may be affected by a variety of histiocytic syndromes. Despite their relative rarity, these histiocytic disorders are important to recognize as specific management approaches are now available. Although some of the histiocytic syndromes are life-threatening and severe, others are indolent and self-limiting. The collaboration between physicians and scientists with expertise in these disorders and grassroots initiatives from patient-led foundations are essential to enable continued progress in the understanding and development of new treatment for these rare lung diseases.

REFERENCES

1. Favara BE, Feller AC, Pauli M, et al. Contemporary classification of histiocytic disorders. The WHO Committee on Histiocytic/Reticulum Cell Proliferations. Reclassification Working Group of the Histiocyte Society. Med Pediatr Oncol 1997;29(3):157–66.
2. Baumgartner I, von Hochstetter A, Baumert B, et al. Langerhans'-cell histiocytosis in adults. Med Pediatr Oncol 1997;28(1):9–14.
3. Basset F, Nezelof C, Ferrans VJ. The histiocytoses. Pathol Annu 1983;18(Pt 2):27–78.
4. Vassallo R, Ryu JH, Schroeder DR, et al. Clinical outcomes of pulmonary Langerhans'-cell histiocytosis in adults. N Engl J Med 2002;346(7):484–90.
5. Gaensler EA, Carrington CB. Open biopsy for chronic diffuse infiltrative lung disease: clinical, roentgenographic, and physiological correlations in 502 patients. Ann Thorac Surg 1980;30(5):411–26.
6. Al-Trabolsi HA, Alshehri M, Al-Shomrani A, et al. "Primary" pulmonary Langerhans cell histiocytosis in a two-year-old child: case report and literature review. J Pediatr Hematol Oncol 2006;28(2):79–81.

7. Vassallo R, Ryu JH, Colby TV, et al. Pulmonary Langerhans'-cell histiocytosis. N Engl J Med 2000; 342(26):1969–78.

8. Hance AJ, Basset F, Saumon G, et al. Smoking and interstitial lung disease. The effect of cigarette smoking on the incidence of pulmonary histiocytosis X and sarcoidosis. Ann N Y Acad Sci 1986; 465:643–56.

9. Howarth DM, Gilchrist GS, Mullan BP, et al. Langerhans cell histiocytosis: diagnosis, natural history, management, and outcome. Cancer 1999;85(10): 2278–90.

10. Mogulkoc N, Veral A, Bishop PW, et al. Pulmonary Langerhans' cell histiocytosis: radiologic resolution following smoking cessation. Chest 1999;115(5): 1452–5.

11. Arico M, Girschikofsky M, Genereau T, et al. Langerhans cell histiocytosis in adults. Report from the International Registry of the Histiocyte Society. Eur J Cancer 2003;39(16):2341–8.

12. Carlson RA, Hattery RR, O'Connell EJ, et al. Pulmonary involvement by histiocytosis X in the pediatric age group. Mayo Clin Proc 1976;51(9):542–7.

13. Colby TV, Lombard C. Histiocytosis X in the lung. Hum Pathol 1983;14(10):847–56.

14. Hirsch MS, Hong CK. Familial pulmonary histiocytosis-X. Am Rev Respir Dis 1973;107(5):831–5.

15. Kambouchner M, Basset F, Marchal J, et al. Three-dimensional characterization of pathologic lesions in pulmonary Langerhans cell histiocytosis. Am J Respir Crit Care Med 2002;166(11):1483–90.

16. Vassallo R, Jensen EA, Colby TV, et al. The overlap between respiratory bronchiolitis and desquamative interstitial pneumonia in pulmonary Langerhans cell histiocytosis: high-resolution CT, histologic, and functional correlations. Chest 2003;124(4): 1199–205.

17. Valladeau J, Dezutter-Dambuyant C, Saeland S. Langerin/CD207 sheds light on formation of Birbeck granules and their possible function in Langerhans cells. Immunol Res 2003;28(2):93–107.

18. Tazi A, Bonay M, Bergeron A, et al. Role of granulocyte-macrophage colony stimulating factor (GM-CSF) in the pathogenesis of adult pulmonary histiocytosis X. Thorax 1996;51(6):611–4.

19. Tazi A, Bonay M, Grandsaigne M, et al. Surface phenotype of Langerhans cells and lymphocytes in granulomatous lesions from patients with pulmonary histiocytosis X. Am Rev Respir Dis 1993;147(6 Pt 1): 1531–6.

20. Burns BF, Colby TV, Dorfman RF. Langerhans cell granulomatosis (histiocytosis X) associated with malignant lymphomas. Am J Surg Pathol 1983;7:529–31.

21. Housini I, Tomashefski JF Jr, Cohen A, et al. Transbronchial biopsy in patients with pulmonary eosinophilic granuloma. Comparison with findings on open lung biopsy. Arch Pathol Lab Med 1994; 118(5):523–30.

22. Nezelof C, Basset F, Rousseau MF. Histiocytosis X histogenetic arguments for a Langerhans cell origin. Biomedicine 1973;18(5):365–71.

23. Banchereau J, Briere F, Caux C, et al. Immunobiology of dendritic cells. Annu Rev Immunol 2000;18: 767–811.

24. Vermaelen K, Pauwels R. Pulmonary dendritic cells. Am J Respir Crit Care Med 2005;172(5):530–51.

25. Zeid NA, Muller HK. Tobacco smoke induced lung granulomas and tumors: association with pulmonary Langerhans cells. Pathology 1995;27(3):247–54.

26. Yousem SA, Colby TV, Chen YY, et al. Pulmonary Langerhans' cell histiocytosis: molecular analysis of clonality. Am J Surg Pathol 2001;25(5):630–6.

27. Willman CL, Busque L, Griffith BB, et al. Langerhans'-cell histiocytosis (histiocytosis X)–a clonal proliferative disease [see comments]. N Engl J Med 1994;331(3):154–60.

28. Roden AC, Hu X, Kip S, et al. BRAF V600E expression in Langerhans cell histiocytosis: clinical and immunohistochemical study on 25 pulmonary and 54 extrapulmonary cases. Am J Surg Pathol 2014; 38(4):548–51.

29. Badalian-Very G, Vergilio JA, Degar BA, et al. Recurrent BRAF mutations in Langerhans cell histiocytosis. Blood 2010;116(11):1919–23.

30. Berres ML, Lim KP, Peters T, et al. BRAF-V600E expression in precursor versus differentiated dendritic cells defines clinically distinct LCH risk groups. J Exp Med 2015;212(2):281.

31. Chakraborty R, Hampton OA, Shen X, et al. Mutually exclusive recurrent somatic mutations in MAP2K1 and BRAF support a central role for ERK activation in LCH pathogenesis. Blood 2014; 124(19):3007–15.

32. Diamond EL, Durham BH, Haroche J, et al. Diverse and targetable kinase alterations drive histiocytic neoplasms. Cancer Discov 2016;6(2):154–65.

33. Mendez JL, Nadrous HF, Vassallo R, et al. Pneumothorax in pulmonary Langerhans cell histiocytosis. Chest 2004;125(3):1028–32.

34. Schonfeld N, Dirks K, Costabel U, et al. A prospective clinical multicentre study on adult pulmonary Langerhans' cell histiocytosis. Sarcoidosis Vasc Diffuse Lung Dis 2012;29(2):132–8.

35. Lacronique J, Roth C, Battesti JP, et al. Chest radiological features of pulmonary histiocytosis X: a report based on 50 adult cases. Thorax 1982; 37(2):104–9.

36. Bonelli FS, Hartman TE, Swensen SJ, et al. Accuracy of high-resolution CT in diagnosing lung diseases. AJR Am J Roentgenol 1998;170(6):1507–12.

37. Brauner MW, Grenier P, Mouelhi MM, et al. Pulmonary histiocytosis X: evaluation with high-resolution CT. Radiology 1989;172(1):255–8.

38. Hartman TE, Tazelaar HD, Swensen SJ, et al. Cigarette smoking: CT and pathologic findings of associated pulmonary diseases. Radiographics 1997; 17(2):377–90.

39. Krajicek BJ, Ryu JH, Hartman TE, et al. Abnormal fluorodeoxyglucose PET in pulmonary Langerhans cell histiocytosis. Chest 2009;135(6): 1542–9.

40. Crausman RS, Jennings CA, Tuder RM, et al. Pulmonary histiocytosis X: pulmonary function and exercise pathophysiology. Am J Respir Crit Care Med 1996;153(1):426–35.

41. Auerswald U, Barth J, Magnussen H. Value of CD-1-positive cells in bronchoalveolar lavage fluid for the diagnosis of pulmonary histiocytosis X. Lung 1991;169(6):305–9.

42. Fruchter O, Fridel L, El Raouf BA, et al. Histological diagnosis of interstitial lung diseases by cryo-transbronchial biopsy. Respirology 2014; 19(5):683–8.

43. Von Essen S, West W, Sitorius M, et al. Complete resolution of roentgenographic changes in a patient with pulmonary histiocytosis X. Chest 1990;98(3): 765–7.

44. Tazi A, de Margerie C, Naccache JM, et al. The natural history of adult pulmonary Langerhans cell histiocytosis: a prospective multicentre study. Orphanet J Rare Dis 2015;10:30.

45. Wolters PJ, Elicker BM. Subacute onset of pulmonary langerhans cell histiocytosis with resolution after smoking cessation. Am J Respir Crit Care Med 2014;190(11):e64.

46. Ninaber M, Dik H, Peters E. Complete pathological resolution of pulmonary Langerhans cell histiocytosis. Respirol Case Rep 2014;2(2): 76–8.

47. Schonfeld N, Frank W, Wenig S, et al. Clinical and radiologic features, lung function and therapeutic results in pulmonary histiocytosis X. Respiration 1993; 60(1):38–44.

48. Benyounes B, Crestani B, Couvelard A, et al. Steroid-responsive pulmonary hypertension in a patient with Langerhans' cell granulomatosis (histiocytosis X). Chest 1996;110(1):284–6.

49. Delobbe A, Durieu J, Duhamel A, et al. Determinants of survival in pulmonary Langerhans' cell granulomatosis (histiocytosis X). Groupe d'Etude en Pathologie Interstitielle de la Societe de Pathologie Thoracique du Nord. Eur Respir J 1996;9(10): 2002–6.

50. Saven A, Piro LD. 2-Chlorodeoxyadenosine: a potent antimetabolite with major activity in the treatment of indolent lymphoproliferative disorders. Hematol Cell Ther 1996;38(Suppl 2):S93–101.

51. Saven A, Burian C. Cladribine activity in adult langerhans-cell histiocytosis. Blood 1999;93(12): 4125–30.

52. Pardanani A, Phyliky RL, Li CY, et al. 2-Chlorodeoxyadenosine therapy for disseminated Langerhans cell histiocytosis. Mayo Clin Proc 2003; 78(3):301–6.

53. Dimopoulos MA, Theodorakis M, Kostis E, et al. Treatment of Langerhans cell histiocytosis with 2 chlorodeoxyadenosine. Leuk Lymphoma 1997; 25(1–2):187–9.

54. Aerni MR, Christine Aubry M, Myers JL, et al. Complete remission of nodular pulmonary Langerhans cell histiocytosis lesions induced by 2-chlorodeoxyadenosine in a non-smoker. Respir Med 2008; 102(2):316–9.

55. Epaud R, Ducou Le Pointe H, Fasola S, et al. Cladribine improves lung cysts and pulmonary function in a child with histiocytosis. Eur Respir J 2015;45(3): 831–3.

56. Grobost V, Khouatra C, Lazor R, et al. Effectiveness of cladribine therapy in patients with pulmonary Langerhans cell histiocytosis. Orphanet J Rare Dis 2014;9:191.

57. Haroche J, Cohen-Aubart F, Emile JF, et al. Dramatic efficacy of vemurafenib in both multisystemic and refractory Erdheim-Chester disease and Langerhans cell histiocytosis harboring the BRAF V600E mutation. Blood 2013;121(9): 1495–500.

58. Chaowalit N, Pellikka PA, Decker PA, et al. Echocardiographic and clinical characteristics of pulmonary hypertension complicating pulmonary Langerhans cell histiocytosis. Mayo Clin Proc 2004;79(10): 1269–75.

59. Le Pavec J, Lorillon G, Jais X, et al. Pulmonary Langerhans cell histiocytosis-associated pulmonary hypertension: clinical characteristics and impact of pulmonary arterial hypertension therapies. Chest 2012;142(5):1150–7.

60. May A, Kane G, Yi E, et al. Dramatic and sustained responsiveness of pulmonary Langerhans cell histiocytosis-associated pulmonary hypertension to vasodilator therapy. Respir Med Case Rep 2015; 14:13–5.

61. Etienne B, Bertocchi M, Gamondes JP, et al. Relapsing pulmonary Langerhans cell histiocytosis after lung transplantation. Am J Respir Crit Care Med 1998;157(1):288–91.

62. Sharma R, Maplethorpe R, Wilson G. Effect of pregnancy on lung function in adult pulmonary Langerhans cell histiocytosis. J Matern Fetal Neonatal Med 2006;19(1):67–8.

63. Scherbaum WA, Seif FJ. Spontaneous transient remission of disseminated histiocytosis X during pregnancy. J Cancer Res Clin Oncol 1995;121(1): 57–60.

64. Neumann MP, Frizzera G. The coexistence of Langerhans' cell granulomatosis and malignant lymphoma may take different forms: report of seven

cases with a review of the literature. Hum Pathol 1986;17(10):1060–5.

65. Egeler RM, Neglia JP, Arico M, et al. The relation of langerhans cell histiocytosis to acute leukemia, lymphomas, and other solid tumors. Hematol Oncol Clin North Am 1998;12(2):369–78.

66. Haroche J, Charlotte F, Arnaud L, et al. High prevalence of BRAF V600E mutations in Erdheim-Chester disease but not in other non-Langerhans cell histiocytoses. Blood 2012; 120(13):2700–3.

67. Munoz J, Janku F, Cohen PR, et al. Erdheim-Chester disease: characteristics and management. Mayo Clin Proc 2014;89(7):985–96.

68. Egan AJ, Boardman LA, Tazelaar HD, et al. Erdheim-Chester disease: clinical, radiologic, and histopathologic findings in five patients with interstitial lung disease. Am J Surg Pathol 1999;23(1): 17–26.

69. Arnaud L, Pierre I, Beigelman-Aubry C, et al. Pulmonary involvement in Erdheim-Chester disease: a single-center study of thirty-four patients and a review of the literature. Arthritis Rheum 2010;62(11): 3504–12.

70. Rush WL, Andriko JA, Galateau-Salle F, et al. Pulmonary pathology of Erdheim-Chester disease. Mod Pathol 2000;13(7):747–54.

71. Diamond EL, Dagna L, Hyman DM, et al. Consensus guidelines for the diagnosis and clinical management of Erdheim-Chester disease. Blood 2014; 124(4):483–92.

72. Tzoulis C, Schwarzlmuller T, Gjerde IO, et al. Excellent response of intramedullary Erdheim-Chester disease to vemurafenib: a case report. BMC Res Notes 2015;8:171.

73. Cartin-Ceba R, Golbin JM, Yi ES, et al. Intrathoracic manifestations of Rosai-Dorfman disease. Respir Med 2010;104(9):1344–9.

74. Foucar E, Rosai J, Dorfman R. Sinus histiocytosis with massive lymphadenopathy (Rosai-Dorfman disease): review of the entity. Semin Diagn Pathol 1990;7(1):19–73.

75. Nagarjun Rao R, Moran CA, Suster S. Histiocytic disorders of the lung. Adv Anat Pathol 2010;17(1):12–22.

76. Aouba A, Terrier B, Vasiliu V, et al. Dramatic clinical efficacy of cladribine in Rosai-Dorfman disease and evolution of the cytokine profile: towards a new therapeutic approach. Haematologica 2006;91(12 Suppl):ECR52.

77. Tasso M, Esquembre C, Blanco E, et al. Sinus histiocytosis with massive lymphadenopathy (Rosai-Dorfman disease) treated with 2-chlorodeoxyadenosine. Pediatr Blood Cancer 2006; 47(5):612–5.

Pulmonary Alveolar Proteinosis Syndrome

Takuji Suzuki, MD, PhD*, Bruce C. Trapnell, MD

KEYWORDS

- Pulmonary surfactant • GM-CSF • Alveolar macrophages • GM-CSF autoantibody • CSF2RA
- CSF2RB • Whole lung lavage • GM-CSF inhalation therapy

KEY POINTS

- Pulmonary alveolar proteinosis (PAP) is a syndrome characterized by the accumulation of surfactant in alveoli and terminal airways resulting in hypoxemic respiratory failure.
- Surfactant is synthesized and secreted by alveolar type II epithelial cells, and removed by uptake, recycling, and catabolism in these epithelial cells and by uptake and catabolism in alveolar macrophages.
- Autoimmune PAP is related to alveolar macrophage dysfunction caused by the disruption of GM-CSF signaling caused by high levels of anti-GM-CSF autoantibody in the lungs.
- Elevated serum GM-CSF autoantibody is diagnostic for autoimmune PAP in patients with typical history; radiologic findings; bronchoalveolar lavage cytology findings with a milky, turbid appearance; and/or lung biopsy.
- Whole-lung lavage (WLL) is the standard first-line therapy and GM-CSF inhalation for autoimmune PAP is a promising therapy under clinical study.

INTRODUCTION

Pulmonary alveolar proteinosis (PAP) is a rare syndrome characterized by the accumulation of surfactant in alveolar macrophages and alveoli resulting in hypoxemic respiratory failure. In 1958, Rosen and colleagues[1] first reported PAP as a disorder consisting of filling of alveoli by a periodic acid–Schiff (PAS)-positive proteinaceous material, rich in lipid. The accumulated material is now known to be comprised primarily of pulmonary surfactant and smaller amounts of cell debris. PAP is often reported in the medical literature as a disease rather than as a syndrome and by the use of various terms, such as pulmonary alveolar lipoproteinosis, idiopathic PAP, acquired PAP, and congenital PAP.[2] However, it should be noted that PAP is not a single disease. These disorders of surfactant homeostasis are defined in the context of abnormalities of surfactant production or surfactant clearance. Surfactant production disorders are less common, typically occur in neonates and children, and are associated with alveolar wall distortion and varying degrees of accumulation of dysfunctional surfactant. They are caused by genetic mutations in genes that encode surfactant proteins or proteins involved in surfactant lipid metabolism, such as mutation in the SFTPB, SFTPC, ABCA3, or Nkx2.1 genes. Disorders of surfactant clearance are caused by disruption of granulocyte-macrophage colony–stimulating factor (GM-CSF) signaling (primary PAP) or by an underlying disease that impairs alveolar macrophage number or functions including

Disclosure Statement: The authors have nothing to disclose.
Division of Pulmonary Biology, Cincinnati Children's Hospital Medical Center, MLC7029, 3333 Burnet Avenue, Cincinnati, OH 45229, USA
* Corresponding author. Cincinnati Children's Hospital Medical Center, Room 4030, Location R, Cincinnati, OH 45229.
E-mail address: Takuji.Suzuki@cchmc.org

Clin Chest Med 37 (2016) 431–440
http://dx.doi.org/10.1016/j.ccm.2016.04.006

surfactant catabolism (secondary PAP) (**Table 1**). Among these PAP-causing diseases, autoimmune PAP is most common and is a focus of this article.[2–4]

PATHOGENESIS

Pulmonary surfactant maintains lung function by creating an air-liquid interface on the alveolar surface, reducing surface tension and preventing alveolar collapse. It is comprised of 90% lipid (primary phospholipids) and 10% proteins (surfactant protein [SP]-A, -B, -C, and -D). It is also important for host defense against microbial pathogens.[4] Surfactant is synthesized and secreted by alveolar type II epithelial cells, removed by uptake, recycling, and catabolism in these epithelial cells, and by uptake and catabolism in alveolar macrophages. The surfactant pool size is tightly regulated by the balance of secretion and removal by these cells (**Fig. 1**). Studies in $Csf2^{-/-}$ (GM-CSF gene deficient) mice revealed the role of GM-CSF in surfactant homeostasis and suggested the pathogenesis of PAP in 1994.[5,6] This finding

was confirmed by an identical pulmonary phenotype in $Csf2rb^{-/-}$ (GM-CSF receptor beta chain gene deficient) mice.[7,8] These results showed that the catabolism of surfactant in alveolar macrophages requires the presence of GM-CSF in the lungs. Based on these mechanisms, disorders of surfactant clearance are classified as primary PAP, which is caused by disruption of GM-CSF signaling, and secondary PAP, which is associated with an underlying disease that impairs alveolar macrophage functions and/or numbers (see **Table 1**).

Although GM-CSF gene deficiency has never been identified in human patients, neutralizing autoantibodies against GM-CSF in bronchoalveolar lavage (BAL) fluid from patients with "idiopathic" PAP were first reported in 1999.[9] This form of PAP is now classified as autoimmune PAP, which is the most common clinical form of PAP and accounts for 90% of cases. Autoimmune PAP is related to alveolar macrophage dysfunction caused by the disruption of GM-CSF signaling, which is in turn caused by a high level of anti-GM-CSF autoantibody in the lungs. The

Table 1
Classification of diseases and risk factors reported in association with PAP syndrome[a]

PAP Classification	Risk Factor
Primary PAP[b]	GM-CSF autoantibodies[c] *CSF2RA* mutations[d] *CSF2RB* mutations[d]
Secondary PAP[e]	Hematologic diseases[f] Nonhematologic malignancies Immune deficiency/disruption diseases[g] Chronic inflammatory/infectious diseases Toxic inhalation exposures[h] *SLC7A7* mutations *MARS* mutations[i]
Surfactant production disorders[j]	*SFTPB* mutations *SFTPC* mutations *ABCA3* mutations *TTF1* (*NKX2.1*) mutations

[a] Abridged list. The strength of association of risk factors with the occurrence PAP varies widely.
[b] Defined as PAP associated with a primary disruption of GM-CSF signaling.
[c] Neutralizing GM-CSF autoantibodies mediate disease pathogenesis of what is now called autoimmune PAP (previously idiopathic, acquired, other names), which represents ~85% to 90% of all patients with PAP syndrome. The presence of serum GM-CSF autoantibodies is 100% sensitive and specific for this disease.
[d] The associated disease is commonly referred to as hereditary or familial PAP.
[e] Defined as PAP associated with an underlying clinical condition secondarily affecting alveolar macrophage.
[f] Myelodysplastic syndrome is the most common current disease in this category, although many hematologic diseases have been reported in association with PAP.
[g] Includes acquired immunodeficiency syndrome, agammaglobulinemia, amyloidosis, Bechet disease, juvenile dermatomyositis, and Fanconi syndrome.
[h] Includes inorganic dusts (aluminum, cement, silica, titanium, indium), organic dusts (agricultural, bakery flour, fertilizer, sawdust), and fumes (chlorine, cleaning products, gasoline/petroleum, nitrogen dioxide, paint, synthetic plastic fumes, varnish).
[i] Biallelic MARS mutations cause a lung and liver phenotype and are prevalent in a population on Reunion Island.[19]
[j] Defined as PAP associated with genetic mutations resulting in abnormal surfactant protein or lipid production.

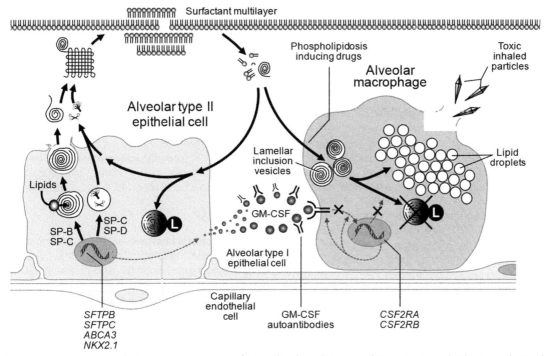

Fig. 1. Regulation of surfactant homeostasis. Surfactant lipids and proteins (SP-A, -B, -C, and -D) are synthesized in alveolar type II epithelial cell, secreted into the intra-alveolar space, and adsorb to surfactant layer at the air-liquid-tissue interface. The primary function of surfactant is to reduce surface tension within the alveolus to limit collapse of small airspaces. Surfactant lipids and proteins are removed by uptake and recycling in type II epithelial cells or by uptake and catabolism in alveolar macrophages. GM-CSF, a critical regulator of surfactant catabolism in alveolar macrophages, functions by binding to hetero-oligomeric receptors on alveolar macrophages and stimulating surfactant catabolism. Impaired GM-CSF signaling by GM-CSF autoantibodies or gene mutations in the GM-CSF receptor (*CSF2RA*, *CSF2RB*) cause alveolar macrophage dysfunction, which leads to impaired clearance and accumulation of surfactant in the lung (primary PAP).

pathogenesis of autoimmune PAP was confirmed in a 2009 study where the adoptive transfer of autoantibodies from patients with PAP into nonhuman primates resulted in PAP.[10] The incidence and prevalence of autoimmune PAP is 0.49 and 6.2 per million, respectively, in the general population according to a Japanese cohort study.[11] Autoimmune PAP is twice as common in males, typically presenting in the third through sixth decades, and is rare in children younger than 10 years of age. Among GM-CSF autoantibody-negative patients with PAP, gene mutations of GM-CSF receptor alpha and beta genes (*CSF2RA* and *CSF2RB*, respectively) were identified.

Disruption of GM-CSF signaling by recessive mutations in *CSF2RA* or *CSF2RB* causes a hereditary form of PAP that is clinically, physiologically, and histologically indistinguishable from autoimmune PAP.[12–16] These genetic forms of PAP are now classified as hereditary PAP. Hereditary PAP probably accounts for less than 1% of cases. Secondary PAP is associated with various underlying

diseases, such as hematologic diseases (myelodysplastic syndrome [MDS], acute myelogenous leukemia, acute lymphoblastic leukemia, chronic myelocytic leukemia, chronic lymphocytic leukemia, aplastic anemia, multiple myeloma, lymphoma, and Waldenström macroglobulinemia), nonhematologic malignancies (lung adenocarcinoma, glioblastoma, melanoma), infectious diseases (cytomegalovirus, *Mycobacterium tuberculosis*, *Nocardia*, *Pneumocystis jirovecii*), immune deficiency/disruption syndromes (acquired immunodeficiency syndrome, amyloidosis, Fanconi syndrome, agammaglobulinemia, Bechet disease, juvenile dermatomyositis, renal tubular acidosis, severe combined immunodeficiency disease), and toxic inhalation exposures (see **Table 1**). Inorganic dust (aluminum, cement, silica, titanium, indium), organic dust (agricultural, bakery flour, fertilizer, sawdust), and fumes (chlorine, cleaning products, gasoline/petroleum, nitrogen dioxide, paint, synthetic plastic fumes, varnish) have also been reported to be associated with secondary PAP. These underlying diseases or conditions are thought to impair alveolar macrophage number or functions including surfactant catabolism.

Hematologic disorders (especially MDS) are the major underlying disease in greater than 75% of cases with adult-onset secondary PAP.[17] Secondary PAP accounts for 8% to 9% of all PAP cases, with an incidence and prevalence of approximately 0.05 and 0.5 per million, respectively. Surfactant production disorders are less common and are caused by genetic mutations in genes that encode surfactant proteins or proteins involved in surfactant lipid metabolism, such as mutations in the *SFTPB*, *SFTPC*, *ABCA3*, or *Nkx2.1* genes. Other genetic defects, such as y+LAT1 (*SLC7A7*) gene mutations, which causes lysinuric protein intolerance,[18] and Methionyl-tRNA synthetase (*MARS*) gene mutations,[19] were reported to be associated with PAP. The precise mechanisms of PAP pathogenesis induced by these gene mutations have not been elucidated.

CLINICAL PRESENTATION

Common symptoms of PAP include exertional dyspnea, cough, fatigue, and weight loss (**Table 2**). Fever (1% in Japanese cohort, 11% in Italian cohort, and 15% in Chinese cohort) and sputum production (4% in Japanese cohort and 1% in Italian cohort) are less common. In 20 patients with hereditary PAP caused by *CSF2RA* mutations and forms of secondary PAP, similar symptoms

have been reported.[17,20] In secondary PAP with MDS, the most common symptoms were fever (45%), dyspnea on exertion (42%), and cough (42%).[21] In autoimmune PAP, a smoking history is commonly present (57% in Japanese cohort, 79% in German cohort, and 64% in Italian cohort), and dust or fume exposure have been reported (26% in Japanese cohort, 54% in German cohort, and 32% in Italian cohort). In several studies, two-thirds of the patients were men (male/female ratio is 2:2).[2,11,22–24] The physical examination is generally unremarkable, but crackles, clubbing, and cyanosis have been reported in some patients.

DIAGNOSIS

PAP syndrome is identified based on a compatible history, typical radiologic findings, BAL cytology and/or lung biopsy findings, and compatible biomarkers. However, diagnosis of the specific PAP-causing disease in secondary PAP syndromes requires further studies. If a patient is suspected to have PAP based on history, radiology studies, and other findings, early anti-GM-CSF autoantibody testing is useful to make the diagnosis of autoimmune PAP, the most common etiology, and can minimize the use of more invasive procedures (see later). A diagnostic algorithm is shown in **Fig. 2**.

Radiographic Findings

A chest radiograph may be a useful screening test for the diagnosis of PAP. The distribution of

Table 2
Clinical presentation in patients with PAP syndrome

Study	Inoue	Bonella	Campo
Geographic location of patients	Japan	Germany	Italy
Number of patients	223	70	73
Disease/disease category			
Autoimmune PAP (%)	100	91	100
Secondary PAP (%)	0	9	0
Symptom/sign	Frequency (% of patients)		
Dyspnea	52	94	67
Cough	23	66	31
Fatigue	0	49	0
Weight loss	0.4	43	0
Fever	1	0	11
Sputum	4	0	1
None	31	0	5
Reference	11	22	23

Only reports with a comprehensive symptom inventory are shown here. Studies with incomplete symptom assessment and symptom frequency in other PAP-causing diseases are found in the text.

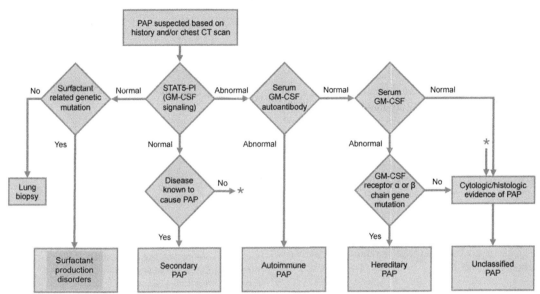

Fig. 2. Algorithm used for the differential diagnosis of PAP syndrome. The diagnosis of PAP is made based on a compatible history, typical radiologic findings, compatible biomarkers, and characteristic lung biopsy or bronchoalveolar lavage cytology findings. Patients with high serum GM-CSF autoantibodies but without underlying diseases known to be associated with PAP are diagnosed with autoimmune PAP. Patients with negative serum GM-CSF autoantibodies and with underlying diseases known to cause PAP are diagnosed with secondary PAP. Patients with negative serum GM-CSF autoantibodies and elevated levels of serum GM-CSF without apparent underlying diseases known to be associated with PAP need further evaluation for hereditary PAP by analyzing GM-CSF receptor gene (*CSF2RA* or *CSF2RB*) mutations. Whole-blood GM-CSF signaling tests, such as the GM-CSF-induced STAT5 phosphorylation index test (STAT5-PI), may support the diagnosis of primary PAP. Surfactant production disorders are diseases caused by the gene mutations of *SFTPB*, *SFTPC*, *ABCA3*, and *NKX2.1*. * Indicates that patients with normal STAT5-PI and no known disease to cause PAP need to be evaluated for cytologic/histologic evidence of PAP. (*From* Trapnell BC, Luisetti M. Pulmonary alveolar proteinosis syndrome. In: Broaddus VC, Mason RJ, Ernst JD, et al, eds. Murray and Nadel's textbook of pulmonary medicine. 6th edition. Philadelphia: Elsevier Saunders; 2015; with permission.)

infiltrates in autoimmune PAP and hereditary PAP is typically bilateral symmetric opacities in the mid- and lower-lung fields (**Fig. 3**A). High-resolution computed tomography (HRCT) shows ground-glass opacities in autoimmune, hereditary, and secondary PAP (**Fig. 3**B). Ground-glass opacities present as a patchy geographic pattern that is distributed in the lower lung fields in autoimmune PAP, whereas ground-glass opacities typically present as a diffuse pattern in secondary PAP. A "crazy paving" appearance (ground-glass opacities superimposed on septal thickening)

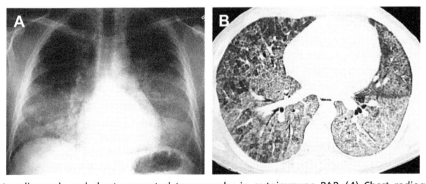

Fig. 3. Chest radiograph and chest computed tomography in autoimmune PAP. (*A*) Chest radiograph shows diffuse, bilateral infiltrates suggestive of pulmonary edema but without findings suggestive of cardiovascular disease. (*B*) Chest computed tomography shows a geographic pattern of ground-glass opacification superimposed on thickened interlobular septa commonly referred to as "crazy paving". (*From* Trapnell BC, Whitsett JA, Nakata K. Pulmonary alveolar proteinosis. N Engl J Med 2003;349:2528; with permission.)

and subpleural sparing are frequently seen in auto-immune PAP, but are less frequently apparent in secondary PAP comprising 12% of 27 cases in one study.[17]

Laboratory Findings

Most of the routine laboratory tests are normal in PAP. The serum level of lactate dehydrogenase (LDH) is typically elevated, although this finding is nonspecific. LDH and Pao_2 are moderately correlated and LDH and alveolar-arterial oxygen gradient ($A-aDO_2$) are more significantly correlated.[2] Levels of other biomarkers including SP-A, SP-B, SP-C, KL-6, MCP-1, CEA, cytokeratin 19, Cyfra 21 to 1, and NSE are increased and some of them correlate with disease severity (see later), although none of these findings are specific or diagnostic for PAP.

Pulmonary Function Testing

Pulmonary function testing is of limited usefulness in diagnosing the severity of PAP lung disease. Increased $A-aDO_2$ correlates better with disease severity. Forced vital capacity (FVC) and forced expiratory volume in 1 second are generally within normal limits. Some patients show decreased FVC, consistent with restrictive physiology.[25] The diffusion capacity of the lung for carbon monoxide (DLCO) is frequently reduced and correlates with disease severity.[11]

Bronchoscopy, Bronchoalveolar Lavage, Microbiologic Culture

Bronchoscopic examination of the airways is unremarkable in PAP but BAL fluid shows a milky, turbid appearance and thick sediment. BAL is emerging as a useful diagnostic tool for PAP (rising from 4% of 410 published cases in 2002 to 83% in a German series in 2011).[2,22] In a Japanese cohort, the diagnosis of PAP was based on HRCT and BAL analysis in 58.7% of patients; HRCT, BAL fluid, and transbronchial lung biopsy in 34.1% of patients; and BAL analysis or transbronchial lung biopsy and video-assisted thoracoscopic surgery in 7.2% of patients.[11] Cytology of PAP BAL fluid reveals PAS stain and oil red O stain positive large foamy macrophages and dirty-appearing sediment. Fungal, mycobacterial, and other infectious etiologies should be ruled out by appropriate staining and culture.

Histopathology

The histopathology of PAP reveals well-preserved alveoli filled with eosinophilic, granular, and PAS-positive material and foamy alveolar macrophages (**Fig. 4**). It is associated with minimal interstitial

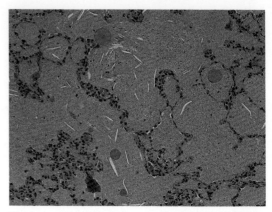

Fig. 4. Lung histopathology in autoimmune PAP. The alveoli are completely filled with amorphous, acellular eosinophilic material. The alveolar architecture is well preserved, and the alveolar walls are essentially unremarkable. (Periodic acid-Schiff (PAS) stain, original magnification ×20).

inflammation or fibrosis. The combined use of BAL analysis and measurement of serum GM-CSF autoantibody obviates histologic confirmation in many cases of suspected PAP.

Biomarkers

In autoimmune PAP, the only disease-specific biomarker that is known to be elevated in serum is the GM-CSF autoantibody (**Fig. 5**). This test is simple, standardized, and can be used to identify the disease in a large number of patients. The reported sensitivity and specificity for autoimmune PAP approaches 100%.[26] GM-CSF autoantibody levels in serum do not correlate with duration of disease, disease severity, pulmonary function (% FVC, % vital capacity, % forced expiratory volume in 1 second, % DLCO), or serum biomarkers (LDH, SP-A, SP-D, CEA, KL-6).[11] The serum GM-CSF autoantibody also does not correlate with age, gender, smoking status, a history of environmental or occupational dust inhalation exposure, or duration of disease in a Japanese series,[11] but shows a weak correlation with age and the duration of disease.[22] GM-CSF autoantibody-negative patients with PAP with an underling disease known to cause PAP are diagnosed with secondary PAP. Serum GM-CSF is elevated in hereditary PAP, likely caused by the absence of receptor-mediated clearance. Although this serum GM-CSF test is not disease specific, the combination of serum GM-CSF autoantibody-negativity and elevated GM-CSF without underlying disease should prompt genetic evaluation for hereditary PAP (see **Fig. 2**).[15] Whole-blood GM-CSF signaling tests, such as the GM-CSF-induced STAT5 phosphorylation index test, may support

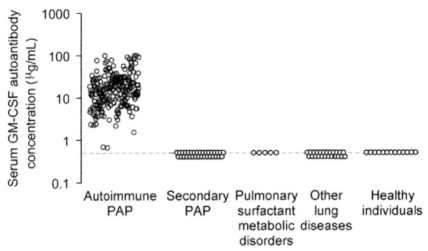

Fig. 5. Serum GM-CSF autoantibody testing and diagnosis of autoimmune PAP. A serum level of GM-CSF autoantibody is specifically elevated in autoimmune PAP. The autoantibodies are not elevated in patients with other forms of PAP or other lung diseases or in normal persons. (*From* Trapnell BC, Luisetti M. Pulmonary alveolar proteinosis syndrome. In: Broaddus VC, Mason RJ, Ernst JD, et al, eds. Murray and Nadel's textbook of pulmonary medicine. 6th edition. Philadelphia: Elsevier Saunders; 2015; with permission.)

the diagnosis of primary PAP.[15] Although elevated in a wide range of other lung diseases, serum levels of LDH, SP-A, SP-B, SP-D, KL-6, CEA, M-CSF, and MCP-1 are elevated in PAP. Serum levels of LDH, KL-6, and CEA are reported to be correlated with some markers of lung function (Pao$_2$, A-aDO$_2$, or % DLCO).[22,25] Cancer biomarkers other than CEA, such as NSE and Cyfra 21 to 1, are also elevated in PAP.[23] The elevation of serum levels of SP-A, SP-D, and KL-6 is also reported in secondary PAP.[17] Although most of these biomarkers are not helpful in establishing a diagnosis, they may be useful in monitoring disease activity in patients with PAP.

NATURAL HISTORY

In a Japanese cohort study, one-third of patients with autoimmune PAP were asymptomatic.[11] In contrast, 5% of patients were asymptomatic in an Italian study.[23] The onset of disease is poorly studied because patients who become symptomatic present for evaluation only after substantial alveolar filling with surfactant has occurred. The natural history of autoimmune PAP generally follows one of three patterns: (1) spontaneous improvement (ranging from 5% to 7%); (2) persistent, unremitting symptoms; or (3) progressive deterioration with respiratory failure. Secondary infection occurs in primary and secondary PAP. The 5-year survival among 231 patients with PAP was 85% without therapy and 94% with whole-lung lavage (WLL) therapy.[2] In this study, 72% of deaths were caused by respiratory failure and 18% were caused by uncontrolled infections. In

the Japanese cohort study, the 5-year survival was 100% and significant infection was found in 4% of patients.[11] The clinical course of secondary PAP is strongly influenced by that of the underlying disease causing PAP and the prognosis is poorer than that of autoimmune PAP. Development of secondary PAP during the course of MDS is an important adverse prognostic risk factor in these patients.[21]

THERAPY
Current Therapy

WLL has been the standard first-line therapy since the 1960s.[27] The WLL procedure is performed under general anesthesia using a double-lumen endotracheal tube to ventilate one lung while repeatedly filling and emptying the other with up to 50 L of saline to physically remove surfactant from the lung. Although many patients with PAP have been treated with WLL (28% in the Chinese cohort, 90% in the German cohort, and 54% in the Italian cohort), the procedures are still not standardized and are highly operator-dependent.[2,22–24] Lobar and segmental lavage performed using a fiberoptic bronchoscope has also been reported. Although segmental BAL may be less effective compared with WLL because of the small lavage volume, one study reported that the two methods seem to be used at similar frequencies in the treatment of patients.[24] For secondary PAP, approach to treatment is often dictated by the underlying disease. For example, it has been reported that secondary PAP improves after hematopoietic stem cell transplantation in patients with hematologic diseases.[28] Therapy for the surfactant production disorders (congenital PAP) is supportive, although successful lung transplantation has been reported.[29] There is no evidence that corticosteroids are effective for autoimmune PAP.[30]

Experimental Approaches

The first treatments with exogenous GM-CSF in patients with PAP were administered subcutaneously.[31] The use of subcutaneous GM-CSF in escalating doses for 6 to 12 months produced an overall response rate of 48%.[32] In this study, 85% of patients receiving subcutaneous GM-CSF had local reactions at the site of injection and other minor adverse events. Aerosolized GM-CSF inhalation therapy has also been tested in PAP.[33] In 35 patients with autoimmune PAP, 62% of patients receiving inhaled GM-CSF therapy had improvement in the $A\text{-}aDO_2$ gradient, whereas serum GM-CSF autoantibody levels were unchanged.[34] Importantly, no serious adverse events occurred in this study.[34] Among these 35 patients, 66% had a durable response to the inhalation therapy and required no further treatments during the 30-month observation period. A low baseline vital capacity seemed to be a prognostic marker for disease recurrence.[35] As another potential therapeutic strategy to reduce the level of GM-CSF autoantibodies, anti-B-cell therapy with rituximab for autoimmune PAP has been reported.[36–38] Plasmapheresis for autoimmune PAP is also a potential approach that can remove GM-CSF autoantibodies.[39] Although some of these experimental approaches are promising, further efficacy and safety studies are necessary before conclusions are drawn about their potential use in the treatment of patients with PAP.

KNOWLEDGE GAPS AND FUTURE RESEARCH

The critical role of GM-CSF signaling in primary PAP (autoimmune and hereditary PAP) pathogenesis has been revealed by effects of GM-CSF autoantibodies or GM-CSF receptor gene (*CSF2RA* or *CSF2RB*) mutations to disrupt the clearance of pulmonary surfactant by alveolar macrophages. However, the molecular mechanisms of PAP pathogenesis beyond the loss of GM-CSF signaling are largely unexplored. Furthermore, the reasons that GM-CSF autoantibodies are produced in autoimmune PAP are not clear. Although smoking history and dust or fume exposure are often observed in patients with autoimmune PAP, the role of these inhalations in autoantibody production has not been elucidated.

Although WLL is a standard therapy for PAP, no clinical practice guidelines have been established. Future studies are needed to define the optimal indications, timing, and conduct of WLL procedure (eg, volume of saline infused, use of mechanical percussion, positioning of the patient). In experimental approaches, a clinical study with inhaled GM-CSF in autoimmune PAP was shown to be safe and effective. However, the mechanisms underlying the therapeutic effect have not been determined. Further studies investigating the optimal dose, timing, duration of administration, and long-term safety are necessary. In hereditary PAP, WLL is also a current standard therapy. Pulmonary macrophage transplantation and gene therapy have shown promising results in a mouse model of hereditary PAP[40] and represent promising future research directions.

ACKNOWLEDGMENTS

The authors thank Paritha Arumugam and Elizabeth Kopras (Cincinnati Children's Hospital Medical Center) for reviewing this manuscript.

REFERENCES

1. Rosen SG, Castleman B, Liebow AA. Pulmonary alveolar proteinosis. N Engl J Med 1958;258: 1123–42.
2. Seymour JF, Presneill JJ. Pulmonary alveolar proteinosis: progress in the first 44 years. Am J Respir Crit Care Med 2002;166:215–35.
3. Trapnell BC, Whitsett JA, Nakata K. Pulmonary alveolar proteinosis. N Engl J Med 2003;349:2527–39.
4. Whitsett JA, Wert SE, Weaver TE. Diseases of pulmonary surfactant homeostasis. Annu Rev Pathol 2015;10:371–93.
5. Dranoff G, Crawford AD, Sadelain M, et al. Involvement of granulocyte-macrophage colony-stimulating factor in pulmonary homeostasis. Science 1994;264: 713–6.
6. Stanley E, Lieschke GJ, Grail D, et al. Granulocyte/macrophage colony-stimulating factor-deficient mice show no major perturbation of hematopoiesis but develop a characteristic pulmonary pathology. Proc Natl Acad Sci U S A 1994;91:5592–6.
7. Nishinakamura R, Nakayama N, Hirabayashi Y, et al. Mice deficient for the IL-3/GM-CSF/IL-5 beta c receptor exhibit lung pathology and impaired immune response, while beta IL3 receptor- deficient mice are normal. Immunity 1995;2:211–22.
8. Robb L, Drinkwater CC, Metcalf D, et al. Hematopoietic and lung abnormalities in mice with a null mutation of the common beta subunit of the receptors for granulocyte-macrophage colony-stimulating

factor and interleukins 3 and 5. Proc Natl Acad Sci U S A 1995;92:9565–9.

9. Kitamura T, Tanaka N, Watanabe J, et al. Idiopathic pulmonary alveolar proteinosis as an autoimmune disease with neutralizing antibody against granulocyte/macrophage colony-stimulating factor. J Exp Med 1999;190:875–80.

10. Sakagami T, Uchida K, Suzuki T, et al. Human GM-CSF autoantibodies and reproduction of pulmonary alveolar proteinosis. N Engl J Med 2009;361: 2679–81.

11. Inoue Y, Trapnell BC, Tazawa R, et al. Characteristics of a large cohort of patients with autoimmune pulmonary alveolar proteinosis in Japan. Am J Respir Crit Care Med 2008;177:752–62.

12. Martinez-Moczygemba M, Doan ML, Elidemir O, et al. Pulmonary alveolar proteinosis caused by deletion of the GM-CSFRalpha gene in the X chromosome pseudoautosomal region 1. J Exp Med 2008;205:2711–6.

13. Suzuki T, Maranda B, Sakagami T, et al. Hereditary pulmonary alveolar proteinosis caused by recessive CSF2RB mutations. Eur Respir J 2011;37: 201–4.

14. Suzuki T, Sakagami T, Rubin BK, et al. Familial pulmonary alveolar proteinosis caused by mutations in CSF2RA. J Exp Med 2008;205:2703–10.

15. Suzuki T, Sakagami T, Young LR, et al. Hereditary pulmonary alveolar proteinosis: pathogenesis, presentation, diagnosis, and therapy. Am J Respir Crit Care Med 2010;182:1292–304.

16. Tanaka T, Motoi N, Tsuchihashi Y, et al. Adult-onset hereditary pulmonary alveolar proteinosis caused by a single-base deletion in CSF2RB. J Med Genet 2011;48:205–9.

17. Ishii H, Tazawa R, Kaneko C, et al. Clinical features of secondary pulmonary alveolar proteinosis: pre-mortem cases in Japan. Eur Respir J 2011;37: 465–8.

18. Parenti G, Sebastio G, Strisciuglio P, et al. Lysinuric protein intolerance characterized by bone marrow abnormalities and severe clinical course. J Pediatr 1995;126:246–51.

19. Hadchouel A, Wieland T, Griese M, et al. Biallelic mutations of Methionyl-tRNA synthetase cause a specific type of pulmonary alveolar proteinosis prevalent on Reunion Island. Am J Hum Genet 2015;96:826–31.

20. Hildebrandt J, Yalcin E, Bresser HG, et al. Characterization of CSF2RA mutation related juvenile pulmonary alveolar proteinosis. Orphanet J Rare Dis 2014;9:171.

21. Ishii H, Seymour JF, Tazawa R, et al. Secondary pulmonary alveolar proteinosis complicating myelodysplastic syndrome results in worsening of prognosis: a retrospective cohort study in Japan. BMC Pulm Med 2014;14:37.

22. Bonella F, Bauer PC, Griese M, et al. Pulmonary alveolar proteinosis: new insights from a single-center cohort of 70 patients. Respir Med 2011;105: 1908–16.

23. Campo I, Mariani F, Rodi G, et al. Assessment and management of pulmonary alveolar proteinosis in a reference center. Orphanet J Rare Dis 2013;8:40.

24. Xu Z, Jing J, Wang H, et al. Pulmonary alveolar proteinosis in China: a systematic review of 241 cases. Respirology 2009;14:761–6.

25. Presneill JJ, Nakata K, Inoue Y, et al. Pulmonary alveolar proteinosis. Clin Chest Med 2004;25:593–613, viii.

26. Uchida K, Nakata K, Carey B, et al. Standardized serum GM-CSF autoantibody testing for the routine clinical diagnosis of autoimmune pulmonary alveolar proteinosis. J Immunol Methods 2014;402:57–70.

27. Beccaria M, Luisetti M, Rodi G, et al. Long-term durable benefit after whole lung lavage in pulmonary alveolar proteinosis. Eur Respir J 2004;23:526–31.

28. Cordonnier C, Fleury-Feith J, Escudier E, et al. Secondary alveolar proteinosis is a reversible cause of respiratory failure in leukemic patients. Am J Respir Crit Care Med 1994;149:788–94.

29. Hamvas A, Nogee LM, Mallory GB Jr, et al. Lung transplantation for treatment of infants with surfactant protein B deficiency. J Pediatr 1997;130:231–9.

30. Akasaka K, Tanaka T, Kitamura N, et al. Outcome of corticosteroid administration in autoimmune pulmonary alveolar proteinosis: a retrospective cohort study. BMC Pulm Med 2015;15:88.

31. Seymour JF, Dunn AR, Vincent JM, et al. Efficacy of granulocyte-macrophage colony-stimulating factor in acquired alveolar proteinosis. N Engl J Med 1996;335:1924–5.

32. Venkateshiah SB, Yan TD, Bonfield TL, et al. An open-label trial of granulocyte macrophage colony stimulating factor therapy for moderate symptomatic pulmonary alveolar proteinosis. Chest 2006;130: 227–37.

33. Tazawa R, Hamano E, Arai T, et al. Granulocyte-macrophage colony-stimulating factor and lung immunity in pulmonary alveolar proteinosis. Am J Respir Crit Care Med 2005;171:1142–9.

34. Tazawa R, Trapnell BC, Inoue Y, et al. Inhaled granulocyte/macrophage-colony stimulating factor as therapy for pulmonary alveolar proteinosis. Am J Respir Crit Care Med 2010;181:1345–54.

35. Tazawa R, Inoue Y, Arai T, et al. Duration of benefit in patients with autoimmune pulmonary alveolar proteinosis after inhaled granulocyte-macrophage colony-stimulating factor therapy. Chest 2014;145: 729–37.

36. Amital A, Dux S, Shitrit D, et al. Therapeutic effectiveness of rituximab in a patient with unresponsive autoimmune pulmonary alveolar proteinosis. Thorax 2010;65:1025–6.

37. Borie R, Debray MP, Laine C, et al. Rituximab therapy in autoimmune pulmonary alveolar proteinosis. Eur Respir J 2009;33:1503–6.

38. Malur A, Kavuru MS, Marshall I, et al. Rituximab therapy in pulmonary alveolar proteinosis improves alveolar macrophage lipid homeostasis. Respir Res 2012;13:46.

39. Kavuru MS, Bonfield TL, Thomassen MJ. Plasmapheresis, GM-CSF, and alveolar proteinosis. Am J Respir Crit Care Med 2003;167:1036 [author reply: 1036–7].

40. Suzuki T, Arumugam P, Sakagami T, et al. Pulmonary macrophage transplantation therapy. Nature 2014; 514:450–4.

Pulmonary Alveolar Microlithiasis

Atsushi Saito, MD, PhD[a,b], Francis X. McCormack, MD[c],*

KEYWORDS

- Pulmonary alveolar microlithiasis • Congenital disease • SLC34A2
- Type II b sodium-phosphate cotransporter (NPT2B) • Phosphate homeostasis

KEY POINTS

- Pulmonary alveolar microlithiasis (PAM) is a genetic lung disorder that is characterized by the accumulation of calcium phosphate deposits in the alveolar spaces of the lung.
- Mutations in the type II sodium phosphate cotransporter, NPT2b, have been reported in patients with PAM.
- Patients typically present without symptoms at a young age, with dense ground glass infiltrates noted on chest radiographs obtained for another purpose.
- PAM progresses gradually, often producing incremental dyspnea on exertion, desaturation in young adulthood, and, ultimately, respiratory insufficiency by late middle age.
- Treatment remains supportive. For patients with end-stage disease, lung transplantation is an option.

INTRODUCTION

Pulmonary alveolar microlithiasis (PAM) is a rare hereditary lung disease in which calcium phosphate deposits (calcospherites) accumulate in the distal airspaces. An Italian scientist, Marcello Malpighi, first described PAM in 1868; Harbitz[1] first carefully detailed the histopathology in 1918. The disease was named "Microlithiasis Alveolaris Pulmonum" by the Hungarian pathologist Puhr[2] in 1933. Since the first description of the disease almost 150 years ago, more than 1000 cases have been reported in the world literature.[3] PAM is often discovered on chest radiographs obtained for other purposes during early adulthood. Patients typically remain asymptomatic until middle age, when pulmonary fibrosis, pulmonary hypertension, and chronic respiratory failure ensue. Chest radiographs reveal diffuse, hyperdense, micronodular shadows producing a characteristic snowstorm appearance.[4] The diagnosis can often be established based on radiographic appearance alone, especially in *patients* with a family history. The recent discovery in patients with PAM of genetic mutations in the SLC34A2 gene, which encodes the sodium-phosphate cotransporter NPT2b (*SLC34A2*, NPT2b, NaPi-2b), has opened a window into PAM disease pathogenesis.[5,6] An animal model has been developed that can serve as a preclinical model for testing candidate therapies, and a worldwide network of rare lung disease clinics has identified potential subjects with PAM for trials. Here the authors review the cause, epidemiology, pathology, clinical features, and potential future treatment strategies for PAM.

EPIDEMIOLOGY

PAM has long been considered to be an autosomal recessive disorder because it transmits horizontally

Disclosure: The authors have nothing to disclose.
[a] Department of Biochemistry, Sapporo Medical University, School of Medicine, Sapporo 0608543, Japan; [b] Department of Respiratory Medicine and Allergology, Sapporo Medical University, School of Medicine, Sapporo 0608556, Japan; [c] Division of Pulmonary, Critical Care, and Sleep Medicine, The University of Cincinnati, MSB 6165, 231 Albert Sabin Way, Cincinnati, OH 45267-0564, USA
* Corresponding author.
E-mail address: frank.mccormack@uc.edu

Clin Chest Med 37 (2016) 441–448
http://dx.doi.org/10.1016/j.ccm.2016.04.007
0272-5231/16/$ – see front matter Published by Elsevier Inc.

and is associated with consanguinity. Most patients with PAM have at least one sibling who is also affected by the disease. Mariotta and colleagues[7] reported that 35.8% of patients with PAM were diagnosed before 20 years of age and 88.2% before 50 years of age. PAM has also been reported in newborns and toddlers, including twins who died within 12 hours of birth,[8] and in octagenarians.[9,10] Familial incidence has been reported in 35% to 50% of cases reported from Japan,[11] Turkey,[12] Italy,[13] and other countries.[14] The frequency of PAM mutations in the Japanese population was determined to be less than 0.008.[6] There is no clear sex predilection for PAM.

PATHOLOGY
Molecular Pathogenesis

In 2006 and 2007, SLC34A2 mutations were identified in patients with PAM by homozygosity mapping.[5,6] The SLC34A2 gene is located on chromosome 4p15 and comprises 13 exons. It encodes a 2280-nt mRNA and a 690 amino acid sodium-phosphate cotransporter called NPT2b. A total of more than 15 different mutations have been described in 30 patients to date (**Fig. 1**).[3] Mutations have been found on multiple exons in patients from Turkey, but mutations seem to cluster in exon 8 in cases from China and in exons 7 and 8 in Japan.[15] The heterogeneity in mutations found is inconsistent with a founder effect, at least in the Turkish and Japanese populations, which have the largest populations studied. Most DNA aberrations found to date are missense mutations that result in protein truncation, but 3 damaging substitutions (G106R, T192K, Y455H) and a nonsense mutation that introduces a premature stop codon have been described.[5,15,16] In the few family studies that have been completed, the disease has demonstrated 100% penetrance in that all those with homozygous mutations are affected.[5] There does not seem to be any genotype/phenotype correlation based on variation in the age of disease onset in large family cohorts.[5] Genetic heterogeneity (ie, more than one gene involved) is not likely

because mutations in SLC34A2 have been identified in almost all patients studied. Almost all mutations identified to date have been homozygous, suggestive of identity by descent.

NPT2b is abundantly expressed in lung, primarily on the surface of alveolar type II cells, where it is thought to function as an exporter of phosphate generated by the metabolism of surfactant phospholipids.[17,18] In the absence of NPT2b activity, phosphate levels likely increase in the alveolar lining fluid and form complexes with calcium, resulting in the formation of lamellated microliths.[19] Alveolar pH, calcium concentrations, and nucleating proteins, lipids, or other molecules likely play an important role in microlith formation; but little is known about the conditions that favor stone initiation and growth. NPT2b is also expressed in the gut, where it functions as the major transporter for the uptake of dietary phosphorus, as well as in the breast, liver, testes, prostate, kidney, pancreas, and ovaries.[20,21]

Other sodium phosphate cotransporters include SLC34 family members NPT2a and NPT2c, which are predominantly expressed in the kidney, and SLC20 family members PIT1 and PIT2, which are ubiquitously expressed. The pulmonary expression of SLC20, NPT2a, and NPT2c transporters has not been well characterized in humans. Recently Saito and colleagues[19] reported expression of Pit1 and Pit2 but not NPT2a or NPT2c in mouse lung. The 3 SLC34 isoforms (NaPi-IIa, b, c) transport a divalent Pi (hydrogen phosphate [HPO_4^{2-}]) on binding of 2 or 3 sodium ions and use the inwardly directed Na+ electrochemical gradient to drive intracellular movement of inorganic phosphate (Pi).[22] The crystal structure has not been solved for any of the sodium-dependent phosphate cotransporters, and the bacterial dicarboxylate transporter has been used as a model for sodium-dependent anion transport.[23] The 3-dimensional (3D) structures of the wild-type NPT2b and 2 naturally occurring mutants were predicted by protein folding recognition with 3-dimensional position specific scoring matrix (Phyre Version 0.2) and molecular dynamics simulations.[15]

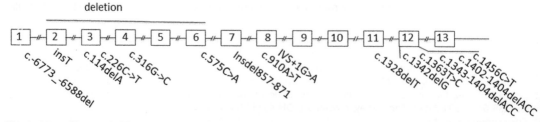

Fig. 1. Map of known SLC34A2 mutations. The SLC34A2 gene comprises 13 exons on chr. 4p15. (*Data from* Castellana G, Carone D, Castellana M. Microlithiasis of seminal vesicles and severe oligoasthenospermia in pulmonary alveolar microlithiasis (PAM): report of an unusual sporadic case. Int J Fertil Steril 2015;9(1):137–40.)

Epithelial deletion of NPT2b in mice resulted in a progressive pulmonary process characterized by diffuse alveolar microlith accumulation, radiographic opacification, restrictive physiology, inflammation, and fibrosis that closely mimic PAM.[19] Expression of NPT2b on the luminal surface of alveolar type II cells was apparent in the wild-type mice and lost in the knockout (KO) mouse (**Fig. 2**A). The concentrations of calcium and phosphorus in alveolar lavage fluids were increased by roughly 10-fold in the NPT2b-deficient animals compared with wild-type mice, whereas serum concentrations of the ions were unchanged in the two groups. The microliths that were isolated were demonstrated to contain calcium phosphate. The KO animals developed an unexpected alveolar phospholipidosis, which has not been reported in humans to the authors' knowledge, and may be related to altered surfactant catabolism due to dysfunction of alveolar macrophages. Filling of alveolar spaces with abundant eosinophilic material has been reported in identical twins with PAM who died within 12 hours of birth, however, which could be consistent with phospholipidosis,[8] as could serum surfactant protein elevations[24] and oil red O–positive alveolar macrophages that have been reported in patients with PAM.[25] Cytokine and surfactant protein elevations in the alveolar lavage and serum of PAM mice

and confirmed in serum from patients with PAM validated serum monocyte chemotactic protein 1 (MCP-1) and surfactant protein D (SP-D) as potential biomarkers (**Fig. 2**B). Microliths introduced by adoptive transfer into the lungs of wild-type mice produced marked macrophage-rich inflammation and elevation of serum MCP-1 that peaked at 1 week and resolved at 1 month, associated with clearance of stones. Microliths isolated by bronchoalveolar lavage readily dissolved in ethylenediaminetetraacetic acid (EDTA), and therapeutic EDTA lavage reduced the burden of stones in the lungs. A low-phosphate diet prevented microlith formation in young animals and reduced serum SP-D, a potential biomarker of lung injury (**Fig. 2**C). The burden of pulmonary calcium deposits in established PAM was also diminished within 4 weeks by a low-phosphate diet challenge. The rapid reversal of an established PAM lesion in the lungs of mice suggests an active transport process that removes calcium, phosphate, or both in a process that may be triggered by vitamin D, FGF23 (fibroblast growth factor 23), or serum levels of calcium or phosphate. These data support a causative role for NPT2b in the pathogenesis of PAM and the use of the PAM mouse model as a preclinical platform for the development of biomarkers and therapeutic strategies.

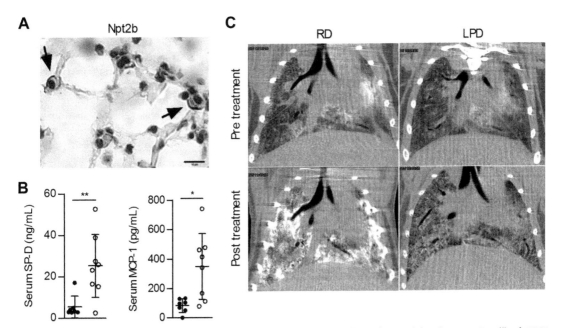

Fig. 2. (*A*) Arrows demonstrate enhanced NPT2b staining in the apical membrane (alveolar type II cell) of AECII of wild-type mice. (*B*) The elevation of human surfactant protein D (SP-D) and monocyte chemotactic protein 1 (MCP-1) in the serum from patients with PAM (*opened circle*) compared with healthy volunteers (*closed circle*). (*C*) Low-phosphate diet (LPD) prevents microlith accumulation in mice. RD, regular diet. Data are expressed as mean ± SD. *P<0.05, **P<0.01. (*From* Saito A, Nikolaidis NM, Amlal H, et al. Modeling pulmonary alveolar microlithiasis by epithelial deletion of the NPT2b sodium phosphate cotransporter reveals putative biomarkers and strategies for treatment. Sci Transl Med 2015;7(313):313ra181; with permission.)

Histology

At autopsy, the lungs from patients with PAM are enlarged, heavy, and nonbouyant.[26] The pleural surface has a studded, fine, granular appearance. Sectioning of the lung reveals a diffusely calcified and gritty surface. Stones isolated from the lung range from 50 to 5000 μm in diameter[27–31] and have a lamellated, onionskin appearance under the microscope. The microliths are primarily composed of calcium phosphate and small amounts of calcium carbonate, magnesium, and iron.[32] Under the microscope, the pulmonary architecture is diffusely altered because of filling of alveoli with multiple microliths.[33] Patchy inflammation is frequently present, especially in patients with a longer duration of illness. Variable degrees of pulmonary fibrosis are often found in the pulmonary interstitium.[27] Evidence of pulmonary hypertension, with increased intimal and medial thickening, is also apparent in advanced cases.[34] Morphometric analysis of CD34 immunostained sections in an autopsy case revealed a significant reduction in the pulmonary capillary beds as a potential mechanism for pulmonary hypertension.[35]

The pathologic changes in PAM are primarily confined to lungs; but occasional reports of extrapulmonary calcifications in the pleura,[36] diaphragm,[37] lumbar sympathetic chain, and testicles[5] have appeared in the literature.

CLINICAL FEATURES
Symptoms and Signs

In early stages, patients with PAM are asymptomatic. Cases of early disease onset or rapid progression are rare. As the disease progresses, symptoms, such as dyspnea on exertion and dry cough, may develop. Asthenia, chest pain, cyanosis, hemoptysis, and pneumothorax have been all been reported. Physical examination may reveal rales and finger clubbing. Subjective complaints are often less severe than radiological findings suggest, a scenario that has been termed *clinical-radiological dissociation*. There is some evidence that smoking and infection may accelerate disease progression.[5]

Clinical Testing

Pulmonary function testing is usually normal in early stages. Reduction in diffusing capacity for carbon monoxide and a restrictive ventilatory impairment develop over time. Echocardiography may reveal evidence of pulmonary hypertension and right heart strain.[38]

Serum phosphate and calcium are typically normal in patients with PAM,[39] as are other hematological and biochemical parameters. In 2 patients, SP-D was found to be elevated in the serum, which could reflect higher alveolar SP-D levels, compromised barrier integrity, or both.[24] Serum MCP-1 was found to be elevated in patients with PAM.[19] These reports suggest the possibility that SP-D and MCP-1 may be useful as diagnostic biomarkers or indicators of disease activity or progression.

Radiology

The routine chest radiograph in patients with PAM typically reveals a fine, sandlike micronodular pattern that is more pronounced in the bases than in the apices (**Fig. 3**A). The vascular tree and the borders of the heart and diaphragm are often obscured (vanishing heart phenomenon),

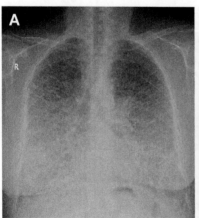
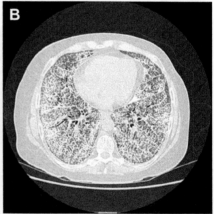

Fig. 3. Chest radiograph (*A*) and high-resolution computed tomography findings (*B*) of a 59-year-old Middle Eastern woman with a history of PAM, showing diffuse opacification in both lungs with hyperdense micronodular, called sand-storm appearance. (*From* Gupta N, McCormack FX. Pulmonary alveolar microlithiasis. Am J Respir Crit Care Med 2013;188(7):e11–2; with permission.)

and air bronchograms coursing through areas of consolidation may be apparent.

High-resolution computed tomography (CT) also reveals widespread, tiny microcalcifications throughout the lungs. Ground-glass opacities and airspace consolidation may occupy a large fraction of the lung fields (**Fig. 3**B).[40,41] Microliths are typically diffusely distributed but may be preferentially deposited in the posterior segments of the lower lobes. The profusion of microliths may be increased in the upper lobes of smokers. Interlobular septal thickening is often apparent and may produce a crazy-paving appearance. A linear radiolucency at the pleural boundaries abutting the heart, diaphragm, and pleura is a characteristic radiological feature of PAM and is likely secondary to the subpleural cystic changes that are often seen at cross-sectional imaging and pathological evaluations.[42] These cystic changes seem to be due to dilation of alveolar ducts.[41] Small apical bullae are another typical feature.

In a radiological study of 13 PAM cases in Brazil, CT findings in decreasing order of prevalence included ground-glass opacities, small parenchymal nodules, and small subpleural nodules in more than 90%; subpleural cysts in 85%; and subpleural linear calcifications, crazy paving pattern, nodular fissure, calcification along interlobular septa, and dense consolidations in 46% to 70%.[43] Intermingled air bronchograms were identified in 6 cases. The lower third of the lungs was predominantly affected, but there was no predominant distribution along the axial or anteroposterior axes.

Extrapulmonary Disease

Deposition of microliths in the external male genitalia has been described in patients with PAM, including deposition in testicles and seminal vesicles associated with hematuria, testicular atrophy, obstructive azoospermia, and infertility.[44–49] Testicular microlithiasis occurs in 0.6% to 9.0% of the male population, and it is associated with most primary testicular malignancies and in about 1% of cases of male infertility.[50–52] Corut and colleagues[5] tested 15 patients with testicular microlithiasis for NPT2b mutations and found 2 mutations that were not conclusively damaging. It is not clear whether NPT2b plays a role in the pathogenesis of testicular microlithiasis.

Associated Diseases

Other diseases that have been reported in patients with PAM include pericardial cyst, lymphocytic interstitial pneumonitis, non-Hodgkin lymphoma, antiphospholipid syndrome, discoid lupus, rheumatoid arthritis, psoriasis, osteopetrosis, Sjögren syndrome, hypertrophic pulmonary osteoarthropathy, and pectus excavatum. It is unclear if there is any association between these disorders and PAM or whether these were chance occurrences. Other heritable diseases that have been reported in patients with PAM may be coincidental, due to cotransmission in families with consanguineous relationships, and include diaphyseal aclasis and autosomal recessive Waardenburg-anophthalmia syndrome.

DIAGNOSIS

The diagnosis of PAM can usually be established radiographically. Bronchoalveolar lavage demonstrating microliths with the typical lamellar structure has been helpful in cases where doubt exists. In some cases, microliths have been recovered in expectorated sputum.[53] Transbronchial biopsy seems to have a reasonable yield and safety profile but is not usually required when the radiographic presentation is typical. In the literature, the diagnosis has been determined by lung biopsy in about 46.9% of cases,[7] likely because the disease is unfamiliar to many physicians. In general, lung biopsy should be reserved for cases where uncertainty persists despite more conservative diagnostic methods. Genotyping for *SLC34A2* gene mutations is commercially available and may be useful for screening family members, with appropriate genetic counseling, but is currently not otherwise clinically informative or necessary for diagnosis.

DIFFERENTIAL DIAGNOSIS

When the chest radiograph demonstrating dense micronodular and ground-glass opacities in asymptomatic patients is first obtained, diagnostic considerations may include miliary tuberculosis (TB), pulmonary alveolar proteinosis, sarcoidosis, healed varicella or variola pneumonia, metastatic calcification, pneumoconioses including silicosis, pulmonary hemosiderosis, or amyloidosis. PAM is perhaps most frequently confused with pulmonary TB, in part because regions where consanguineous marriage is common and TB is highly prevalent frequently overlap. There have been at least 5 cases of concomitant TB in patients with PAM.[3] The crazy-paving pattern that has been described in PAM was once thought to be pathognomonic for pulmonary alveolar proteinosis and can lead to diagnostic confusion.[3,54] However, discrete calcifications visualized within mediastinal window settings distinguish PAM from PAP (pulmonary alveolar proteinosis). In patients who are demonstrated to have diffuse pulmonary calcifications on CT or chest radiograph, the differential includes the many causes of both metastatic and dystrophic pulmonary calcification, which occur in formerly normal lung tissue and damaged lung tissue, respectively.[55] Pulmonary metastatic calcification is most frequently due to chronic renal failure but may also be seen in patients with hyperparathyroidism, mild alkali syndrome, talcosis, amiodarone toxicity, iodinated oil embolism, and aspirated or extravasated contrast material. Dystrophic calcification may occur as a sequela of viral infection due to varicella or variola, granulomatous disease due to TB, histoplasmosis, coccidioidomycosis, or sarcoidosis.

PROGNOSIS

The prognosis of PAM is unclear. In a study of 53 Japanese patients, 34.1% to 42.9% died within 10 to 49 years of diagnosis, at a mean age of 46.2 years. The most common cause of death was respiratory failure. These results suggest a poor long-term prognosis for patients with PAM, including patients discovered to have asymptomatic disease in childhood.[39]

PHARMACOLOGIC TREATMENT OPTIONS
Etidronate

Etidronate is a unique bisphosphonate that not only inhibits osteoclast driven bone resorption, as do many other members of the class, but also inhibits crystal formation and bone mineralization. Etidronate is approved by the Food and Drug Administration for the treatment of Paget disease and heterotopic calcification.[56] In a handful of case studies, etidronate has been reported to improve lung function and reduce radiographic opacification of the lung in patients with PAM.[13,57–60] In other reports, etidronate has been ineffective.[13,61] Further studies will be required to determine if etidronate has a role in the treatment of PAM.

Steroid Hormones

In general, steroid hormone therapy seems to be ineffective for PAM, though a few investigators have reported subjective improvement in some patients.[62,63]

Bronchoalveolar Lavage

Repeated lavage is often used for pulmonary alveolar proteinosis and is a plausible treatment strategy for PAM because the microliths are exclusively localized to the alveolar lumen.

Unfortunately, there is no evidence that this approach has been effective.[64]

Oxygen Therapy and Vaccinations

Supplemental oxygen therapy is prudent for patients who are hypoxemic with rest, exercise, or sleep. Patients with PAM should receive pneumococcal and influenza vaccinations.

SURGICAL TREATMENT OPTIONS
Lung Transplantation

As of 2015, unilateral and bilateral lung transplantation had been reported in 17 patients with PAM,[65–69] without any documented recurrence in the grafts.[33] Comparisons of outcomes of transplant in patients with PAM with those of patients with other lung diseases has not been reported.

SUMMARY

PAM is a genetic lung disorder that is characterized by the accumulation of calcium phosphate deposits in the alveolar spaces of the lung. Mutations in the type II sodium phosphate cotransporter, NPT2b, have been reported in patients with PAM. Patients typically present without symptoms at a young age, with dense ground infiltrates noted on chest radiographs obtained for another purpose, as well as dyspnea on exertion, a restrictive ventilatory defect, and decreased diffusion capacity. Dissociation between radiological findings and clinical symptoms is a clinical feature of PAM. PAM progresses gradually, often producing incremental dyspnea on exertion and desaturation in young adulthood and, ultimately, respiratory insufficiency by late middle age. Extrapulmonary disease is uncommon. Treatment remains supportive, including supplemental oxygen therapy. For patients with end-stage disease, lung transplantation is available as a last resort. Patients are so rare and geographically dispersed that trials are difficult. The recent development of a laboratory animal model has revealed several promising treatment approaches for future trials.

REFERENCES

1. Harbitz F. Extensive calcification of the lungs as a distinct disease. Arch Intern Med 1918;21(1): 139–46.
2. Puhr L. Mikrolithiasis alveolaris pulmonum. Virchows Arch Pathol Anat 1933;290(1):156–60.
3. Castellana G, Carone D, Castellana M. Microlithiasis of seminal vesicles and severe oligoasthenospermia in pulmonary alveolar microlithiasis (PAM): report of an unusual sporadic case. Int J Fertil Steril 2015; 9(1):137–40.

4. Sosman MC, Dodd GD, Jones WD, et al. The familial occurrence of pulmonary alveolar microlithiasis. Am J Roentgenol Radium Ther Nucl Med 1957;77(6): 947–1012.

5. Corut A, Senyigit A, Ugur SA, et al. Mutations in SLC34A2 cause pulmonary alveolar microlithiasis and are possibly associated with testicular microlithiasis. Am J Hum Genet 2006;79(4):650–6.

6. Huqun, Izumi S, Miyazawa H, et al. Mutations in the SLC34A2 gene are associated with pulmonary alveolar microlithiasis. Am J Respir Crit Care Med 2007; 175(3):263–8.

7. Mariotta S, Ricci A, Papale M, et al. Pulmonary alveolar microlithiasis: report on 576 cases published in the literature. Sarcoidosis Vasc Diffuse Lung Dis 2004;21(3):173–81.

8. Caffrey PR, Altman RS. Pulmonary alveolar microlitbiasis occurring in premature twins. J Pediatr 1965;66:758–63.

9. Tiedjen KU, Kosberg R, Kruger G. Pulmonary microlithiasis following iodine lipiodol lymphography? Radiologe 1986;26(10):460–3 [in German].

10. Chang AR. Pulmonary alveolar microlithiasis. Pathology 1980;12(2):164–7, 282–163.

11. Hagiwara K, Johkoh T, Tachibana T. Pulmonary alveolar microlithiasis. In: McCormack F, Panos R, Trapnell B, editors. Molecular Basis of Pulmonary Disease. Series Respiratory Medicine Ed Sharon Rounds. New York: Springer; 2010. p. 325–8.

12. Ucan ES, Keyf AI, Aydilek R, et al. Pulmonary alveolar microlithiasis: review of Turkish reports. Thorax 1993;48(2):171–3.

13. Mariotta S, Guidi L, Mattia P, et al. Pulmonary microlithiasis. Report of two cases. Respiration 1997; 64(2):165–9.

14. Castellana G, Gentile M, Castellana R, et al. Pulmonary alveolar microlithiasis: clinical features, evolution of the phenotype, and review of the literature. Am J Med Genet 2002;111(2):220–4.

15. Yang W, Wang Y, Pu Q, et al. Elevated expression of SLC34A2 inhibits the viability and invasion of A549 cells. Mol Med Rep 2014;10(3):1205–14.

16. Ma T, Ren J, Yin J, et al. A pedigree with pulmonary alveolar microlithiasis: a clinical case report and literature review. Cell Biochem Biophys 2014;70(1): 565–72.

17. Hashimoto M, Wang DY, Kamo T, et al. Isolation and localization of type IIb Na/Pi cotransporter in the developing rat lung. Am J Pathol 2000;157(1):21–7.

18. Traebert M, Hattenhauer O, Murer H, et al. Expression of type II Na-P(i) cotransporter in alveolar type II cells. Am J Physiol 1999;277(5 Pt 1):L868–73.

19. Saito A, Nikolaidis NM, Amlal H, et al. Modeling pulmonary alveolar microlithiasis by epithelial deletion of the Npt2b sodium phosphate cotransporter reveals putative biomarkers and strategies for treatment. Sci Transl Med 2015;7(313):313ra181.

20. Sabbagh Y, O'Brien SP, Song W, et al. Intestinal npt2b plays a major role in phosphate absorption and homeostasis. J Am Soc Nephrol 2009;20(11): 2348–58.

21. Schiavi SC, Tang W, Bracken C, et al. Npt2b deletion attenuates hyperphosphatemia associated with CKD. J Am Soc Nephrol 2012;23(10):1691–700.

22. Bacconi A, Virkki LV, Biber J, et al. Renouncing electroneutrality is not free of charge: switching on electrogenicity in a Na+-coupled phosphate cotransporter. Proc Natl Acad Sci U S A 2005; 102(35):12606–11.

23. Mancusso R, Gregorio GG, Liu Q, et al. Structure and mechanism of a bacterial sodium-dependent dicarboxylate transporter. Nature 2012;491(7425):622–6.

24. Takahashi H, Chiba H, Shiratori M, et al. Elevated serum surfactant protein A and D in pulmonary alveolar microlithiasis. Respirology 2006;11(3):330–3.

25. Monabati A, Ghayumi MA, Kumar PV. Familial pulmonary alveolar microlithiasis diagnosed by bronchoalveolar lavage. A case report. Acta Cytol 2007;51(1):80–2.

26. Chalmers AG, Wyatt J, Robinson PJ. Computed tomographic and pathological findings in pulmonary alveolar microlithiasis. Br J Radiol 1986;59(700): 408–11.

27. Moran CA, Hochholzer L, Hasleton PS, et al. Pulmonary alveolar microlithiasis. A clinicopathologic and chemical analysis of seven cases. Arch Pathol Lab Med 1997;121(6):607–11.

28. Portnoy LM, Amadeo B, Hennigar GR. Pulmonary alveolar microlithiasis. An unusual case (associated with milk-alkali syndrome). Am J Clin Pathol 1964;41: 194–201.

29. Siddiqui NA, Fuhrman CR. Best cases from the AFIP: pulmonary alveolar microlithiasis. Radiographics 2011;31(2):585–90.

30. Kawakami M, Sato S, Takishima T. Electron microscopic studies on pulmonary alveolar microlithiasis. Tohoku J Exp Med 1978;126(4):343–61.

31. Barnard NJ, Crocker PR, Blainey AD, et al. Pulmonary alveolar microlithiasis. A new analytical approach. Histopathology 1987;11(6):639–45.

32. Pracyk JB, Simonson SG, Young SL, et al. Composition of lung lavage in pulmonary alveolar microlithiasis. Respiration 1996;63(4):254–60.

33. Samano MN, Waisberg DR, Canzian M, et al. Lung transplantation for pulmonary alveolar microlithiasis: a case report. Clinics (Sao Paulo) 2010;65(2):233–6.

34. Ghosh GC, Kategeri B, Chatterjee K, et al. Pulmonary alveolar microlithiasis: a rare cause of right heart failure. BMJ Case Rep 2013;2013 [pii:bcr2013010218].

35. Terada T. Pulmonary alveolar microlithiasis with cor pulmonale: an autopsy case demonstrating a marked decrease in pulmonary vascular beds. Respir Med 2009;103(11):1768–71.

36. Malhotra B, Sabharwal R, Singh M, et al. Pulmonary alveolar microlithiasis with calcified pleural plaques. Lung India 2010;27(4):250–2.

37. Pant K, Shah A, Mathur RK, et al. Pulmonary alveolar microlithiasis with pleural calcification and nephrolithiasis. Chest 1990;98(1):245–6.

38. Prakash UB, Barham SS, Rosenow EC 3rd, et al. Pulmonary alveolar microlithiasis. A review including ultrastructural and pulmonary function studies. Mayo Clin Proc 1983;58(5):290–300.

39. Tachibana T, Hagiwara K, Johkoh T. Pulmonary alveolar microlithiasis: review and management. Curr Opin Pulm Med 2009;15(5):486–90.

40. Cluzel P, Grenier P, Bernadac P, et al. Pulmonary alveolar microlithiasis: CT findings. J Comput Assist Tomogr 1991;15(6):938–42.

41. Sumikawa H, Johkoh T, Tomiyama N, et al. Pulmonary alveolar microlithiasis: CT and pathologic findings in 10 patients. Monaldi Arch Chest Dis 2005;63(1):59–64.

42. Felson B. Thoracic calcifications. Dis Chest 1969; 56(4):330–43.

43. Francisco FA, Rodrigues RS, Barreto MM, et al. Can chest high-resolution computed tomography findings diagnose pulmonary alveolar microlithiasis? Radiol Bras 2015;48(4):205–10.

44. Coetzee T. Pulmonary alveolar microlithiasis with involvement of the sympathetic nervous system and gonads. Thorax 1970;25(5):637–42.

45. Sandhyamani S, Verma K, Sharma SK, et al. Pulmonary alveolar microlithiasis. Indian J Chest Dis Allied Sci 1982;24(1):33–5.

46. Arslan A, Yalin T, Akan H, et al. Pulmonary alveolar microlithiasis associated with calcifications in the seminal vesicles. J Belge Radiol 1996;79(3):118–9.

47. Qublan HS. Azoospermia associated with testicular and pulmonary microlithiasis. J Diagn Med Sonogr 2003;19:192–4.

48. Kanat F, Teke T, Imecik O. Pulmonary alveolar microlithiasis with epididymal and periurethral calcifications causing obstructive azospermia. Int J Tuberc Lung Dis 2004;8(10):1275.

49. Castellana G, Castellana R, Carone D, et al. Microlitiasi alveolare polmonare associata a microlitiasi delle vescichette seminali. Rass Pat App Respir 2010;25:206–10.

50. Kim B, Winter TC 3rd, Ryu JA. Testicular microlithiasis: clinical significance and review of the literature. Eur Radiol 2003;13(12):2567–76.

51. Middleton WD, Teefey SA, Santillan CS. Testicular microlithiasis: prospective analysis of prevalence and associated tumor. Radiology 2002;224(2):425–8.

52. Miller FN, Sidhu PS. Does testicular microlithiasis matter? A review. Clin Radiol 2002;57(10):883–90.

53. Chatterji R, Gaude GS, Patil PV. Pulmonary alveolar microlithiasis: diagnosed by sputum examination and transbronchial biopsy. Indian J Chest Dis Allied Sci 1997;39(4):263–7.

54. Gasparetto EL, Tazoniero P, Escuissato DL, et al. Pulmonary alveolar microlithiasis presenting with crazy-paving pattern on high resolution CT. Br J Radiol 2004;77(923):974–6.

55. Belem LC, Zanetti G, Souza AS Jr, et al. Metastatic pulmonary calcification: state-of-the-art review focused on imaging findings. Respir Med 2014; 108(5):668–76.

56. Watts NB, Harris ST, Genant HK, et al. Intermittent cyclical etidronate treatment of postmenopausal osteoporosis. N Engl J Med 1990;323(2):73–9.

57. Kumazoe H, Matsunaga K, Nagata N, et al. "Reversed halo sign" of high-resolution computed tomography in pulmonary sarcoidosis. J Thorac Imaging 2009;24(1):66–8.

58. Ozcelik U, Gulsun M, Gocmen A, et al. Treatment and follow-up of pulmonary alveolar microlithiasis with disodium editronate: radiological demonstration. Pediatr Radiol 2002;32(5):380–3.

59. Ozcelik U, Yalcin E, Ariyurek M, et al. Long-term results of disodium etidronate treatment in pulmonary alveolar microlithiasis. Pediatr Pulmonol 2010; 45(5):514–7.

60. Zompatori M, Poletti V, Battista G, et al. Bronchiolitis obliterans with organizing pneumonia (BOOP), presenting as a ring-shaped opacity at HRCT (the atoll sign). A case report. Radiol Med 1999;97(4):308–10.

61. Jankovic S, Pavlov N, Ivkosic A, et al. Pulmonary alveolar microlithiasis in childhood: clinical and radiological follow-up. Pediatr Pulmonol 2002; 34(5):384–7.

62. Ganesan N, Ambroise MM, Ramdas A, et al. Pulmonary alveolar microlithiasis: an interesting case report with systematic review of Indian literature. Front Med 2015;9(2):229–38.

63. Flynn A, Agastyaraju AD. Pulmonary alveolar microlithiasis. Int J Case Rep Imag 2013;4(2):108–10.

64. Palombini BC, da Silva Porto N, Wallau CU, et al. Bronchopulmonary lavage in alveolar microlithiasis. Chest 1981;80(2):242–3.

65. Jackson KB, Modry DL, Halenar J, et al. Single lung transplantation for pulmonary alveolar microlithiasis. J Heart Lung Transplant 2001;20(2):226.

66. Stamatis G, Zerkowski HR, Doetsch N, et al. Sequential bilateral lung transplantation for pulmonary alveolar microlithiasis. Ann Thorac Surg 1993; 56(4):972–5.

67. Borrelli R, Fossi A, Volterrani L, et al. Right single-lung transplantation for pulmonary alveolar microlithiasis. Eur J Cardiothorac Surg 2014;45(2):e40.

68. Bonnette P, Bisson A, el Kadi NB, et al. Bilateral single lung transplantation. Complications and results in 14 patients. Eur J Cardiothorac Surg 1992;6(10): 550–4.

69. Edelman JD, Bavaria J, Kaiser LR, et al. Bilateral sequential lung transplantation for pulmonary alveolar microlithiasis. Chest 1997;112(4):1140–4.

Primary Ciliary Dyskinesia

Michael R. Knowles, MD[a],*, Maimoona Zariwala, PhD[b], Margaret Leigh, MD[c]

KEYWORDS

- Primary ciliary dyskinesia • Kartagener syndrome • Nasal nitric oxide • Genetic testing

KEY POINTS

- Primary ciliary dyskinesia (PCD) is a recessive genetically heterogeneous disorder of motile cilia with chronic otosinopulmonary disease and organ laterality defects in ~50% of cases.
- The prevalence of PCD is difficult to determine, because there has historically been no readily available and standardized diagnostic approach.
- Recent diagnostic advances through measurement of nasal nitric oxide and genetic testing has allowed rigorous diagnoses and determination of a robust clinical phenotype, which includes neonatal respiratory distress, daily nasal congestion, and wet cough starting early in life, along with organ laterality defects.
- There is early onset of lung disease in PCD with abnormal airflow mechanics and radiographic abnormalities detected in infancy and early childhood.
- The treatment of PCD is not fully standardized, but PCD Foundation consensus recommendations on diagnosis, monitoring, and treatment of PCD have recently been published.

INTRODUCTION

Primary ciliary dyskinesia (PCD) is a genetically heterogeneous recessive disorder of motile cilia associated with respiratory distress in term neonates, chronic otosinopulmonary disease, male infertility, and organ laterality defects in ~50% of cases.[1-4] This syndrome was initially recognized based on the triad of chronic sinusitis, bronchiectasis, and situs inversus (Kartagener syndrome)[5] and Afzelius[6] later recognized that these patients had immotile cilia and defective ciliary ultrastructure. Over time, it was recognized that most patients had stiff, uncoordinated, and/or ineffective ciliary beat, and the term PCD was used to distinguish this ciliary genetic disorder from secondary or acquired ciliary defects.

Even though PCD has an estimated incidence of 1 per 10,000 to 20,000 births, based on population surveys of situs inversus and bronchiectasis,[7,8] it is difficult to determine the prevalence of PCD in the United States, largely because of suboptimal diagnostic approaches.[9] Further, many physicians do not appreciate and recognize the key clinical features, particularly in infants and children;

Disclosures: None relevant to this publication.

Grant Support: National Institutes of Health (NIH), number U54HL096458, 5R01HL071798; the Genetic Disorders of Mucociliary Clearance (U54HL096458) is a part of the National Center for Advancing Translational Sciences (NCATS) Rare Diseases Clinical Research Network (RDCRN). RDCRN is an initiative of the Office of Rare Diseases Research (ORDR). NCATS funded through a collaboration between NCATS and NHLBI; CTSA NIH/NCATS UNC ULTR000083; CTSA NIH/NCATS Colorado UL1TR000154; Intramural Research Program of NIH/NIAID.

[a] Department of Medicine, Marsico Lung Institute/UNC CF Research Center, School of Medicine, University of North Carolina at Chapel Hill, Chapel Hill, NC 27599, USA; [b] Department of Pathology and Laboratory Medicine, Marsico Lung Institute/UNC CF Research Center, School of Medicine, University of North Carolina at Chapel Hill, Chapel Hill, NC 27599, USA; [c] Department of Pediatrics, Marsico Lung Institute/UNC CF Research Center, School of Medicine, University of North Carolina at Chapel Hill, Chapel Hill, NC 27599, USA

* Corresponding author. 7214 Marsico Hall, Chapel Hill, NC 27599-7248.

E-mail address: michael_knowles@med.unc.edu

however, recent advances in defining the clinical phenotype are likely to increase the level of awareness for PCD.[10,11] Moreover, better definition of genotype/phenotype will also facilitate recognition of the early onset and severity of clinical disease in children with PCD.[2,4,11,12]

Laboratory diagnostic capabilities have recently benefited from the development of nasal nitric oxide (nNO) as a new test for PCD.[13] Analysis of ciliary ultrastructure is improving; however, it is now recognized that ~30% of patients with PCD have normal ciliary electron micrographs, which precludes diagnosis by ciliary EM. Genetic testing is also becoming feasible, because there are now 35 genes with PCD-causing genetic mutations,[14,15] which likely accounts for ~70% of PCD.

There are no validated PCD-specific therapies, and the treatment of PCD has not been standardized; however, recently published PCD Foundation consensus recommendations on diagnosis, monitoring, and treatment of PCD provide guidelines for clinical care.[15]

This article provides an overview of the rapidly evolving state of the art for PCD, including a focus on the diagnosis and treatment of PCD, and a summary of the progress that promises to revolutionize the identification and treatment of patients with PCD.[1–4,11–15]

STRUCTURE AND FUNCTION OF MOTILE CILIA

Cilia are evolutionarily conserved organelles and motile respiratory cilia have a complex (9 + 2) axonemal structure to generate functional ciliary motility.[16,17] Motile cilia have microtubules composed of alpha and beta monomers of tubulin (**Fig. 1**).[17] Outer dynein arms (ODAs) and inner dynein arms (IDAs) are present along the length of the peripheral microtubules (doublets), and contain enzymes for ATP hydrolysis.[16,17] Nexin-dynein regulatory complexes (nexin links) connect the doublets, and radial spokes connect the doublets to the central pair for structural support during cilia bending.[18] Mutations in genes necessary for the biogenesis of cilia, or genes encoding the axonemal structure and/or functional components of motile cilia, can result in PCD.

During early development, each cell in the embryonic ventral node contains a single motile cilium. This specialized cilium has 9 peripheral doublets and dynein arms, but lacks the central pair of microtubules (9 + 0 axonemal structure).[17] Functionally, this cilium has a rotary motion, which drives a vectorial movement and laterality of organ lateralization during embryogenesis.[19] When nodal ciliary function is absent, organ lateralization is random. Mutations in genes that encode for components of the central apparatus (central pair, radial spokes) do not cause laterality defects.[1,14,15]

In addition to motile cilia, most cells of the body have a single nonmotile (sensory or primary) cilium that has specialized receptors to sense the local environment, and that play a key role in planar cell polarity.[20] Mutations in genes encoding proteins for sensory cilia cause disorders involving multiple organs (eg, Bardet-Biedl syndrome, nephronophthisis, retinitis pigmentosa, and Joubert syndrome).[20]

The function of normal motile cilia is to clear mucus as well as bacteria and toxic substances from the conducting airways.[21,22] ATP hydrolysis in dynein arms induces sliding of adjacent axonemal structures, and generates the complex ciliary waveform in human airways.[16–18,23] Several hundred cilia per cell beat in a coordinated fashion, which generates coordinated vectorial flow from planar orientation.[24] The cilia beat in plane, and the forward (power) stroke is more rapid and extends slightly higher into the mucus layer than the recovery stroke.[23] Ciliary beating is regulated by multiple signaling molecules, including cyclic AMP, cyclic GMP, and NO.[16]

ULTRASTRUCTURAL AND FUNCTIONAL DIAGNOSTIC TESTS

The diagnosis of PCD is delayed in both European and North American children (median age of diagnosis, 5.5 years and 5.0 years, respectively).[1] Because most institutions do not have adequate resources for a rigorous diagnostic evaluation for PCD, referral to specialized centers may be beneficial. This recommendation includes patients with situs inversus with any respiratory disease, or unexplained neonatal respiratory distress, as well as bronchiectasis without a defined cause, and/or a family history of PCD. For adults, all men with abnormal spermatozoal movement should be evaluated for PCD if they have respiratory symptoms. Several medical disorders and phenotypes may coexist with PCD, including complex congenital heart disease, laterality defects, retinitis pigmentosa, hydrocephalus, pectus excavatum, and scoliosis.[1–4]

In the evaluation of patients with chronic respiratory disease, it is critical to identify phenotypic features that characterize PCD, compared with other diseases.[11,15] Neonatal respiratory distress is a common feature (>80%) and a useful marker of PCD (**Box 1**), particularly for infants or children who have not developed bronchiectasis, and represents a special challenge for diagnosis.[11,15,25,26] Laterality defects are fairly specific

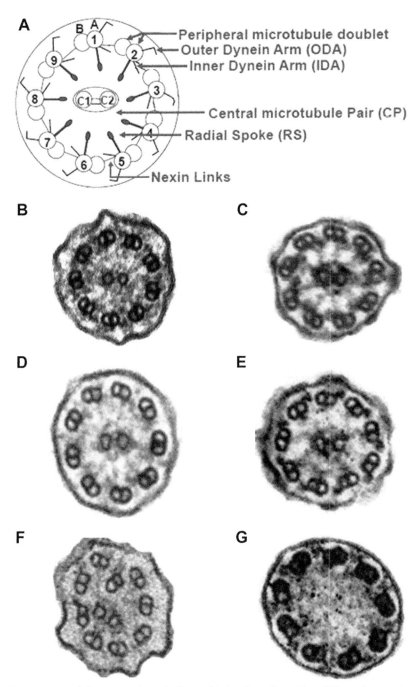

Fig. 1. Ciliary ultrastructure. (*A*) Cross section of cilium with 9 + 2 configuration. Ciliary ultrastructure by EM from (*B*) normal subject and (*C–G*) patients with PCD. (*A*) The 9 + 2 structure is shown with individual components of the axonemal structure. (*B*) Normal EM. (*C*) Outer dynein arm (ODA) defect, as seen in DNAH5 mutations. (*D*) ODA + inner dynein arm (IDA) defect, as seen in DNAAF1 mutations. (*E, F*) IDA defect alone, and IDA defect with microtubular disorganization, as seen in CCDC39 mutations. (*G*) Missing central pair (CP), as seen in ~12% of cilia with RSPH1 mutations.

for distinguishing children with PCD from other children with chronic respiratory symptoms. The early onset and persistence of respiratory symptoms may help distinguish PCD from disorders with more episodic respiratory symptoms.[11,12,15] In PCD, the chronic nasal congestion and wet cough occur daily throughout the year. Chronic otitis media often develops in the first months of

---

Box 1
Consensus-based PCD diagnostic criteria by age

Newborns (0–1 month of age)

- Situs inversus totalis and unexplained neonatal respiratory distress (NRD) at term birth, plus at least 1 of the following:
- Diagnostic ciliary ultrastructure electron micrographs or 2 mutations in PCD-associated gene

Children (1 month to 5 years)

- Two or more major PCD clinical criteria (NRD,[a] wet cough, nasal congestion, laterality defect), plus at least 1 of the following (nasal nitric oxide not included in this age group, because it is not yet sufficiently tested):
- Diagnostic ciliary ultrastructure on electron micrographs
- Two mutations in 1 PCD-associated gene
- Persistent and diagnostic ciliary waveform abnormalities on high-speed videomicroscopy, on multiple occasions

Children (5–18 years of age) and adults

- Two or more PCD clinical criteria (NRD,[a] wet cough, nasal congestion, laterality defect), plus at least 1 of the following:
- Nasal nitric oxide during plateau less than 77 nL/min on 2 occasions, greater than 2 months apart (with CF excluded)
- Diagnostic ciliary ultrastructure on electron micrographs
- Two mutations in 1 PCD-associated gene
- Persistent and diagnostic ciliary waveform abnormalities on high-speed videomicroscopy, on multiple occasions

Pediatric pulmonology.[15]

[a] In term neonates.

---

life, and is persistent, despite antibiotics and/or use of tympanostomy tubes.[11,12] If bronchiectasis is identified in a young child, and cystic fibrosis (CF) has been ruled out, PCD is highly likely.[25–27] In summary, the typical clinical phenotype in PCD includes

- Neonatal respiratory distress and/or
- Chronic, persistent lower respiratory symptoms (early onset and persistent wet cough); and/or
- Chronic, persistent upper respiratory symptoms (nasal congestion and otitis media); and/or
- Laterality defect (situs inversus or ambiguus) (see **Box 1**)

The presence of any 2 of these 4 hallmark clinical features provides a strong clinical phenotype for PCD, assuming that CF has been excluded.[11,15]

Electron microscopy (EM) to identify ciliary ultrastructural defects historically has been the test used to confirm a diagnosis of PCD, but this approach is no longer the sole gold standard for diagnosis, because at least 30% of patients with PCD have normal ultrastructure.[1–4,14,15] For patients with PCD with ultrastructural defects, most involve the absence or shortening of ODAs (38.5%), or an ODA defect in conjunction with an IDA defect (10.5%) (see **Fig. 1**). Isolated IDA defects occur in only a small fraction of confirmed PCD (<1%), and false-positive EM diagnoses are common with IDA defects.[9,28] Before an isolated IDA defect can be used to validate a diagnosis of PCD, a ciliary biopsy for EM must be repeated when the nasal epithelium is healthy.[28] Most validated IDA defects have associated central apparatus abnormalities (~14% of PCD), and these abnormalities occur in only 5% to 20% of cilia (see **Fig. 1**). Central apparatus defects associated with IDA defects include microtubular disorganization and transposition of outer doublets into the center of cilia cross sections, and frequently reflect mutations in *CCDC39* or *CCDC40*.[29,30] Ciliary disorientation (misalignment of the central pair) is a secondary change, and is no longer used as a diagnostic ultrastructural feature.[31] A few patients have absent, or only a few, cilia on multiple biopsies (oligocilia), and recent studies show that some of these cases reflect mutations in *CCNO* or *MCIDAS*.[32,33] A recent report suggested that ultrastructure of respiratory epithelia with inclusions of basal bodies, and microvilli and cilia, is a variant form of PCD,[34] but follow-up studies in several of those patients showed that these EM findings are not specific for PCD (M. Leigh and S. Sagel, personal communication, 2016). The limitations of EM testing of cilia was highlighted by the experience in our North American Rare Disease Consortium, in which as many as 15% to 20% of the patients referred with a supposedly confirmed diagnosis of PCD (based on ciliary ultrastructure) had a false-positive diagnosis of PCD.[35,36] To optimize the use of ciliary EM for diagnosis, many EM cross sections (multiple sections containing high-quality images of at least 20 unique cilia) should be examined by experienced readers, using a quantitative approach to interpretation.[9] EM analysis is more successful in biopsies from adults versus children, likely because of limitations in obtaining adequate scrape biopsies from narrow airways.[35,37] Acquired (secondary) ciliary defects result from airway damage, from recurrent infections, and can sometimes be difficult to differentiate from PCD. In addition, at least 30% of patients with a strong PCD clinical phenotype and low nNO have normal ciliary EM. For example, a recent study showed that 22% of 61 such patients had PCD-causing mutations in *DNAH11*.[38] Thus, normal ciliary ultrastructure cannot rule out PCD.

Evaluations of ciliary motility from fresh biopsies of respiratory epithelium has been used to confirm a diagnosis of PCD, particularly in Europe. However, substantial limitations preclude reliance on this as the sole diagnostic approach. In this regard, secondary effects on ciliary function create problems and recognition of more subtle motility defects requires experienced investigators.[18,39] It is also now clear that standard light microscopic analysis is not sufficient, because many patients with PCD have ciliary movement.[40] Even with high-speed video microscopy (HSVM), there is overlap of ciliary beat frequency between PCD and disease control and normal subjects, and there is no standardized protocol for interpretation of HSVM.[41,42] There have been multiple approaches to try to improve accuracy of HSVM, but these modifications do not eliminate all of the limitations.[43–45] A recent publication touted the use of automated identification of abnormal ciliary motion,[46] but this approach has not been independently validated, and should not be used to diagnose PCD. It is also now clear through genetic testing that many forms of PCD have no, or only subtle, abnormalities of ciliary ultrastructure and/or beat frequency and waveform. Therefore, these biological assays of ciliary function are not sensitive for detecting the growing range of ciliary phenotypes in PCD.

nNO levels in patients with PCD are low (<77 nL/min), relative to normal values (range 125–867 nL/min; mean, 287 nL/min); thus, nNO can be a useful test for PCD if performed correctly.[1,9,13,47] Nasal NO is measured by aspirating nasal air through a catheter placed at the opening of 1 nostril and analyzed by an NO analyzer.[48] Exhaled air from the lower airways has a much lower concentration of NO than the nose; thus, maneuvers must be instituted to close the soft palate to limit contamination of nasal air by air from the lower airways.[48] This approach has been validated in adults and children more than 5 years of age,[13,49] but is less feasible in younger children. For infants and young children, one study measured nNO during tidal breathing[50]; however, it should be noted that nNO values during tidal breathing are ~40% lower in healthy subjects than values obtained at plateau during palate closure. It is critical to recognize that low nNO levels are seen in some patients with CF.[9,13,47] Therefore, CF needs to be ruled out by sweat testing or *CFTR* genetic studies if nNO is low. Because nNO values can be low during acute viral infections, acute sinusitis, and panbronchiolitis, measurements should be performed when respiratory status is stable, and should be confirmed on a separate day.[1,13,15] Although nNO has previously been used in a limited number of specialized PCD centers, there is a growing number of these specialized centers in North America (see the PCD Foundation Web site; www.pcdfoundation. org). With standardization, and definition of appropriate cutoff values,[13] nNO measurement is becoming more widely used as a diagnostic test for PCD (see **Box 1**).[15]

Fluorescence-labeled antibodies have been used to show the absence of cilia axonemal and cytoplasmic preassembly proteins, but only a few laboratories are using this approach.[51,52] Measurement of mucociliary clearance in the lung has been used in some cases, but is not reliable, because it is confounded by involuntary cough and bronchiectasis from other causes.[53] There is no role for the nasal saccharine clearance test as a diagnostic method, because of multiple limitations in performance and interpretation of the test.

GENETIC TESTING FOR DIAGNOSIS

PCD is a mendelian recessive and genetically heterogeneous disorder. Between 1999 and 2012, PCD-causing mutations were described in 14 genes.[1,2,4,14,15] Since early 2012, there has been extensive genetic discovery, through exome sequencing, whereby PCD-causing mutations in 21 additional genes have been published (**Table 1**).[1,2,4,14,15] Most (81%) of the mutations are loss-of-function changes (nonsense, frameshift, or defective splice sites), and ~19% are conservative missense changes or in-frame del-dup (deletion-duplication). Based on studies of genetic mutations in patients with PCD in our North American Rare Disease Consortium, and a review of the published literature, it is estimated that ~75% of the mutations are private, occurring in only 1 family/patient, but ~25% are seen in multiple unrelated families/patients (founder, or recurrent mutations). Mutations in 5 genes (*DNAH5, DNAH11, DNAI1, CCDC39, CCDC40*) are the most prevalent in PCD, and ~26% of these mutations are recurrent.[14] There are also more than 20 mutations that are associated with specific ethnic groups or geographic locations.[4,14] It is estimated that ~65% to 70% of patients with PCD can be identified as having 2 mutations in one of these 35 published PCD genes.[14] The feasibility of testing a multigene panel of PCD genes at a reasonable cost is becoming a reality, as several Clinical Laboratory Improvement Amendments–approved laboratories and companies have recently begun to offer such services (see the PCD Foundation Web site; www.pcdfoundation.org).[15] This type of genetic testing will revolutionize the diagnostic approach in PCD and lead to early identification and initiation of clinical monitoring and treatment.

The role of PCD-associated genes in normal ciliary biogenesis and function, and the effect of mutations on cilia structure and function, are detailed in several reviews,[1,2,4,14] and key points are summarized here. There is strong correlation between mutations in specific genes and effect on ciliary ultrastructure (see **Table 1**). Although most PCD-associated genes code for proteins in the ciliary axonemes, there are 10 PCD-associated genes that have a functional role in the cytoplasm in preassembly of the cilia components, and mutations in these genes lead to loss of both ODA and IDA (see **Table 1**). There is strong correlation between mutations in genes that lead to ultrastructural dynein arm defects and the development of situs abnormalities, but mutations in genes that code for central apparatus, radial spoke, or nexin link proteins are not associated with organ laterality defects. Genetic discovery has also provided the opportunity to examine ciliary electron micrographs from multiple patients with mutations in the same PCD-causing gene, which has allowed recognition of unusual changes, such as (1) radial spoke genes, in which as many as 80% of ciliary EM cross sections are normal; and (2) IDA defects associated with microtubular disorganization, which may affect only 10% of ciliary cross sections, and reflect mutations in *CCDC39* and *CCDC40*.[29,30] Except for *RSPH1*[54] (discussed later) biallelic loss-of-function mutations routinely lead to low nNO levels (<77 nL/min).[13] Pathogenic mutations in DNAH11 in patients with PCD with normal ciliary ultrastructure provide confirmation that PCD can occur in the absence of ciliary EM defects.[38] In addition, the ciliary beat frequency in patients with mutations in some genes (eg, *DNAH11, RSPH4A*,

Table 1
Mutations in genes that cause PCD; associations with ciliary ultrastructure and organ laterality defects

Ciliary EM	Genes	Laterality Defects
ODA defect	*DNAH5, DNAI1, DNAI2, DNAL1, NME8, CCDC114, CCDC151, ARMC4*	Yes
ODA + IDA defect	*DNAAF1, DNAAF2, DNAAF3, LRRC6, C21orf59, DNAAF5 (HEATR2), ZMYND10, DYX1C1 (DNAAF4), SPAG1, CCDC103*	Yes
IDA defect + MTD	*CCDC39, CCDC40*	Yes
RS/CP defect[a]	*RSPH1, RSPH3, RSPH4A, RSPH9, HYDIN*	No
Nexin Link defect[a]	*CCDC164 (DRC1), CCDC65 (DRC2), GAS8 (DRC4)*	No
Normal EM	*DNAH11*	Yes
EM not available	*DNAH1, DNAH8*	Yes (*DNAH1*), unknown (*DNAH8*)
Oligocilia	*CCNO, MCIDAS*	No
PCD + XLMR[a]	*OFD1*	Yes[b]
PCD + XLRP[a]	*RPGR*	No

Abbreviations: CP, central pair; RS, radial spoke.
[a] Difficult to discern EM defect (appears normal); PCD with x-linked syndromes.
[b] Unpublished data from genetic disorders of Mucociliary Clearance Consortium.

RSPH9, RSPH1) with mostly normal EM can be normal (or higher than normal), and the waveforms can appear normal, or have only subtle defects.[14]

Identification of genetic causes of PCD has uncovered unique genotype/phenotype relationships. Patients with PCD with mutations in *RSPH1* have milder disease with less neonatal respiratory distress (50% vs the usual 80%), later onset of clinical symptoms, subtle EM defects and changes in ciliary waveform, better forced expiratory volume in 1 second (FEV$_1$; percentage of predicted) versus age-matched and gender-matched patients with PCD with axonemal defects, and borderline (or normal) nasal NO levels.[54,55] The milder disease is thought to reflect some residual ciliary function associated with a partially intact radial spoke system.[55] In contrast, patients with PCD with mutations in *CCDC39* or *CCDC40* have more severe disease with a higher prevalence of neonatal respiratory distress, earlier onset and severity of clinical symptoms, lower body mass index, and worse FEV$_1$ than other patients with PCD, as well as a greater extent of bronchiectasis.[56] The mechanism of worse disease with mutations in *CCDC39* and *CCDC40* is not known, although the authors speculate that these genes may play some role in lung host defense that extends beyond ciliary function.

EARLY FEATURES OF CLINICAL DISEASE

The clinical features of PCD reflect defective function of motile cilia in the conducting airways, paranasal sinuses, middle ear (eustachian tube), and the reproductive tract, as well as specialized motile cilia in the ventral node during embryogenesis (see **Box 1**).[1–4] Manifestations of PCD occur early in life, and the clinical phenotype gives strong insight into the likelihood of PCD, based on systematic analysis of patients in our rare disease consortium.[11]

The earliest manifestations of PCD occur in the neonatal period, because more than 80% of full-term neonates with PCD have respiratory distress. Signs include tachypnea and increased work of breathing, and affected individuals typically require supplemental oxygen for a few hours to weeks.[12,57] These infants are often diagnosed with transient tachypnea of the newborn or neonatal pneumonia, but the clinical presentation in PCD is different with (1) later onset of respiratory distress (12 hours of age), (2) longer duration of required oxygen therapy, and (3) higher frequency of atelectasis and/or lobar collapse.[57] This neonatal presentation of respiratory distress indicates that normal ciliary function plays a critical role in the clearance of fetal lung fluid at birth, although the mechanism is unknown. Unexplained respiratory distress and radiographic abnormalities, along with supplemental oxygen requirements in a full-term infant, should raise suspicion for PCD, particularly in neonates with situs inversus.

Infants and children with PCD typically have year-round wet cough and daily nasal congestion (rhinitis) starting soon after birth.[1–4,11] Chronic otitis media that causes temporary or permanent hearing loss and recurrent sinusitis is common. Sinusitis is sometimes not recognized in young children because radiographic imaging is not performed. Bronchiectasis occurs in some infants and preschoolers.[12,25–27] Chest computed tomography (CT) scans show various abnormalities, including atelectasis, mucous plugging, air trapping, and thickened airway walls.[26,27,58] These respiratory manifestations overlap with other common early childhood diseases; thus, the diagnosis of PCD is frequently missed, despite the presence of typical clinical features, even when situs inversus is present. This lack of recognition of cardinal clinical features in PCD highlights the importance of education for many pertinent subspecialties, including neonatology, pulmonology, otolaryngology, and cardiology, as well as primary care.

LUNG DISEASE

Nearly all infants and children with PCD have a year-round daily wet cough, which compensates, in part, for defective mucociliary clearances. Despite the daily cough, infections occur in the lower airways, and there is age-dependent development of bronchiectasis, which is universal in adults with PCD.[1,12,25,47,58]

Respiratory bacteriology of children with PCD is dominated by *Haemophilus influenzae, Staphylococcus aureus,* and *Streptococcus pneumoniae.*[12] Unlike CF, children with PCD, including infants/preschoolers, also intermittently culture *Pseudomonas aeruginosa,* which evolves into chronic airway infection in teenagers and young adults with PCD.[12,47,59] Many patients culture more than 1 type of bacteria in the same sample. Nontuberculous mycobacteria (NTM) are present in 15% of adults with PCD, but there is a lower prevalence in children.[1,15,47]

In contrast with the perceptions of many clinicians, the severity of lung disease in children with PCD is substantial. Abnormal lung function develops early in life, because many infants and young children show abnormal airflow mechanics.[60–63] The range of FEV$_1$ in PCD is heterogeneous at age 6 to 8 years, because some young patients with PCD have obstructive airways disease that is worse than that of patients with CF at the same age. Patients with PCD have evidence of airflow obstruction in small airways (ie, decreased maximum midexpiratory flow) and ventilation inhomogeneity, as measured through multiple breath washout.[60–64] Cross-sectional and longitudinal data show that airflow obstruction worsens with increasing age.[61–63] However, airways disease does not progress as rapidly in late childhood and early adulthood compared with CF, which may relate to preservation of cough clearance. One longitudinal study showed that lung function remains stable in patients with PCD who received regular monitoring and treatment.[62]

Radiographic studies using high-resolution chest CT show that lung disease in PCD begins in infancy or early childhood. Findings include subsegmental atelectasis, mucous plugging, air trapping, ground-glass opacity, and peribronchial thickening. Bronchiectasis can occur during infancy, and ~50% to 75% of older pediatric patients and nearly all adults with PCD have bronchiectasis with worse disease in the middle lobe and lingula, as well as basilar regions.[25–27,49,58] Chest CT is more sensitive for detecting early lung disease in PCD, compared with lung function testing by spirometry.[60] MRI of the chest may be as effective as chest CT in defining the extent and severity of lung disease in PCD, which is an intriguing option for longitudinal evaluation and research.[65]

NONPULMONARY MANIFESTATIONS

Situs abnormalities are present in more than 50% of pediatric patients, which may aid earlier recognition of PCD. Laterality defects reflect abnormal function of the specialized (9 + 0) motile cilium during embryogenesis.[19] At least 12% of patients with PCD have situs ambiguous, and these patients have a 200-fold increased probability of having structural congenital heart disease compared with the general population with heterotaxy.[66–68] Some patients with situs ambiguous have heterotaxia syndromes, which include polysplenia (left isomerism) and asplenia (right isomerism). Taken together, these clinical characteristics show a strong association between defective cilia and congenital heart disease. Patients with heterotaxy and congenital heart disease have increased respiratory complications after cardiac surgery, which suggests that some of these patients may have PCD.[69,70] Studies in mice with mutations in motile cilia confirm that cilia are required for normal heart development.[71]

Almost all men with PCD are infertile, secondary to dysmotility of spermatozoa, or rarely

azoospermia. A few men with PCD have adequate sperm motility and have fathered children.[72] Women with PCD have impaired ciliary function in the fallopian tubes, which may lead to reduced fecundity and/or a history of ectopic pregnancies.[73]

Pectus excavatum occurs in as many as 10% of patients with PCD, versus 0.3% in the general population.[58] The authors and others have also reported a high prevalence of scoliosis (5%–10%) in PCD[1]; thus, PCD should be considered in patients with pectus excavatum and/or scoliosis and unexplained sinopulmonary disease.

MANAGEMENT OF LUNG DISEASE

Respiratory symptoms and lung disease in PCD begin early in life, and reflect defective mucociliary clearance, which is the key innate pulmonary defense mechanism.[21] No validated PCD-specific therapies are available; therefore, therapies for PCD are extrapolated from other diseases, such as CF and non-CF bronchiectasis, particularly as relates to antibiotic therapy and macrolides as antiinflammatory agents.[15,74–78] A recent state-of-the-art publication provides consensus recommendations from the PCD Foundation for monitoring and management of lung disease in PCD.[15] Clinic visits at least twice per year are recommended for monitoring lung function and respiratory microbiology, including NTM. Chest imaging studies are also indicated to periodically monitor the extent of disease. Preventive measures include infection control training and routine immunizations, as well as pneumococcal and influenza vaccines.

Multiple studies show that systemic antibiotics are effective at treating worsening respiratory symptoms (exacerbations) in CF and non-CF bronchiectasis, including some patients with PCD.[76] Antibiotics should be chosen based on respiratory cultures. Unexpectedly, preliminary studies of inhaled antibiotics in non-CF bronchiectasis did not show benefit with respect to lung function, although there was a reduction of neutrophil elastase activity in sputum in some studies.[78,79] One controlled study (12 months long) of inhaled gentamicin in non-CF bronchiectasis showed a striking reduction in the frequency of exacerbations, as well as reductions in the burden of bacteria and markers of pulmonary and systemic inflammation.[80] It is noteworthy that 1 study in patients with non-CF bronchiectasis showed high rates of eradication for patients who develop airway infection with P aeruginosa.[75]

Stimulation of chloride (and liquid) secretion by an inhaled P2Y2 receptor agonist has been reported to improve cough clearance of radiolabeled particles in a small study of adults with PCD.[81] More recently, nebulized 7% hypertonic saline improved lung function and quality of life (QOL), and reduced antibiotic use in non-CF bronchiectasis in a 3-month study.[82] The therapeutic concept is that stimulation of cough and increased hydration of airway secretions with hypertonic saline (or other osmotic agents) can benefit cough clearance. By analogy, hydrating airway secretions may benefit cough clearance in PCD, even though defective mucociliary clearance persists. Dornase alfa has not been shown to improve pulmonary status in non-CF bronchiectasis, even though it is beneficial in CF. Adults with non-CF bronchiectasis taking dornase alfa for 24 weeks experienced more pulmonary exacerbations and a greater decline in FEV_1 compared with the placebo group.[83]

Oral macrolides are clearly effective in CF through antiinflammatory mechanisms, resulting in improvement in lung function and reduction in exacerbations. In non-CF bronchiectasis, similar data are emerging in small studies with regard to reducing exacerbations.[74,77] In contrast with CF, most patients with non-CF bronchiectasis have bacterial infections other than *P aeruginosa*; therefore, the mechanism of action for macrolides in non-CF bronchiectasis could relate, in part, to antibiotic effect. Patients with PCD should not receive chronic oral macrolides unless they have been tested and shown to not harbor NTM.[74,77] The widespread use of inhaled or systemic corticosteroids in non-CF bronchiectasis has not been validated by standardized clinical studies.

Resection of severely affected lung in PCD is occasionally useful, but should be undertaken only after careful consideration and consultation with PCD experts, because PCD affects all regions of the lung. The selection of patients for resection should focus on those with severe localized bronchiectasis and recurrent febrile relapses or severe hemoptysis, despite aggressive medical management.[84] Patients with end-stage PCD lung disease are candidates for lung transplant, and a modest number of transplants have been successfully performed.

Some key goals for the PCD community to develop the requisite capabilities for performing therapeutic clinical trials have recently been achieved. Specifically, there is now expanded capability to perform genetic testing for the diagnosis of PCD at a reasonable cost, which will expand the pool of patients with a confirmed diagnosis of PCD. There is also an increasing number of PCD clinical sites to perform those clinical trials. Further, there is a published QOL instrument as an

outcome measure in PCD adults[85] and another QOL instrument for pediatric patients is close to being finalized. Therefore, the PCD community is poised to do therapeutic studies for lung disease in PCD (discussed later, and see the PCD Foundation Web site; www.pcdfoundation.org).

MANAGEMENT OF OTOLARYNGOLOGIC MANIFESTATIONS

Otitis media with effusion affects almost all children with PCD, but there is no consensus for management, even though this disorder has implications for conductive hearing loss, delayed speech and language development, and cholesteatoma formation.[12,15,86] Clinicians who support the use of tympanostomy tubes suggest that hearing may be improved long term in some patients, and otorrhea can be controlled.[86] In contrast, the European Respiratory Society consensus statement recommends against placement of tubes for chronic otitis media in PCD, because resultant otorrhea is problematic, and spontaneous resolution of chronic otitis media may occur in the teenage years.[87,88] Acute episodes of otitis media should be treated by standard approaches, but the question of surgical intervention remains. It should be recognized that chronic otitis media may persist into adulthood, and conductive hearing loss (glue ear) occurs in some patients. Therefore, audiology assessments, hearing aids, and communication assistance should be used.

Sinus disease is a major problem in PCD. Initial management may include nasal steroids, nasal lavage, and intermittent courses of systemic antibiotics. Polyps may require surgery, and functional endoscopic sinus surgery is helpful in many patients who are refractory to medical therapy, particularly if there is good postsurgical treatment to maintain adequate drainage.[89,90]

FUTURE DIRECTIONS

Although treatment of patients with PCD has not been standardized, the recent PCD Foundation consensus statement on diagnosis and management offers specific guidance for clinicians. It is hoped that this will improve clinical care, including regular surveillance of clinical status, lung function, and respiratory microbiology, and allow antibiotic treatment targeted to specific pathogens. A multidisciplinary approach to management of chronic disease is well recognized to benefit long-term outcomes, particularly for rare diseases, such as CF. The PCD Foundation is developing a national registry, and there is an ever-growing network of certified PCD clinical centers, which should alleviate some of the inconsistency in care. This network will also facilitate discovery of additional PCD genes, and allow more extensive studies of genotype/phenotype in PCD. Further, this network will also facilitate the identification of patients with PCD for participation in prospective clinical trials, and provide geographically dispersed sites for these therapeutic trials (see the PCD Foundation Web site for further information; www.pcdfoundation.org). In summary, there has been striking progress in the understanding of PCD over the past 15 years, and this is being rapidly translated into more available and effective clinical care.

ACKNOWLEDGMENTS

The authors thank all of the patients with PCD and family members for their participation. They acknowledge the Genetic Disorders of Mucociliary Clearance Consortium and the principal investigators and research coordinators that are part of the Rare Disease Clinical Research Network. The authors thank Ms Elizabeth Godwin for administrative support and Ms Alexandra Infanzon for editorial assistance. They are also grateful to the PCD Foundation, and Ms Michele Manion, founder of the US PCD Foundation.

REFERENCES

1. Knowles MR, Daniels LA, Davis SD, et al. Primary ciliary dyskinesia. Recent advances in diagnostics, genetics, and characterization of clinical disease. Am J Respir Crit Care Med 2013;188: 913–22.
2. Lobo J, Zariwala MA, Noone PG. Primary ciliary dyskinesia. Semin Respir Crit Care Med 2015;36: 169–79.
3. Praveen K, Davis EE, Katsanis N. Unique among ciliopathies: primary ciliary dyskinesia, a motile cilia disorder. F1000Prime Rep 2015;7:36.
4. Horani A, Ferkol TW, Dutcher SK, et al. Genetics and biology of primary ciliary dyskinesia. Paediatr Respir Rev 2016;18:18–24.
5. Kartagener M. Zur pathogenese der bronkiektasien: bronkiektasien bei situs viscerum inversus. Beitr Klin Tuberk 1933;82:489–501.
6. Afzelius BA. A human syndrome caused by immotile cilia. Science 1976;193:317–9.
7. Torgersen J. Transposition of viscera, bronchiectasis and nasal polyps; a genetical analysis and a contribution to the problem of constitution. Acta Radiol 1947;28:17–24.
8. Katsuhara K, Kawamoto S, Wakabayashi T, et al. Situs inversus totalis and Kartagener's syndrome in a Japanese population. Chest 1972;61:56–61.
9. Lucas JS, Leigh MW. Diagnosis of primary ciliary dyskinesia: searching for a gold standard. Eur Respir J 2014;44:1418–22.
10. Hosie PH, Fitzgerald DA, Jaffe A, et al. Presentation of primary ciliary dyskinesia in children: 30 years' experience. J Paediatr Child Health 2015; 51:722–6.
11. Leigh MW, Ferkol TW, Davis SD, et al. Clinical features and associated likelihood of primary ciliary dyskinesia in children and adolescents. Ann Am Thorac Soc 2016. [Epub ahead of print].
12. Sagel SD, Davis SD, Campisi P, et al. Update of respiratory tract disease in children with primary ciliary dyskinesia. Proc Am Thorac Soc 2011;8:438–43.
13. Leigh MW, Hazucha MJ, Chawla KK, et al. Standardizing nasal nitric oxide measurement as a test for primary ciliary dyskinesia. Ann Am Thorac Soc 2013; 10:574–81.
14. Zariwala MA, Knowles MR, Leigh MW. Primary ciliary dyskinesia. In: Pagon RA, Adam MP, Ardinger HH, et al, editors. GeneReviews® [Internet]. Seattle (WA); 1993. Updated September 2015.
15. Shapiro AJ, Zariwala MA, Ferkol T, et al. Diagnosis, monitoring, and treatment of primary ciliary dyskinesia: PCD foundation consensus recommendations based on state of the art review. Pediatr Pulmonol 2016;51(2):115–32.
16. Salathe M. Regulation of mammalian ciliary beating. Annu Rev Physiol 2007;69:401–22.
17. Satir P, Christensen ST. Overview of structure and function of mammalian cilia. Annu Rev Physiol 2007;69:377–400.
18. Chilvers MA, Rutman A, O'Callaghan C. Ciliary beat pattern is associated with specific ultrastructural defects in primary ciliary dyskinesia. J Allergy Clin Immunol 2003;112:518–24.
19. Basu B, Brueckner M. Cilia multifunctional organelles at the center of vertebrate left-right asymmetry. Curr Top Dev Biol 2008;85:151–74.
20. Hildebrandt F, Benzing T, Katsanis N. Ciliopathies. N Engl J Med 2011;364:1533–43.
21. Knowles MR, Boucher RC. Mucus clearance as a primary innate defense mechanism for mammalian airways. J Clin Invest 2002;109:571–7.
22. Tilley AE, Walters MS, Shaykhiev R, et al. Cilia dysfunction in lung disease. Annu Rev Physiol 2015;77:379–406.
23. Sears PR, Thompson K, Knowles MR, et al. Human airway ciliary dynamics. Am J Physiol Lung Cell Mol Physiol 2013;304:L170–83.
24. Mitchell B, Stubbs JL, Huisman F, et al. The PCP pathway instructs the planar orientation of ciliated cells in the Xenopus larval skin. Curr Biol 2009;19: 924–9.
25. Boon M, Vermeulen FL, Gysemans W, et al. Lung structure-function correlation in patients with primary ciliary dyskinesia. Thorax 2015;70:339–45.

26. Santamaria F, Montella S, Tiddens HA, et al. Structural and functional lung disease in primary ciliary dyskinesia. Chest 2008;134:351–7.

27. Jain K, Padley SP, Goldstraw EJ, et al. Primary ciliary dyskinesia in the paediatric population: range and severity of radiological findings in a cohort of patients receiving tertiary care. Clin Radiol 2007;62: 986–93.

28. O'Callaghan C, Rutman A, Williams GM, et al. Inner dynein arm defects causing primary ciliary dyskinesia: repeat testing required. Eur Respir J 2011; 38:603–7.

29. Merveille AC, Davis EE, Becker-Heck A, et al. CCDC39 is required for assembly of inner dynein arms and the dynein regulatory complex and for normal ciliary motility in humans and dogs. Nat Genet 2011;43:72–8.

30. Becker-Heck A, Zohn IE, Okabe N, et al. The coiled-coil domain containing protein CCDC40 is essential for motile cilia function and left-right axis formation. Nat Genet 2011;43:79–84.

31. Jorissen M, Willems T. The secondary nature of ciliary (dis)orientation in secondary and primary ciliary dyskinesia. Acta Otolaryngol 2004;124:527–31.

32. Wallmeier J, Al-Mutairi DA, Chen CT, et al. Mutations in CCNO result in congenital mucociliary clearance disorder with reduced generation of multiple motile cilia. Nat Genet 2014;46:646–51.

33. Boon M, Wallmeier J, Ma L, et al. MCIDAS mutations result in a mucociliary clearance disorder with reduced generation of multiple motile cilia. Nat Commun 2014;5:4418.

34. Wartchow EP, Jaffe R, Mierau GW. Ciliary inclusion disease: report of a new primary ciliary dyskinesia variant. Pediatr Dev Pathol 2014;17:465–9.

35. Olin JT, Burns K, Carson JL, et al. Diagnostic yield of nasal scrape biopsies in primary ciliary dyskinesia: a multicenter experience. Pediatr Pulmonol 2011; 46:483–8.

36. Daniels LA, Baker B, Minnix SL, et al. The diagnostic dilemma of primary ciliary dyskinesia: findings and experience of the genetic disorders of mucociliary clearance consortium. Am J Respir Crit Care Med 2011;183:A1217.

37. Papon JF, Coste A, Roudot-Thoraval F, et al. A 20-year experience of electron microscopy in the diagnosis of primary ciliary dyskinesia. Eur Respir J 2010;35:1057–63.

38. Knowles MR, Leigh MW, Carson JL, et al. Mutations of DNAH11 in patients with primary ciliary dyskinesia with normal ciliary ultrastructure. Thorax 2012;67:433–41.

39. Chilvers MA, Rutman A, O'Callaghan C. Functional analysis of cilia and ciliated epithelial ultrastructure in healthy children and young adults. Thorax 2003; 58:333–8.

40. Santamaria F, de Santi MM, Grillo G, et al. Ciliary motility at light microscopy: a screening technique for ciliary defects. Acta Paediatr 1999;88:853–7.

41. Thomas B, Rutman A, O'Callaghan C. Disrupted ciliated epithelium shows slower ciliary beat frequency and increased dyskinesia. Eur Respir J 2009;34: 401–4.

42. Olm MA, Kogler JE Jr, Macchione M, et al. Primary ciliary dyskinesia: evaluation using cilia beat frequency assessment via spectral analysis of digital microscopy images. J Appl Physiol (1985) 2011; 111:295–302.

43. Hirst RA, Rutman A, Williams G, et al. Ciliated air-liquid cultures as an aid to diagnostic testing of primary ciliary dyskinesia. Chest 2010;138:1441–7.

44. Smith CM, Hirst RA, Bankart MJ, et al. Cooling of cilia allows functional analysis of the beat pattern for diagnostic testing. Chest 2011;140:186–90.

45. Jackson CL, Goggin PM, Lucas JS. Ciliary beat pattern analysis below 37 degrees C may increase risk of primary ciliary dyskinesia misdiagnosis. Chest 2012;142:543–4 [author reply: 544–5].

46. Quinn SP, Zahid MJ, Durkin JR, et al. Automated identification of abnormal respiratory ciliary motion in nasal biopsies. Sci Transl Med 2015;7:299ra124.

47. Noone PG, Leigh MW, Sannuti A, et al. Primary ciliary dyskinesia: diagnostic and phenotypic features. Am J Respir Crit Care Med 2004;169: 459–67.

48. American Thoracic Society, European Respiratory Society. ATS/ERS recommendations for standardized procedures for the online and offline measurement of exhaled lower respiratory nitric oxide and nasal nitric oxide, 2005. Am J Respir Crit Care Med 2005;171:912–30.

49. Kouis P, Papatheodorou SI, Yiallouros PK. Diagnostic accuracy of nasal nitric oxide for establishing diagnosis of primary ciliary dyskinesia: a meta-analysis. BMC Pulm Med 2015;15:153.

50. Mateos-Corral D, Coombs R, Grasemann H, et al. Diagnostic value of nasal nitric oxide measured with non-velum closure techniques for children with primary ciliary dyskinesia. J Pediatr 2011;159: 420–4.

51. Mitchison HM, Schmidts M, Loges NT, et al. Mutations in axonemal dynein assembly factor DNAAF3 cause primary ciliary dyskinesia. Nat Genet 2012; 44:381–9. S1–2.

52. Frommer A, Hjeij R, Loges NT, et al. Immunofluorescence analysis and diagnosis of primary ciliary dyskinesia with radial spoke defects. Am J Respir Cell Mol Biol 2015;53:563–73.

53. Marthin JK, Mortensen J, Pressler T, et al. Pulmonary radioaerosol mucociliary clearance in diagnosis of primary ciliary dyskinesia. Chest 2007;132:966–76.

54. Knowles MR, Ostrowski LE, Leigh MW, et al. Mutations in RSPH1 cause primary ciliary dyskinesia

with a unique clinical and ciliary phenotype. Am J Respir Crit Care Med 2014;189:707–17.

55. Lin J, Yin W, Smith MC, et al. Cryo-electron tomography reveals ciliary defects underlying human RSPH1 primary ciliary dyskinesia. Nat Commun 2014;5: 5727.

56. Davis SD, Ferkol TW, Rosenfeld M, et al. Clinical features of childhood primary ciliary dyskinesia by genotype and ultrastructural phenotype. Am J Respir Crit Care Med 2015;191:316–24.

57. Mullowney T, Manson D, Kim R, et al. Primary ciliary dyskinesia and neonatal respiratory distress. Pediatrics 2014;134:1160–6.

58. Kennedy MP, Noone PG, Leigh MW, et al. High-resolution CT of patients with primary ciliary dyskinesia. AJR Am J Roentgenol 2007;188:1232–8.

59. Alanin MC, Nielsen KG, von Buchwald C, et al. A longitudinal study of lung bacterial pathogens in patients with primary ciliary dyskinesia. Clin Microbiol Infect 2015;21(1093):e1091–7.

60. Maglione M, Bush A, Montella S, et al. Progression of lung disease in primary ciliary dyskinesia: is spirometry less accurate than CT? Pediatr Pulmonol 2012;47:498–504.

61. Marthin JK, Petersen N, Skovgaard LT, et al. Lung function in patients with primary ciliary dyskinesia: a cross-sectional and 3-decade longitudinal study. Am J Respir Crit Care Med 2010;181: 1262–8.

62. Ellerman A, Bisgaard H. Longitudinal study of lung function in a cohort of primary ciliary dyskinesia. Eur Respir J 1997;10:2376–9.

63. Hellinckx J, Demedts M, De Boeck K. Primary ciliary dyskinesia: evolution of pulmonary function. Eur J Pediatr 1998;157:422–6.

64. Green K, Buchvald FF, Marthin JK, et al. Ventilation inhomogeneity in children with primary ciliary dyskinesia. Thorax 2012;67:49–53.

65. Montella S, Maglione M, Bruzzese D, et al. Magnetic resonance imaging is an accurate and reliable method to evaluate non-cystic fibrosis paediatric lung disease. Respirology 2012;17:87–91.

66. Brueckner M. Heterotaxia, congenital heart disease, and primary ciliary dyskinesia. Circulation 2007;115: 2793–5.

67. Shapiro AJ, Davis SD, Ferkol T, et al. Laterality defects other than situs inversus totalis in primary ciliary dyskinesia: insights into situs ambiguus and heterotaxy. Chest 2014;146:1176–86.

68. Harrison MJ, Shapiro AJ, Kennedy MP. Congenital heart disease and primary ciliary dyskinesia. Paediatr Respir Rev 2016;18:25–32.

69. Swisher M, Jonas R, Tian X, et al. Increased postoperative and respiratory complications in patients with congenital heart disease associated with heterotaxy. J Thorac Cardiovasc Surg 2011;141:637–44, 644.e1–3.

70. Brueckner M. Impact of genetic diagnosis on clinical management of patients with congenital heart disease: cilia point the way. Circulation 2012;125: 2178–80.

71. Francis RJ, Christopher A, Devine WA, et al. Congenital heart disease and the specification of left-right asymmetry. Am J Physiol Heart Circ Physiol 2012;302:H2102–11.

72. Munro NC, Currie DC, Lindsay KS, et al. Fertility in men with primary ciliary dyskinesia presenting with respiratory infection. Thorax 1994;49: 684–7.

73. Halbert SA, Patton DL, Zarutskie PW, et al. Function and structure of cilia in the fallopian tube of an infertile woman with Kartagener's syndrome. Hum Reprod 1997;12:55–8.

74. Wong C, Jayaram L, Karalus N, et al. Azithromycin for prevention of exacerbations in non-cystic fibrosis bronchiectasis (EMBRACE): a randomised, double-blind, placebo-controlled trial. Lancet 2012;380: 660–7.

75. White L, Mirrani G, Grover M, et al. Outcomes of *Pseudomonas* eradication therapy in patients with non-cystic fibrosis bronchiectasis. Respir Med 2012;106:356–60.

76. King PT, Holmes PW. Use of antibiotics in bronchiectasis. Rev Recent Clin Trials 2012;7:24–30.

77. Masekela R, Green RJ. The role of macrolides in childhood non-cystic fibrosis-related bronchiectasis. Mediators Inflamm 2012;2012:134605.

78. Polineni D, Davis SD, Dell SD. Treatment recommendations in primary ciliary dyskinesia. Paediatr Respir Rev 2016;18:39–45.

79. Evans DJ, Bara AI, Greenstone M. Prolonged antibiotics for purulent bronchiectasis in children and adults. Cochrane Database Syst Rev 2007;(2):CD001392.

80. Murray MP, Govan JR, Doherty CJ, et al. A randomized controlled trial of nebulized gentamicin in non-cystic fibrosis bronchiectasis. Am J Respir Crit Care Med 2011;183:491–9.

81. Noone PG, Bennett WD, Regnis JA, et al. Effect of aerosolized uridine-5'-triphosphate on airway clearance with cough in patients with primary ciliary dyskinesia. Am J Respir Crit Care Med 1999;160: 144–9.

82. Kellett F, Robert NM. Nebulised 7% hypertonic saline improves lung function and quality of life in bronchiectasis. Respir Med 2011;105:1831–5.

83. O'Donnell AE, Barker AF, Ilowite JS, et al. Treatment of idiopathic bronchiectasis with aerosolized recombinant human DNase I. rhDNase Study Group. Chest 1998;113:1329–34.

84. Smit HJ, Schreurs AJ, Van den Bosch JM, et al. Is resection of bronchiectasis beneficial in patients with primary ciliary dyskinesia? Chest 1996;109: 1541–4.

85. Lucas JS, Behan L, Dunn Galvin A, et al. A quality-of-life measure for adults with primary ciliary dyskinesia: QOL-PCD. Eur Respir J 2015; 46:375–83.

86. Campbell R. Managing upper respiratory tract complications of primary ciliary dyskinesia in children. Curr Opin Allergy Clin Immunol 2012;12:32–8.

87. Barbato A, Frischer T, Kuehni CE, et al. Primary ciliary dyskinesia: a consensus statement on diagnostic and treatment approaches in children. Eur Respir J 2009;34:1264–76.

88. Pruliere-Escabasse V, Coste A, Chauvin P, et al. Otologic features in children with primary ciliary dyskinesia. Arch Otolaryngol Head Neck Surg 2010;136:1121–6.

89. Min YG, Shin JS, Choi SH, et al. Primary ciliary dyskinesia: ultrastructural defects and clinical features. Rhinology 1995;33:189–93.

90. Parsons DS, Greene BA. A treatment for primary ciliary dyskinesia: efficacy of functional endoscopic sinus surgery. Laryngoscope 1993;103: 1269–72.

Lymphocytic Interstitial Pneumonia

Tanmay S. Panchabhai, MD[a], Carol Farver, MD[b,c], Kristin B. Highland, MD, MSCR[d],*

KEYWORDS

- Pulmonary lymphoproliferative disorders • Cystic lung disease • Pseudolymphoma
- Interstitial lung disease in HIV-positive patients • Polyclonal lymphoid lung infiltrates
- Interstitial lung disease • Interstitial lung disease in Sjögren syndrome

KEY POINTS

- Lymphocytic interstitial pneumonia (LIP) is a clinicopathologic entity on the spectrum of benign pulmonary lymphoproliferative disorders.
- Common associations of LIP include autoimmune disorders (Sjögren syndrome, rheumatoid arthritis, systemic lupus erythematosus), dysgammaglobulinemia, infections (human immunodeficiency virus and Epstein-Barr virus), and genetic predisposition.
- Thin-walled cysts in random distribution are the characteristic abnormality, along with other imaging features of ground-glass opacities, poorly defined centrilobular and subpleural nodules, reticulonodular opacities, and alveolar consolidation with air bronchograms (in advanced disease).
- The key pathologic features of LIP include dense polyclonal interstitial lymphocytic infiltrates with widened interlobular/alveolar septa.
- Features that indicate pulmonary lymphoma instead of LIP include dense infiltrates distorting the lung architecture with invasion or destruction of vessel walls and airways, gammopathy, hypogammaglobulinemia, pleural infiltration, and clonality of immunoglobulin heavy chain gene rearrangements.

INTRODUCTION

Lymphocytic interstitial pneumonia (LIP), a clinicopathologic condition, involves an inflammatory pulmonary reaction of the bronchus-associated lymphoid tissue (BALT). This inflammatory reaction culminates in cellular expansion and infiltration of the interstitium by reactive T and B lymphocytes, plasma cells, and histiocytes.[1–6] Carrington and Liebow[7] first suggested LIP in a 1966 abstract that detailed the pulmonary disorders of 4 adults and 1 child who had massive lymphoid infiltrates of the lung. Several years later, these investigators published their experience with a series of 17 additional patients in an article entitled, "Diffuse Pulmonary Lymphoreticular Infiltrates Associated with Dysproteinaemia"[1] and offered a more concrete description allowing LIP to be differentiated from other lymphocytic infiltrative disorders (**Box 1**).

Disclosures: None.
[a] Department of Medicine, Norton Thoracic Institute, St. Joseph's Hospital and Medical Center, Creighton University School of Medicine, Phoenix Regional Campus, 500 West Thomas Road, Suite 500, Phoenix, AZ 85013, USA; [b] Department of Anatomic Pathology, Pathology and Laboratory Medicine Institute, Cleveland Clinic, 9500 Euclid Avenue, Cleveland, OH 44195, USA; [c] Department of Pathology, Cleveland Clinic Lerner College of Medicine of Case Western Reserve University School of Medicine, Cleveland Clinic, 9500 Euclid Avenue, L25, Cleveland, OH 44195, USA; [d] Department of Pulmonary Medicine, Respiratory Institute, Cleveland Clinic, 9500 Euclid Avenue, A90, Cleveland, OH 44195, USA
* Corresponding author.
E-mail address: highlak@ccf.org

Clin Chest Med 37 (2016) 463–474
http://dx.doi.org/10.1016/j.ccm.2016.04.009

PATHOGENESIS

The precise pathogenesis of LIP is unknown; it is thought to be in the spectrum of benign pulmonary lymphoproliferative disorders (**Table 1**).[8] LIP represents a nonspecific response to multiple stimuli[3,9] and has been linked to several diverse systemic and infectious disorders that are associated with dysgammaglobulinemia and lymphocytic infiltration (**Table 2**). LIP is most commonly associated with Sjögren syndrome,[10] followed by infectious causes; mainly human immunodeficiency virus (HIV) and Epstein-Barr virus (EBV).[3]

The association of LIP with dysgammaglobulinemia was highlighted in the landmark article by Liebow and Carrington.[1] Subsequently, dysproteinemia has been identified in roughly 80% of patients. Most of these patients had a polyclonal hypergammaglobulinemia, although hypogammaglobulinemia has also been reported in approximately 10% of cases.[1,8,11,12] Patients with monoclonal proliferations are more likely to have low-grade non-Hodgkin lymphomas.[13] It is not known whether dysgammaglobulinemia is the initiating event in the cause of LIP, or whether other precipitating factors (eg, viral) cause the

Table 1
Lymphoproliferative disorders of the lung

Disorder	Common Features	Age at Onset (y)	Signs and Symptoms
Angioimmunoblastic lymphadenopathy	Multicompartment mediastinal adenopathy; may have lung masses or infiltrates. Can involve the pleura	50–70	Moderate to severe
Castleman disease	Solitary mass in the middle or posterior mediastinum, occasional calcification	20–30	None
Follicular bronchiolitis	Bronchiolar tree-in-bud pattern with centrilobular nodules and mosaicism from air trapping	30–70 (depending on underlying disorder)	Moderate
Immunoglobulin G4–related disease	Ground-glass opacities to large masslike densities	Variable	No symptoms to mild disease
Infectious mononucleosis	Mediastinal adenopathy, rarely interstitial pulmonary infiltrates	10–20	Mild
Lymphoid interstitial pneumonia	Poorly defined interstitial or alveolar opacities or both	40–70	None to severe
Lymphomatoid granulomatosis	Poorly defined interstitial or alveolar opacities or both	30–50	Moderate to severe
Nodular lymphoid hyperplasia	Solitary mass lesion or alveolar infiltrate	30–70	None
Posttransplant lymphoproliferative disorder	Solitary or multiple lung masses	Variable	None to mild

Adapted from Bragg DG, Chor PJ, Murray KA, et al. Lymphoproliferative disorders of the lung: histopathology, clinical manifestations, and imaging features. AJR Am J Roentgenol 1994;163(2):274.

Table 2
Studies revealing conditions associated with LIP

Disease	Author, Year
Allogenic bone marrow transplant	Perreault et al,[70] 1985
Autoerythrocyte sensitization syndrome	DeCoteau et al,[71] 1974
Autoimmune hemolytic anemia	Kokosi et al,[48] 2015 Liebow & Carrington,[1] 1973
Castleman disease	Hare et al,[44] 2012 Torii et al,[53] 1994
Celiac sprue	Neil et al,[72] 1986
Chronic active hepatitis	Helman et al,[73] 1977
Common variable immunoglobulin deficiency	Matsubara et al,[34] 2008 Church et al,[74] 1981 Levinson et al,[75] 1976
Drugs (eg, diphenylhydantoin)	Chamberlain et al,[76] 1986
Epstein-Barr virus	Abdarbashi & Abrudescu,[4] 2013 Grieco & Chinoy-Acharya,[21] 1985
Familial	Launay et al,[30] 2006
Hashimoto disease	Miyamoto et al,[18] 2000
Human immunodeficiency virus	Abdarbashi & Abrudescu,[4] 2013 Oldham et al,[22] 1989 Grieco & Chinoy-Acharya,[21] 1985
Human T-cell lymphotropic virus type I	Setoguchi et al,[77] 1991
Hypothyroidism	Cha et al,[12] 2006
Idiopathic plasmacytic lymphadenopathy with hypergammaglobulinemia	Torii et al,[53] 1994
Juvenile rheumatoid arthritis	Uziel et al,[78] 1998
Legionella pneumonia	Dicicco & Anderson,[79] 1994
Monoclonal hyperimmunoglobulinemia	Ichikawa et al,[33] 1994
Myasthenia gravis	Montes et al,[15] 1968
Pernicious anemia	Levinson et al,[75] 1976
Polyclonal hyperglobulinemia	Ichikawa et al,[33] 1994 Garcia & Young,[5] 2013
Polymyositis	Cha et al,[12] 2006
Primary biliary cirrhosis	Weissman & Becker,[80] 1983
Pulmonary alveolar microlithiasis	Ratjen et al,[81] 1992
Pulmonary alveolar proteinosis	Bakhos et al,[82] 1996
Rheumatoid arthritis	Matsuyama et al,[19] 2003 Miyamoto et al,[18] 2000 Cha et al,[12] 2006
Sjögren syndrome	Bonner et al,[83] 1973 Weisbrot,[84] 1976 Faguet et al,[85] 1978 Abdarbashi & Abrudescu,[4] 2013 Garcia & Young,[5] 2013
Systemic lupus erythematosus	Kim et al,[20] 2011 Garcia & Young,[5] 2013

immunologic abnormalities that in turn perpetrate damage.[14] It has been previously postulated that the infiltrating plasma cells largely produce excess immunoglobulin.[1,15] However, more recent evidence suggests that increased B-cell numbers were found to precede hypergammaglobulinemia suggesting that B-cell activation is a precursor to abnormal plasma cell activity.[16]

Associations with numerous autoimmune phenomena suggest that LIP is itself an autoimmune disease, and LIP is included in the provisional criteria for autoimmune-featured interstitial lung disease.[3,11,17] Approximately 25% of LIP cases are associated with Sjögren syndrome, and it is estimated that 1% of patients with Sjögren syndrome develop LIP during the course of the disease.[3,8,11] The disorder in the lungs of patients with LIP is similar to the lymphocytic infiltration seen in the lacrimal and salivary glands of patients with Sjögren syndrome. LIP has also been described in patients with rheumatoid arthritis, systemic lupus erythematosus, and polymyositis.[5,6,12,18–20]

LIP has been strongly associated with infectious triggers as well. It may represent a specific pulmonary reaction to HIV infection,[3,4,21,22] because more severe infiltrates on imaging are associated with better survival and probably indicate the ability to sustain a more vigorous response to HIV. Likewise, radiographic resolution of LIP in the absence of antiretroviral or corticosteroid therapy is an ominous predictor of worsening immunosuppression.[3,22] LIP is particularly common in children with HIV[23,24] and is considered an acquired immunodeficiency syndrome (AIDS)–defining illness in individuals younger than 13 years of age. In addition, nearly 50% of patients with HIV with diffuse infiltrative lymphocytosis syndrome (DILS) have been found to have LIP.[25–27] DILS is clinically and histologically similar to Sjögren syndrome, although infiltrates are composed predominantly of CD8+ (cluster of differentiation 8) as opposed to CD4+ (cluster of differentiation 4) lymphocytes. Data also suggest that EBV infection in the setting of a dysregulated host immune system allows cellular proliferation.[3,28] Simultaneous infection with EBV and HIV results in increased proliferation of BALT and increases the risk of development of LIP.[3]

There is also evidence of a genetic predisposition to the development of LIP. Several familial cohorts[29,30] have indicated an autosomal dominant with incomplete penetrance pattern of inheritance, although specific genetic polymorphisms have yet to be identified. Abnormal expression of HLA-DR (human leukocyte antigen-D related) in nonimmune cells with resultant exaggerated production of transforming growth factor-beta has been reported to play a role in the pathogenesis of LIP in some patients.[31]

EPIDEMIOLOGY

The incidence and prevalence of LIP are unknown. It more commonly affects women than men (male to female ratio of 1:2.75).[12] Men are more likely to develop idiopathic LIP, whereas women are more likely to have LIP related to an autoimmune disorder.[12] There is no racial preponderance in children; most HIV-positive adults with LIP are black, whereas most HIV-negative adults with LIP are white.[1,3,11,22] Three-quarters of reported patients had no history of smoking.

The average age at diagnosis for non–HIV-related LIP is between 30 and 50 years, although both pediatric and geriatric cases have been reported.[12,13,32] HIV-related LIP occurs most commonly in children, with 16% to 50% of children infected with HIV developing LIP within the second or third year of life.[23,24]

CLINICAL PRESENTATION

The onset of LIP is generally insidious, with symptom duration ranging from 2 months to 12 years before evaluation and typically in excess of 3 years.[8,11,12] LIP may be diagnosed incidentally,[33,34] although most patients become symptomatic with dyspnea on exertion and nonproductive cough.[4,31–33] Patients may also experience pleuritic chest pain[4,32] and systemic symptoms such as fever, weight loss, fatigue, and night sweats.[13,35] Physical examination is generally notable for crackles[12,14,15,32] on pulmonary auscultation, although a prolonged expiratory phase with wheezing has also been described.[15] The presence of clubbing has rarely been reported.[14,15,22] Extrapulmonary findings, such as peripheral lymphadenopathy, hepatomegaly, or splenomegaly, are uncommon and should prompt further investigation for possible lymphoma or other diagnoses.[1,11,21]

RADIOGRAPHIC MANIFESTATIONS

Chest radiography is neither sensitive nor specific for LIP. If findings are present, they generally include bilateral and basilar reticular or reticulonodular opacities[3,33,36] and ill-defined nodules.[37,38] As the disease progresses, cellular infiltrates expand into the alveolar spaces and appear as fluffy alveolar infiltrates, with or without air bronchograms.[11,22,39]

High-resolution computed tomography (HRCT) of the chest characteristically shows areas of ground-glass attenuation and poorly defined centrilobular and subpleural nodules of varying sizes (Figs. 1–3, Box 2).[40,41] Although the process is diffuse, LIP has a propensity to be most severe in the perilymphatic interstitium along bronchovascular bundles, interlobular septa, and the pleura (see Figs. 1–3).[40–42] Other HRCT findings associated with LIP include thickening of bronchovascular bundles (Fig. 2), interlobular septal

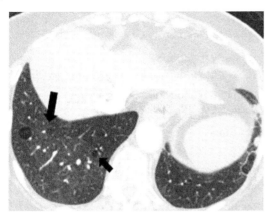

Fig. 1. Computed tomogram of the chest showing perivascular cysts (*small black arrow*) with ground-glass opacities (*long black arrow*) in a patient with LIP.

Fig. 3. Computed tomogram of the chest showing perivascular cysts (*black arrows*) in a patient with LIP.

thickening, and lymph node enlargement.[3,40,41,43,44] LIP should also be considered in the differential diagnosis when the reverse halo sign is seen on imaging.[45]

Thin-walled cysts are a characteristic abnormality on HRCT, and may be seen in as many as 80% of patients.[33,40,41,44] Cysts are typically few, have a random distribution deep within the lung parenchyma, are often bordered by an eccentric vessel, involve less than 10% of the lung, and are superimposed on ground-glass opacities (see **Fig. 2**).[33,40,41,46,47] The size and shape of the cysts, as well as the thickness of the cyst wall, are variable. Most are multiseptated with normal surrounding lung parenchyma. Cysts are usually less than 3 cm, although cysts as large as 10 cm have been reported.[35,40,41,46] The presence of cysts may help differentiate LIP from lymphoma.[46]

Cysts may result from ischemia caused by vascular obstruction, postobstructive bronchiolar ectasia, or bronchiolar compression as a result of peribronchiolar lymphocytic infiltration and subsegmental overinflation caused by a check-valve mechanism.[3,6,33,40,41,48]

Features seen on HRCT may vary depending on the associated underlying disease. Cysts are typically seen in association with underlying Sjögren syndrome and are often the predominant finding.[44] Pulmonary amyloidosis is occasionally seen in association with LIP, also in the context of Sjögren syndrome.[49] The presence of large soft tissue or calcified pulmonary nodules in conjunction with LIP should raise this suspicion. In patients with

Box 2 **Features of LIP on HRCT**
Ground-glass opacities
Uniform or patchy areas
Bilateral
Poorly defined nodules
Centrilobular
Subpleural
Thin-walled cystic air spaces
1 to 30 mm in diameter
Less than 10% lung parenchyma
Interstitial thickening
Peribronchovascular
Interlobular
Mediastinal lymph node enlargement
Data from Refs.[40,41,44]

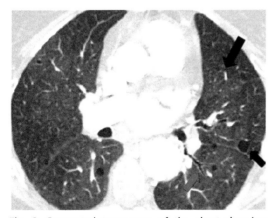

Fig. 2. Computed tomogram of the chest showing perivascular cysts (*small black arrow*) with extensive ground-glass opacities (*long black arrow*) and bronchial wall thickening (*red arrow*) in a patient with LIP.

congenital immunodeficiencies, LIP most often appears on computed tomography as patchy ground-glass opacification, whereas in patients with AIDS it typically manifests with multiple nodules.[44] Bronchiectasis is a common finding in HIV-positive children with LIP,[50,51] but is uncommon in other forms of LIP. Pleural involvement, dense consolidation, and honeycombing are unusual in all forms of LIP.[13,36,51]

PULMONARY FUNCTION TESTS

In most patients with LIP, pulmonary function tests typically show a restrictive ventilatory defect with an associated decrease in the diffusion capacity.[6,8] Concomitant airflow obstruction may occur either from bronchiolar compression and narrowing from the infiltrative process, or from concomitant follicular bronchiolitis.[33,52] Normal pulmonary function tests, including normal blood gas analyses, have been reported.[33,34]

DIAGNOSIS

Bronchoalveolar lavage is useful for ruling out underlying infection, but is otherwise nonspecific in patients with LIP. Typical findings include an increased total white blood cell count with a lymphocytosis and normal CD4/CD8 ratio.[12,34,51,53]

Transbronchial biopsy is seldom an adequate diagnostic tool; surgical lung biopsy is required to confirm the diagnosis in most patients.[12,51] This test may not be necessary in HIV-positive children with classic symptoms and radiographic patterns.[23] Pleural effusions should be tapped and may be helpful if sufficient fluid is present for immunophenotypic flow cytometric analysis to rule out lymphoma.

A thorough evaluation (**Box 3**) for an underlying autoimmune or immunodeficiency state should be conducted after a histopathologic diagnosis of LIP is established. Idiopathic LIP is exceedingly rare[12,48,51,54] and such cases in the literature have largely been reclassified as either low-grade B-cell lymphoma[2,51,55] or cellular nonspecific interstitial pneumonia (NSIP).[3,48,51,54]

PATHOLOGIC FEATURES

LIP is characterized by the presence of dense interstitial lymphocytic infiltrates, which expand and widen interlobular and alveolar septa.[56] The infiltrates are generally polymorphous and are composed of small lymphocytes[57] admixed with variable numbers of plasma cells, immunoblasts, macrophages, and occasional histiocytes. Granulomas and giant cells may be seen but are not

---

Box 3
Suggested laboratory evaluation for LIP

Antinuclear antibody

Anti–cyclic citrullinated peptide antibody

Complete blood count

Complete metabolic panel

EBV titers

HIV

Human T-cell lymphotropic virus

Quantitative immunoglobulins

Rheumatoid factor

Serum protein electrophoresis

Anti–Sjögren syndrome–related antigen A (anti-Ro)

Anti–Sjögren syndrome–related antigen B (anti-La)

Thyroid function studies

Urine protein electrophoresis

---

common (**Fig. 4**).[3,57,58] T cells that express CD3 are most prominent in the interstitium, whereas nodular lymphoid aggregates of B lymphocytes that express CD20 form germinal centers in up to 50% of patients with the idiopathic and connective tissue–associated forms of LIP and less commonly in HIV.[56,59] This pattern is present in the areas surrounding the lymphatic channels, such as the alveolar septa (corresponding with ground-glass opacities seen on HRCT), interstitial septa, peribronchovascular regions (corresponding with centrilobular nodules on HRCT), and subpleural lung zones (**Figs. 4 and 5**).[56,59] The small airways and blood vessels may be infiltrated by this inflammatory infiltrate but no necrosis or angiodestruction is seen.[60] Multinucleated giant cells and/or poorly formed nonnecrotizing granulomas are present in most patients with LIP, but they are usually inconspicuous and loosely arranged.[8,56,57,61,62] Lung cysts, commonly seen on imaging studies, are not seen in pathologic specimens. These cysts most likely are imaging features that are the result of peribronchiolar cellular infiltration leading to stenosis, air trapping, and distal airway dilatation.[8,33,36] Later in the course of the disease, LIP can show variable amounts of interstitial fibrosis and honeycombing, but this is an uncommon pathologic feature.[8] Immunohistochemical examination, molecular studies, or both are necessary to show polyclonality in the lymphoid population, thereby distinguishing LIP from lymphoma.[60,61] Infectious causes must also be diligently excluded.

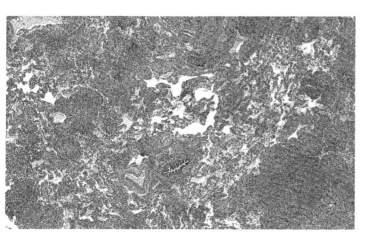

Fig. 4. Lung, wedge biopsy. The lung parenchyma is diffusely involved by a marked inflammatory infiltrate that expands the interstitium (hematoxylin and eosin, original magnification ×30).

There is an overlap between the disorders of follicular bronchiolitis and LIP. LIP can be accompanied by follicular bronchiolitis, but follicular bronchiolitis usually lacks extensive alveolar septal infiltration.[44,56,57] For this reason, the term diffuse lymphoid hyperplasia (DLH) can be used when both entities are present.[51] Nodular lymphoid hyperplasia (NLH), formerly known as pseudolymphoma (a term no longer used), and LIP have similar cellular infiltrates, causing some clinicians to postulate that LIP may be its interstitial counterpart. In general, both DLH and NLH may be difficult to distinguish from a low-grade marginal zone lymphoma of the BALT type and require immunohistochemical and molecular studies to exclude this.[3,42,62]

The pathologic differential diagnosis for LIP includes cellular NSIP and hypersensitivity pneumonitis (HP). HP usually has a more bronchocentric pattern and has loosely formed granulomas or

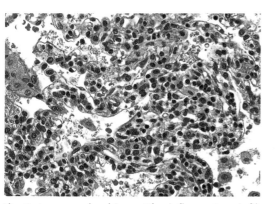

Fig. 5. Lung, wedge biopsy. The inflammatory infiltrate is composed of a mononuclear cell infiltrate of lymphocytes and plasma cells. The adjacent alveoli have scattered alveolar macrophages (hematoxylin and eosin, original magnification ×400).

giant cells around the airways and in the alveolar walls. LIP has a more diffuse and exuberant infiltrate. Granulomas, if present in LIP, are a minor component. Also, organizing pneumonia is much more commonly seen in HP than in LIP.[51] Cellular NSIP can be difficult to distinguish from LIP because both diffusely involve the alveoli without predilection for the airways.[3,63] However, the infiltrate is usually more expansive in LIP.

LYMPHOCYTIC INTERSTITIAL PNEUMONIA AND LYMPHOMA: DIFFERENTIATING FEATURES

Multiple pathologic and radiographic features help distinguish lymphoma from LIP, but immunohistochemical and molecular techniques may be the most useful methods for differentiation (**Box 4**). The presence of a monoclonal gammopathy or hypogammaglobulinemia should raise suspicion for a lymphoproliferative disorder.[48,53] Immunochemical studies and flow cytometry performed on the lung tissue can help distinguish between the polyclonal populations of lymphocytes seen in LIP and the monotypic cell population associated with malignant lymphoproliferative disorders.[3] For an unequivocal diagnosis of LIP, polyclonality in the lymphoid tissue should be established. On reevaluation, many of the historical cases of lymphoma were originally misclassified as LIP.[61,62] It is now estimated that only approximately 5% of LIP cases progress to lymphoma.[61,62]

TREATMENT AND PROGNOSIS

The course of LIP is variable and unpredictable. Patients may have a fairly benign or asymptomatic presentation,[33] and spontaneous remission has been reported, even in patients who are initially symptomatic.[21] Others have complications that

---

Box 4
Features indicating lymphoma instead of LIP (see also Fig. 6)

Pathologic features

Distortion of lung architecture with prominent lymphatic distribution

Dense infiltrate, sometimes a confluent proliferation, with prominent airway and vessel infiltration

Dense bands of hyalinizing fibrosis; amyloid may be present

Frequent lymphoepithelial lesions

Pleural infiltration

Intranuclear B-lymphocyte inclusions (Dutcher bodies)

Immunohistochemistry consists of predominantly B cells and monoclonal pattern of kappa and lambda light chain expression

Immunoglobulin heavy chain gene rearrangement studies show monoclonal B-cell pattern

Rearrangements of the MALT1 gene may be identified

Radiologic features

Consolidation

Large nodules (>10 mm)

Pleural effusions

Absence of cysts

Data from Hare SS, Souza CA, Bain G, et al. The radiological spectrum of pulmonary lymphoproliferative disease. Br J Radiol 2012;85(1015):848–64; and Honda O, Johkoh T, Ichikado K, et al. Differential diagnosis of lymphocytic interstitial pneumonia and malignant lymphoma on high-resolution CT. AJR Am J Roentgenol 1999;173(1):71–4.

---

lead to morbidity and mortality, including superimposed infections, progressive pulmonary fibrosis, and (rarely) transformation into lymphoma.[3,4,42,64]

There are no controlled clinical trials in LIP and treatment regimens have not been well established. Management of LIP should focus on controlling the underlying disease process.[51] It remains unclear whether treatment alters the natural course of LIP[2,3] and it is difficult to predict which patients will respond to treatment. Nevertheless,

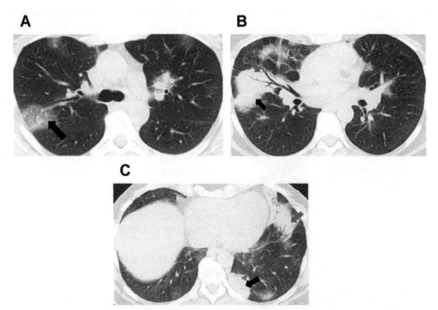

Fig. 6. Computed tomograms of the chest in a patient with NLH showing ground-glass opacities (*A, long black arrow*), dense consolidation (*B, C, short black arrows*), and air bronchograms (*B, C, red arrows*). Similar findings can also be seen in patients with lymphoma.

LIP has generally been regarded as steroid responsive with symptomatic and/or radiographic stabilization or improvement seen in 50% to 60% of patients, but relapses occur.[3,43] A recommended regimen is prednisone, 0.75 to 1.0 mg/kg/d (based on ideal body weight and not to exceed 100 mg/d) for 8 to 12 weeks or until stabilization followed by a slow taper to 0.25 mg/kg/d for another 6 to 12 weeks.[65,66]

Other immunosuppressive agents, such as hydroxychloroquine,[5] azathioprine,[65] cyclosporine A,[12] mycophenolate,[4,20] cyclophosphamide,[20,65] rituximab,[66] tumor necrosis factor antagonists,[20,67] and chlorambucil,[65] have been used with variable results. The number of patients treated with these agents is too small to allow any definitive conclusions regarding efficacy. Progression to fibrosis with honeycombing occurs in only a handful of LIP cases, and there are no reports on the utility of antifibrotic medications in preventing or decelerating this process.

In some patients with HIV, highly active antiretroviral therapy may result in clinical and radiographic improvement or resolution of LIP.[45,68] In a patient with common variable immunoglobulin deficiency, treatment with immunoglobulin was shown to help stabilize disease,[34] but LIP has also been reported to develop after intravenous immunoglobulin replacement therapy.[69] Lung transplant has been reported in 2 patients with LIP without evidence of recurrence of LIP in the transplanted lung on limited follow-up.[12,35]

Mortality in HIV-positive patients does not seem to be adversely affected by the presence of LIP.[3,25] Nevertheless, the reported 5-year mortality is 33% to 50% for all types of LIP despite treatment,[3,4,12] with reported median survival times ranging from 5 years[3] to 11.5 years.[12]

SUMMARY

LIP is a rare benign lymphoproliferative disorder confined to the lungs, typically associated with an underlying disorder. In establishing a diagnosis, it is important to identify the underlying disorder (eg, connective tissue disease, infection) and to differentiate LIP from malignant pulmonary lymphoproliferative disorders (eg, lymphoma). Demonstrating polyclonality with immunohistochemistry is the key to differentiating between LIP and lymphoma, but radiologic features such as dense consolidation, large nodules (>10 mm), pleural effusions, and absence of cysts can also indicate a diagnosis of lymphoma. Although sparse data regarding treatment options exist, steroid-based regimens are most commonly used; there is also anecdotal support for a variety of alternative agents, including azathioprine, mycophenolate mofetil, and rituximab. Whether such therapy alters the course and natural history of disease remains to be established, but survival is also likely influenced by the underlying disorder.

REFERENCES

1. Liebow AA, Carrington CB. Diffuse pulmonary lymphoreticular infiltrations associated with dysproteinemia. Med Clin North Am 1973;57(3):809–43.
2. Nicholson AG. Lymphocytic interstitial pneumonia and other lymphoproliferative disorders in the lung. Semin Respir Crit Care Med 2001;22(4):409–22.
3. Swigris JJ, Berry GJ, Raffin TA, et al. Lymphoid interstitial pneumonia: a narrative review. Chest 2002; 122(6):2150–64.
4. Abdarbashi P, Abrudescu A. Rare case of idiopathic lymphocytic interstitial pneumonia exhibits good response to mycophenolate mofetil. Respir Med Case Rep 2013;9:27–9.
5. Garcia D, Young L. Lymphocytic interstitial pneumonia as a manifestation of SLE and secondary Sjogren's syndrome. BMJ Case Rep 2013. [Epub ahead of print].
6. Gupta N, Vassallo R, Wikenheiser-Brokamp KA, et al. Diffuse cystic lung disease. Part II. Am J Respir Crit Care Med 2015;192(1):17–29.
7. Carrington CB, Liebow AA. Lymphocytic interstitial pneumonia. Am J Pathol 1966;48:36a.
8. Koss MN, Hochholzer L, Langloss JM, et al. Lymphoid interstitial pneumonia: clinicopathological and immunopathological findings in 18 cases. Pathology 1987;19(2):178–85.
9. Fishback N, Koss M. Update on lymphoid interstitial pneumonitis. Curr Opin Pulm Med 1996;2(5): 429–33.
10. Vitali C, Tavoni A, Viegi G, et al. Lung involvement in Sjogren's syndrome: a comparison between patients with primary and with secondary syndrome. Ann Rheum Dis 1985;44(7):455–61.
11. Strimlan CV, Rosenow EC 3rd, Weiland LH, et al. Lymphocytic interstitial pneumonitis. Review of 13 cases. Ann Intern Med 1978;88(5):616–21.
12. Cha SI, Fessler MB, Cool CD, et al. Lymphoid interstitial pneumonia: clinical features, associations and prognosis. Eur Respir J 2006;28(2):364–9.
13. Bragg DG, Chor PJ, Murray KA, et al. Lymphoproliferative disorders of the lung: histopathology, clinical manifestations, and imaging features. AJR Am J Roentgenol 1994;163(2):273–81.
14. Young RC Jr, Tillman RL, Burton AF, et al. Lymphoid interstitial pneumonia with polyclonal gammopathy. A case report. J Natl Med Assoc 1969;61(4):310–4.
15. Montes M, Tomasi TB Jr, Noehren TH, et al. Lymphoid interstitial pneumonia with monoclonal gammopathy. Am Rev Respir Dis 1968;98(2): 277–80.

16. Thomas H, Risma KA, Graham TB, et al. A kindred of children with interstitial lung disease. Chest 2007; 132(1):221–30.

17. Fischer A, Antoniou KM, Brown KK, et al. An official European Respiratory Society/American Thoracic Society research statement: interstitial pneumonia with autoimmune features. Eur Respir J 2015;46(4): 976–87.

18. Miyamoto H, Azuma A, Taniguchi Y, et al. Interstitial pneumonia complicated by Sjogren's syndrome, Hashimoto's disease, rheumatoid arthritis and primary biliary cirrhosis. Intern Med 2000;39(11):970–5.

19. Matsuyama N, Ashizawa K, Okimoto T, et al. Pulmonary lesions associated with Sjogren's syndrome: radiographic and CT findings. Br J Radiol 2003; 76(912):880–4.

20. Kim JY, Park SH, Kim SK, et al. Lymphocytic interstitial pneumonia in primary Sjogren's syndrome: a case report. Korean J Intern Med 2011;26(1):108–11.

21. Grieco MH, Chinoy-Acharya P. Lymphocytic interstitial pneumonia associated with the acquired immune deficiency syndrome. Am Rev Respir Dis 1985;131(6):952–5.

22. Oldham SA, Castillo M, Jacobson FL, et al. HIV-associated lymphocytic interstitial pneumonia: radiologic manifestations and pathologic correlation. Radiology 1989;170(1 Pt 1):83–7.

23. Rubinstein A, Morecki R, Goldman H. Pulmonary disease in infants and children. Clin Chest Med 1988;9(3):507–17.

24. Nesheim SR, Lindsay M, Sawyer MK, et al. A prospective population-based study of HIV perinatal transmission. AIDS 1994;8(9):1293–8.

25. Itescu S, Winchester R. Diffuse infiltrative lymphocytosis syndrome: a disorder occurring in human immunodeficiency virus-1 infection that may present as a sicca syndrome. Rheum Dis Clin North Am 1992;18(3):683–97.

26. Kazi S, Cohen PR, Williams F, et al. The diffuse infiltrative lymphocytosis syndrome. Clinical and immunogenetic features in 35 patients. AIDS 1996;10(4): 385–91.

27. Williams FM, Cohen PR, Jumshyd J, et al. Prevalence of the diffuse infiltrative lymphocytosis syndrome among human immunodeficiency virus type 1-positive outpatients. Arthritis Rheum 1998;41(5): 863–8.

28. Malamou-Mitsi V, Tsai MM, Gal AA, et al. Lymphoid interstitial pneumonia not associated with HIV infection: role of Epstein-Barr virus. Mod Pathol 1992; 5(5):487–91.

29. O'Brodovich HM, Moser MM, Lu L. Familial lymphoid interstitial pneumonia: a long-term follow-up. Pediatrics 1980;65(3):523–8.

30. Launay F, Guillaume JM, Gennari JM, et al. Polyarthritis and familial pulmonary fibrosis in a child. Joint Bone Spine 2006;73(2):212–4.

31. Koga M, Umemoto Y, Nishikawa M, et al. A case of lymphoid interstitial pneumonia in a 3-month-old boy not associated with HIV infection: immunohistochemistry of lung biopsy specimens and serum transforming growth factor-beta 1 assay. Pathol Int 1997;47(10):698–702.

32. Martinez Garcia MA, de Rojas MD, Nauffal Manzur MD, et al. Respiratory disorders in common variable immunodeficiency. Respir Med 2001;95(3): 191–5.

33. Ichikawa Y, Kinoshita M, Koga T, et al. Lung cyst formation in lymphocytic interstitial pneumonia: CT features. J Comput Assist Tomogr 1994;18(5):745–8.

34. Matsubara M, Koizumi T, Wakamatsu T, et al. Lymphoid interstitial pneumonia associated with common variable immunoglobulin deficiency. Intern Med 2008;47(8):763–7.

35. Silva CI, Flint JD, Levy RD, et al. Diffuse lung cysts in lymphoid interstitial pneumonia: high-resolution CT and pathologic findings. J Thorac Imaging 2006; 21(3):241–4.

36. Jawad H, Walker CM, Wu CC, et al. Cystic interstitial lung diseases: recognizing the common and uncommon entities. Curr Probl Diagn Radiol 2014; 43(3):115–27.

37. Fraser RG, Pare JAP, Pare PD, et al. Miscellaneous lymphoproliferative and myeloproliferative disorders. Neoplastic diseases of the lungs. In: Bralow L, editor. Diagnosis of diseases of the chest. 3rd edition. Philadelphia: WB Saunders; 1990. p. 1568–70.

38. Julsrud PR, Brown LR, Li CY, et al. Pulmonary processes of mature-appearing lymphocytes: pseudolymphoma, well-differentiated lymphocytic lymphoma, and lymphocytic interstitial pneumonitis. Radiology 1978;127(2):289–96.

39. Feigin DS, Siegelman SS, Theros EG, et al. Nonmalignant lymphoid disorders of the chest. AJR Am J Roentgenol 1977;129(2):221–8.

40. Johkoh T, Ichikado K, Akira M, et al. Lymphocytic interstitial pneumonia: follow-up CT findings in 14 patients. J Thorac Imaging 2000;15(3):162–7.

41. Johkoh T, Muller NL, Pickford HA, et al. Lymphocytic interstitial pneumonia: thin-section CT findings in 22 patients. Radiology 1999;212(2):567–72.

42. Kradin RL, Mark EJ. Benign lymphoid disorders of the lung, with a theory regarding their development. Hum Pathol 1983;14(10):857–67.

43. Dixon S, Benamore R. The idiopathic interstitial pneumonias: understanding key radiological features. Clin Radiol 2010;65(10):823–31.

44. Hare SS, Souza CA, Bain G, et al. The radiological spectrum of pulmonary lymphoproliferative disease. Br J Radiol 2012;85(1015):848–64.

45. Freeman MD, Grajo JR, Karamsadkar ND, et al. Reversed halo sign on CT as a presentation of lymphocytic interstitial pneumonia. J Radiol Case Rep Oct 2013;7(10):51–6.

46. Honda O, Johkoh T, Ichikado K, et al. Differential diagnosis of lymphocytic interstitial pneumonia and malignant lymphoma on high-resolution CT. AJR Am J Roentgenol 1999;173(1):71–4.

47. Watanabe M, Naniwa T, Hara M, et al. Pulmonary manifestations in Sjogren's syndrome: correlation analysis between chest computed tomographic findings and clinical subsets with poor prognosis in 80 patients. J Rheumatol 2010;37(2):365–73.

48. Kokosi MA, Nicholson AG, Hansell DM, et al. Rare idiopathic interstitial pneumonias: LIP and PPFE and rare histologic patterns of interstitial pneumonias: AFOP and BPIP. Respirology 2015;21(4): 600–14.

49. Jeong YJ, Lee KS, Chung MP, et al. Amyloidosis and lymphoproliferative disease in Sjogren syndrome: thin-section computed tomography findings and histopathologic comparisons. J Comput Assist Tomogr 2004;28(6):776–81.

50. Amorosa JK, Miller RW, Laraya-Cuasay L, et al. Bronchiectasis in children with lymphocytic interstitial pneumonia and acquired immune deficiency syndrome. Plain film and CT observations. Pediatr Radiol 1992;22(8):603–6 [discussion: 606–7].

51. Tian X, Yi ES, Ryu JH. Lymphocytic interstitial pneumonia and other benign lymphoid disorders. Semin Respir Crit Care Med 2012;33(5):450–61.

52. Halprin GM, Ramirez J, Pratt PC. Lymphoid interstitial pneumonia. Chest 1972;62(4):418–23.

53. Torii K, Ogawa K, Kawabata Y, et al. Lymphoid interstitial pneumonia as a pulmonary lesion of idiopathic plasmacytic lymphadenopathy with hyperimmuno-globulinemia. Intern Med 1994;33(4):237–41.

54. Travis WD, Costabel U, Hansell DM, et al. An official American Thoracic Society/European Respiratory Society statement: update of the international multi-disciplinary classification of the idiopathic interstitial pneumonias. Am J Respir Crit Care Med 2013; 188(6):733–48.

55. Herbert A, Walters MT, Cawley MI, et al. Lymphocytic interstitial pneumonia identified as lymphoma of mucosa associated lymphoid tissue. J Pathol 1985;146(2):129–38.

56. Nicholson AG, Wotherspoon AC, Diss TC, et al. Reactive pulmonary lymphoid disorders. Histopathology 1995;26(5):405–12.

57. Guinee DG Jr. Update on nonneoplastic pulmonary lymphoproliferative disorders and related entities. Arch Pathol Lab Med 2010;134(5):691–701.

58. Koss MN. Pulmonary lymphoid disorders. Semin Diagn Pathol 1995;12(2):158–71.

59. Cottin V, Donsbeck AV, Revel D, et al. Nonspecific interstitial pneumonia. Individualization of a clinico-pathologic entity in a series of 12 patients. Am J Respir Crit Care Med 1998;158(4):1286–93.

60. Travis WD, Galvin JR. Non-neoplastic pulmonary lymphoid lesions. Thorax 2001;56(12):964–71.

61. Colby TV, Carrington CB. Pulmonary lymphomas: current concepts. Hum Pathol 1983;14(10):884–7.

62. Colby TV, Carrington CB. Lymphoreticular tumors and infiltrates of the lung. Pathol Annu 1983;18(Pt 1):27–70.

63. Katzenstein ALA. Primary lymphoid lung lesions. In: Katzenstein ALA, editor. Katzenstein and Askin's surgical pathology of non-neoplastic lung disease. 4 edition. Philadelphia: Elsevier Saunders; 2006. p. 237–60.

64. Banerjee D, Ahmad D. Malignant lymphoma complicating lymphocytic interstitial pneumonia: a monoclonal B-cell neoplasm arising in a polyclonal lymphoproliferative disorder. Hum Pathol 1982; 13(8):780–2.

65. Devauchelle-Pensec V, Pennec Y, Morvan J, et al. Improvement of Sjogren's syndrome after two infusions of rituximab (anti-CD20). Arthritis Rheum 2007;57(2):310–7.

66. Schwarz MI. Lymphoplasmacytic interstitial pneumonia. In: Schwarz MI, King TE Jr, editors. Interstitial lung disease. St Louis (MO): Mosby Year Book; 1988. p. 405–12.

67. Yum HK, Kim ES, Ok KS, et al. Lymphocytic interstitial pneumonitis associated with Epstein-Barr virus in systemic lupus erythematosus and Sjogren's syndrome. Complete remission with corticosteroid and cyclophosphamide. Korean J Intern Med 2002; 17(3):198–203.

68. Bach MC. Zidovudine for lymphocytic interstitial pneumonia associated with AIDS. Lancet 1987; 2(8562):796.

69. Davies CW, Juniper MC, Gray W, et al. Lymphoid interstitial pneumonitis associated with common variable hypogammaglobulinaemia treated with cyclosporin A. Thorax 2000;55(1):88–90.

70. Perreault C, Cousineau S, D'Angelo G, et al. Lymphoid interstitial pneumonia after allogeneic bone marrow transplantation. A possible manifestation of chronic graft-versus-host disease. Cancer 1985;55(1):1–9.

71. DeCoteau WE, Tourville D, Ambrus JL, et al. Lymphoid interstitial pneumonia and autoerythrocyte sensitization syndrome. A case with deposition of immunoglobulins on the alveolar basement membrane. Arch Intern Med 1974;134(3):519–22.

72. Neil GA, Lukie BE, Cockcroft DW, et al. Lymphocytic interstitial pneumonia and abdominal lymphoma complicating celiac sprue. J Clin Gastroenterol 1986;8(3 Pt 1):282–5.

73. Helman CA, Keeton GR, Benatar SR. Lymphoid interstitial pneumonia with associated chronic active hepatitis and renal tubular acidosis. Am Rev Respir Dis 1977;115(1):161–4.

74. Church JA, Isaacs H, Saxon A, et al. Lymphoid interstitial pneumonitis and hypogammaglobulinemia in children. Am Rev Respir Dis 1981;124(4):491–6.

75. Levinson AI, Hopewell PC, Stites DP, et al. Coexistent lymphoid interstitial pneumonia, pernicious anemia, and agammaglobulinemia. Arch Intern Med 1976;136(2):213–6.

76. Chamberlain DW, Hyland RH, Ross DJ. Diphenylhydantoin-induced lymphocytic interstitial pneumonia. Chest 1986;90(3):458–60.

77. Setoguchi Y, Takahashi S, Nukiwa T, et al. Detection of human T-cell lymphotropic virus type I-related antibodies in patients with lymphocytic interstitial pneumonia. Am Rev Respir Dis 1991;144(6):1361–5.

78. Uziel Y, Hen B, Cordoba M, et al. Lymphocytic interstitial pneumonitis preceding polyarticular juvenile rheumatoid arthritis. Clin Exp Rheumatol 1998;16(5):617–9.

79. Dicicco BS, Anderson G. Lymphocytic interstitial pneumonitis following legionnaire's pneumonia. Chest 1994;105(1):325.

80. Weissman E, Becker NH. Interstitial lung disease in primary biliary cirrhosis. Am J Med Sci 1983;285(3):21–7.

81. Ratjen FA, Schoenfeld B, Wiesemann HG. Pulmonary alveolar microlithiasis and lymphocytic interstitial pneumonitis in a ten year old girl. Eur Respir J 1992;5(10):1283–5.

82. Bakhos R, Gattuso P, Arcot C, et al. Pulmonary alveolar proteinosis: an unusual association with *Mycobacterium avium-intracellulare* infection and lymphocytic interstitial pneumonia. South Med J 1996;89(8):801–2.

83. Bonner H Jr, Ennis RS, Geelhoed GW, et al. Lymphoid infiltration and amyloidosis of lung in Sjogren's syndrome. Arch Pathol 1973;95(1):42–4.

84. Weisbrot IM. Lymphomatoid granulomatosis of the lung, associated with a long history of benign lymphoepithelial lesions of the salivary glands and lymphoid interstitial pneumonitis. Report of a case. Am J Clin Pathol 1976;66(5):792–801.

85. Faguet GB, Webb HH, Agee JF, et al. Immunologically diagnosed malignancy in Sjogren's pseudolymphoma. Am J Med 1978;65(3):424–9.

Birt-Hogg-Dubé Syndrome

Nishant Gupta, MD[a],*, Bernie Y. Sunwoo, MBBS[b], Robert M. Kotloff, MD[c]

KEYWORDS

- Birt-Hogg-Dubé syndrome • Diffuse cystic lung disease • Fibrofolliculomas • Folliculin
- Pneumothorax • Pleurodesis • Renal cancer

KEY POINTS

- Birt-Hogg-Dubé syndrome (BHD) is a rare autosomal dominant disorder caused by mutations in the *Folliculin (FLCN)* gene and is characterized by the formation of fibrofolliculomas, kidney tumors, pulmonary cysts, and recurrent pneumothoraces.
- Alterations in energy and nutrient sensing through the mammalian target of rapamycin pathway, or impaired cell-cell adhesions, are some of the putative mechanisms responsible for the formation of renal tumors and pulmonary cysts in BHD.
- Patients with BHD are at an increased risk for development of recurrent pneumothoraces, and pleurodesis is recommended after the first episode of pneumothorax.
- Demonstration of fibrofolliculomas on a skin biopsy, or detection of a pathogenic *FLCN* mutation, confirm the diagnosis of BHD in patients with clinical suspicion of the disease.
- Patients with BHD are at a high risk for development of renal cancers, and routine screening for renal tumors should be performed in all adult patients with BHD.

INTRODUCTION

Birt-Hogg-Dubé syndrome (BHD) is a rare autosomal dominant disorder characterized by the formation of hair follicle tumors, kidney tumors, pulmonary cysts, and recurrent spontaneous pneumothoraces. BHD is caused by inactivating mutations in the *folliculin (FLCN)* gene located on chromosome 17.[1] The first description of BHD was actually provided by Hornstein and Knickenberg[2] in 1975. The investigators reported a case of 2 siblings with perifollicular fibromas, along with a family history of similar skin lesions in the father. One of the siblings also had multiple colon polyps and subsequently went on to develop colon cancer. This finding led the investigators to speculate about the association between perifollicular fibromas and intestinal polyps.[2] In 1977, Birt and colleagues[3] provided the first description of the autosomal dominant inheritance of this disorder and diagnosed the characteristic skin lesions as fibrofolliculomas. In this review, the authors provide a concise overview of the genetics, pathogenesis, clinical features, diagnosis, and management of BHD with a focus on pulmonary aspects of the disease.

GENETICS AND PATHOGENESIS

Huge strides have been made over the past 15 years in our understanding of the genetics and molecular mechanisms behind the various manifestations of BHD. In 2001, using genome-wide linkage analysis, the BHD gene locus was

Disclosures: The authors have nothing to disclose.
[a] Division of Pulmonary, Critical Care and Sleep Medicine, University of Cincinnati, 231 Albert Sabin Way, MSB Room 6053, ML 0564, Cincinnati, OH 45267, USA; [b] Division of Pulmonary, Critical Care, Allergy and Sleep Medicine, University of California, San Francisco, 2330 Post Street, Room 420, San Francisco, CA 94115, USA; [c] Department of Pulmonary Medicine, Cleveland Clinic, 9500 Euclid Avenue A90, Cleveland, OH 44195, USA
* Corresponding author.
E-mail address: guptans@ucmail.uc.edu

Clin Chest Med 37 (2016) 475–486
http://dx.doi.org/10.1016/j.ccm.2016.04.010
0272-5231/16/$ – see front matter Published by Elsevier Inc.

chestmed.theclinics.com

mapped to the pericentromeric region of chromosome 17p by 2 independent investigators.[4,5] In 2002, Nickerson and colleagues[6] performed recombination analysis, narrowed the BHD locus to a 700kb region on chromosome 17p11.2, and discovered protein-truncating mutations in a highly conserved protein, folliculin, in affected individuals with BHD. In 2005, Schmidt and colleagues[7] performed direct gene sequencing of the BHD gene in 30 affected families; combined with their prior data,[6] they were able to identify germline mutations in 84% of the affected families. Greater than 50% of patients in their analysis had a cytosine insertion or deletion in a hypermutable polycytosine tract in exon 11, thus, suggesting this region to be a mutation hotspot for BHD.[7] Most of these mutations were loss-of-function mutations, resulting in premature truncation of the protein folliculin. This observation led the investigators to conclude that *FLCN* likely acts as a tumor suppressor gene.[7] Approximately 150 unique mutations in the *FLCN* gene are now reported to be associated with the development of BHD.[8]

Folliculin and Its Role as a Tumor Suppressor

Multiple studies have now established the role of *FLCN* as a tumor suppressor gene. *Flcn* heterozygous knockout mice and rats with *Flcn* mutations are known to develop renal cell carcinoma.[9–12] Somatic frameshift mutations in the *FLCN* gene have been identified in greater than 50% of cases of renal tumors in BHD, suggesting a 2-hit model of renal tumorigenesis in patients with BHD, strongly supporting the tumor suppressor function of the *FLCN* gene.[13] In vitro studies performed on BHD tumor-established cell lines also demonstrate that loss of *FLCN* leads to development of renal cell carcinoma, and the tumorigenic properties are lost after restoring normal copies of *FLCN*.[14]

Mechanism of Action of Folliculin in Tumor Formation

Phenotypic similarities between BHD and tuberous sclerosis complex (TSC) had suggested a possible role of folliculin in energy, metabolism, and nutrient sensing via the mammalian target of rapamycin (mTOR) pathway.[15] Consistent with this observation was the sequential discovery of 2 folliculin interacting proteins, Folliculin Interacting Protein-1, and -2 (FNIP1 and FNIP2).[15,16] Both FNIP1 and FNIP2 interact with the carboxy-terminal of *FLCN* and regulate mTOR activity through modulation of 5′ AMP-activated protein kinase (AMPK), a key molecule for energy sensing that negatively regulates

mTOR activity.[15,16] In a recent study, Fnip1 and Fnip2 were shown to be critical regulators of *Flcn* function in suppressing renal tumors in a murine model of BHD.[17] Hasumi and colleagues[9] showed activation of the Phosphatidylinositol-3-kinase (PI3)-AKT pathway and upregulation of mTORC1 and mTORC2 in a mouse model of renal tumors associated with BHD and suggested a possible therapeutic role of combined mTORC1 and mTORC2 inhibition. Activation of the mTOR pathway in renal tumors associated with BHD has been suggested by other studies as well.[11] However, conflicting evidence suggesting abnormal mTOR inhibition in BHD-associated renal tumors has also been reported in yeast as well as mouse models of BHD.[18,19] In another study, both mTOR activation and mTOR inhibition have been reported,[20] leading to the suggestion of context- or cell-dependent activity of folliculin on mTOR activity.[21]

Numerous other mechanisms have been linked with the functioning of folliculin besides regulation of the mTOR activity.[21] Multiple studies have identified lysosomes as a site of action for folliculin, indicating a critical role for folliculin in the amino acid–dependent activation of mTOR via its direct interaction with the Ras-related GTP (Rag) family of GTPases.[22,23] Nookala and colleagues[24] reported the crystal structure of the folliculin carboxy-terminal domain and demonstrated that it is distantly related to *d*ifferentially expressed in *n*ormal cells and *n*eoplasia domain proteins, a family of Rab guanine nucleotide exchange factors (GEFs). Further, they were able to demonstrate that folliculin has GEF activity in vitro and suggested a role of folliculin in vesicle membrane trafficking. Folliculin downregulation has been linked to activation of an oncogenic transcription factor, Transcription Factor E3 (TFE3),[25] as well as deregulation of genes involved in transforming growth factor β signaling.[14] Finally, p0071 (plakophilin-4) has been identified as a folliculin-interacting protein; *FLCN* loss has been linked to dysregulated RhoA signaling and alterations in cell-cell adhesion.[26,27]

Role of Folliculin in Formation of Pulmonary Cysts

The mechanism by which *FLCN* loss leads to formation of lung cysts is not well established. Murine models of *Flcn* loss have not been successful in replicating formation of pulmonary cysts similar to the human phenotype.[1] Increased mTOR activity,[28] impaired cell-cell adhesion,[29] and increased vulnerability of the alveolar-septal regions to the mechanical forces of respiratory cycle[30] are some of the postulated mechanisms behind formation of pulmonary cysts in patients with

BHD. In a recent study, Goncharova and colleagues[31] demonstrated a relationship of *FLCN* with the E-cadherin-LKB1-AMPK pathway. In a murine model of BHD, the investigators demonstrated that loss of *Flcn* leads to alterations in the E-cadherin-dependent epithelial cell-cell junctions, impairment of LKB1-AMPK signaling, and caspase-dependent apoptosis of lung alveolar epithelial cells and alveolar airspace enlargement.[31] Increased cell-cell adhesions have been demonstrated in *FLCN*-deficient human bronchial epithelial cells with a trend towards increased elastance after exposing *Flcn* heterozygous mice to mechanical ventilation.[29] How increased cell-cell adhesion leads to cyst formation and how alterations in E-cadherin-LKB1-AMPK pathway explain a predominantly basilar location of lung cysts are some of the questions that remain unanswered.

CLINICAL MANIFESTATIONS

There is great phenotypic variability in the clinical features of BHD; patients can present with any combination of skin, pulmonary, or renal findings. *FLCN* gene mutations have been reported in patients presenting with pulmonary cysts and/or pneumothoraces without any skin or renal involvement.[32–34] A summary of the clinical and radiographic features of BHD is provided in **Table 1**.

Pulmonary

Pulmonary involvement is common in BHD, manifesting as pulmonary cysts and the development of pneumothoraces. Multiple and bilateral pulmonary cysts are seen in greater than 80% of patients with BHD.[5,7,35–37] Pulmonary cysts have been reported in patients of widely varying age, from teenagers to 85 year olds, but are more commonly seen in the fourth to fifth decades.[38–40] There is no known sex predilection. The role of cigarette smoking remains unclear, although more severe cystic changes have been reported in smokers compared with nonsmokers in a small case series.[41] The natural history of pulmonary cysts in BHD is unclear, but small studies have suggested no significant change in the number or size of cysts by imaging over a period of up to 66 months.[41–43]

Patients with BHD are typically asymptomatic from a pulmonary perspective until the development of a pneumothorax. Patients with BHD have a 50-fold increased risk of developing a spontaneous pneumothorax after adjusting for age, with a median age of pneumothorax occurrence of 38 years.[35,36]

Table 1
Characteristic clinical, radiological, and pathologic features of Birt-Hogg-Dubé syndrome

Organ System	Clinical Features	Radiology	Pathology
Skin	Multiple, small, dome-shaped, whitish papules most commonly visualized on the face, neck, and upper torso, typically appearing after 20 y of age	None	Fibrofolliculoma: multiple anastomosing strands of 2–4 epithelial cells emanating from a central aberrant hair follicle, encapsulated by a thick connective tissue stroma
Pulmonary	Increased predisposition to development of spontaneous pneumothoraces, with a median age of pneumothorax of 38 y	Basilar predominant, thin-walled cysts surrounded by a normal-appearing lung parenchyma; cysts are frequently lentiform in shape and have a predilection for the subpleural regions	Basilar predominant cysts surrounded by normal lung parenchyma lacking evidence of neoplastic cell proliferations or significant inflammation; histopathologically, BHD cysts potentially indistinguishable from emphysema
Renal	High risk for development of renal cancers, with a mean age of diagnosis of 50 y; frequently, bilateral and multifocal tumors	Bilateral, multifocal renal tumors of varying sizes	Renal cancers of varying histology, with hybrid oncocytic and chromophobe renal cell, and chromophobe renal cell being the most common

24–38% of patients with BHD experience at least one pneumothorax, and patients with a family history of pneumothorax have an increased risk of developing pneumothorax as compared with those without a family history.[7,35,36,44,45] BHD is characterized by an extremely high recurrence rate of pneumothoraces. Approximately 75% of patients with BHD experience a recurrent pneumothorax following a sentinel event.[35] The presence and number of pulmonary cysts, cyst size, and cyst volume have been identified as risk factors for the development of pneumothorax in BHD.[35] However, pneumothorax has been reported in BHD in the absence of radiographically visible cysts.[46] Small studies from China and Holland have suggested that BHD may be the cause of 5% to 10% of apparent primary spontaneous pneumothoraces.[47,48]

Parenchyma surrounding the pulmonary cysts in BHD is largely normal. It is not surprising, therefore, that the limited data on pulmonary function testing in BHD have demonstrated preserved or minimally impaired lung function.[39,41,49] In a retrospective study of 14 patients with BHD, Tobino and colleagues[49] demonstrated normal mean spirometric values (forced expiratory volume in the first second of expiration percent predicted 86.2 ±13.5%) and a mild decrease in diffusing capacity for carbon monoxide adjusted for alveolar volume (73.6 ±10.4%). Consequently, patients with BHD typically function well in the absence of pneumothorax. The recognition of *FLCN* as a tumor suppressor gene and the known association with renal tumors has raised the possibility of increased risk of pulmonary malignancies in BHD. Despite case reports of adenocarcinoma, low-grade adenomatous hyperplasia, and pulmonary histiocytoma in BHD, no clear association with lung cancer has been established to date.[32,39,41,50,51]

Renal

Patients with BHD are at increased risk of developing bilateral, multifocal, renal cell cancers. In 1993, Roth and colleagues[52] reported the first case of bilateral, multifocal chromophobe renal cell cancer in a patient with BHD. A few years later, Toro and colleagues[53] studied 3 kindreds with BHD and found renal cell cancers of varying histology in 7 out of 13 patients. Zbar and colleagues[36] confirmed the association between BHD and renal cell cancer in a subsequent study. In this study, 111 patients with known *FLCN* mutations were compared with 112 unaffected family members. The investigators found a 7-fold higher risk of renal cell cancer in patients with BHD. Multifocal and bilateral tumors were seen frequently; chromophobe renal cell carcinoma was the most common subtype, followed by oncocytic and clear cell tumors.[36]

Subsequent studies have revealed that the prevalence of renal tumors in patients with BHD varies between 27% and 34%, with a mean age at diagnosis of approximately 50 years.[45,54] Most renal cancers associated with BHD tend to follow an indolent course, and only a few cases of metastatic spread are reported in the literature.[55] Renal cysts are seen quite frequently in patients with BHD; however, it is unclear if the prevalence is higher than that of the general population.[55]

Cutaneous

Birt and colleagues[3] described the classic skin findings of BHD as a triad of fibrofolliculomas, trichodiscomas, and acrochordons. Acrochordons, or skin tags, are not specific to BHD and can be seen quite frequently in the general population. Fibrofolliculomas and trichodiscomas have been suggested to be part of a morphologic spectrum.[55,56] Thus, the characteristic skin lesion associated with BHD is a fibrofolliculoma, a benign hair follicle tumor. Fibrofolliculomas typically appear after 20 years of age[55] and present as multiple, small, dome-shaped, whitish papules most commonly visualized on the face, neck, and upper torso (**Fig. 1**A, B).[36,53] Angiofibromas have been described as a cutaneous manifestation of BHD.[57] However, cutaneous angiofibromas are characteristically seen in patients with TSC, and the presence of TSC must be carefully excluded before diagnosing BHD based on the presence of angiofibromas. Multiple oral mucosal papules and multiple lipomas are some of the other cutaneous findings reported to be associated with BHD.[53]

Other Clinical Manifestations

In the first report of BHD, Hornstein and Knickenberg[2] speculated about the association of BHD with intestinal polyps and an increased risk of colon cancer. However, the association between BHD and colon cancer has not been validated uniformly in subsequent studies. In a large study aimed at evaluating this relationship, Zbar and colleagues[36] found no difference in the incidence of colon cancer in patients with BHD when compared with unaffected family members. The prevalence of colon polyps was also similar in both groups. On the other hand, in a study of 149 patients with BHD, Nahorski and colleagues[58] found a higher incidence of colon cancer compared with

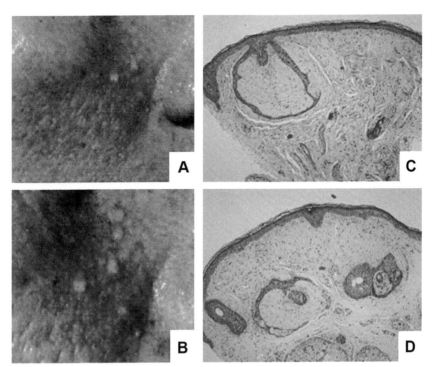

Fig. 1. Characteristic skin findings associated with BHD. (*A, B*) Facial photograph of a patient with BHD showing multiple dome-shaped, whitish papules consistent with fibrofolliculomas in the nasolabial fold area. (*C, D*) Histologic sections of a fibrofolliculoma from a patient with BHD showing cords of mantle epithelium emanating from a central aberrant hair follicle, encapsulated by a thick connective tissue stroma (Hematoxylin and Eosin stain, original magnification ×10). (*Courtesy of* [*C* and *D*] Dr Kerith Spicknall, Department of Dermatology, University of Cincinnati, Cincinnati, OH.)

the general population, especially in older age groups. These contrasting results likely represent differences in environmental exposures and *FLCN* allelic heterogeneity and might point towards a genotype-phenotype correlation in patients with BHD.[58]

A variety of other malignant and nonmalignant conditions, such as parathyroid adenomas,[59] thyroid tumors,[3] parotid oncocytomas,[60] lung cancer,[51] breast cancer,[61] multiple lipomas,[53,59] and so forth, have been reported to be associated with BHD in case reports and small case series. However, evidence of causality between BHD and these conditions is lacking.

RADIOGRAPHIC FEATURES OF BIRT-HOGG-DUBÉ SYNDROME
Pulmonary

Radiographic features demonstrated on high-resolution computed tomography (HRCT) scan of the chest often provide essential clues to the presence of BHD. The pulmonary cysts in BHD are multiple, bilateral, and vary in number; but the total extent of pulmonary cyst involvement usually encompasses less than 30% of the total lung

field.[37,43,62] Tobino and colleagues[43] evaluated the CT characteristics of pulmonary cysts in 12 patients with BHD and found that the greatest number of pulmonary cysts were seen in the lower medial (58.0 ±12.6%) and lower lateral (27.2 ±9.6%) zones followed by the upper medial (11.1 ±5.4%) and upper lateral (3.8 ±3.6%) zones with 40.5 ±12.3% of the cysts bordering the pleura. Pulmonary cysts were often seen abutting or including the proximal aspect of the lower lobe pulmonary arteries or veins.[43] The pulmonary cysts in BHD are thin walled and vary in size but are often small (<1 cm). They also vary in shape and can be irregularly shaped and multiseptated.[37] Thus, the HRCT pattern in BHD can be characterized as a profusion of round-lentiform shaped, thin-walled pulmonary cysts of various sizes, predominantly distributed in the basilar and subpleural regions of the lung (**Fig. 2**).

The cyst characteristics mentioned earlier can help distinguish BHD from other diffuse cystic lung diseases (DCLDs), such as lymphangioleiomyomatosis (LAM), pulmonary Langerhans cell histiocytosis, amyloidosis, light chain deposition disease, lymphoid interstitial pneumonia, cystic metastases, infectious entities, such as *Pneumocystis*,

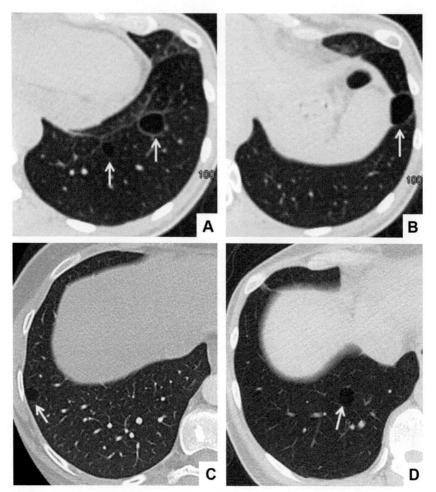

Fig. 2. Characteristic HRCT chest findings in BHD. (*A–D*) All 4 images show a basilar distribution of round-lentiform cysts (*arrows*). Note the subpleural predilection of cysts in BHD (*arrows*) (*B, C*).

and other causes.[38,63,64] Bullous changes seen in emphysema can also produce HRCT patterns that mimic the DCLDs. In a recent analysis, expert radiologists were able to accurately diagnose BHD and differentiate it from other DCLDs in greater than 90% of cases based on HRCT features alone.[63]

Renal

The characteristic radiologic finding of renal involvement in BHD is the presence of bilateral, multifocal renal tumors of varying sizes (**Fig. 3**). The renal tumors in BHD are often multifocal, bilateral, and typically enhance markedly after contrast material administration. The solid nature of the tumors distinguishes them from Von Hippel-Lindau–associated renal tumors, which often have cystic components.[65,66] Because LAM shares both cystic lung disease and renal tumors in common with BHD, differentiating between the two disorders can at times be difficult.

With respect to the renal manifestations, the presence of a fat-containing renal tumor on abdominal MRI or CT is characteristic of an angiomyolipoma, seen in patients with LAM but not BHD.[1]

HISTOPATHOLOGIC FEATURES OF BIRT-HOGG-DUBÉ SYNDROME
Pulmonary

In general, the histologic features of pulmonary cysts in BHD tend to be indistinguishable from those of emphysema.[38,67] In a recent study, Kumasaka and colleagues[30] evaluated the histopathologic features of 229 cysts from 50 patients with BHD and found that the cysts in BHD are surrounded by normal lung parenchyma lacking evidence of neoplastic cell proliferations or significant inflammation, have a basilar distribution, and frequently abut the interlobular septa, which differs from the apical, centrilobular-predominant pattern of emphysema. Further characterization

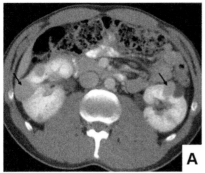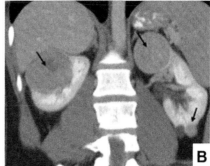

Fig. 3. Abdominal CT scans depicting the presence of bilateral, multifocal renal tumors (*arrows*) in a patient with BHD. (*Courtesy of* Dr Linehan WM, MD, Bethesda, MD; and *Adapted from* Schmidt LS, Linehan WM. Molecular genetics and clinical features of Birt-Hogg-Dube syndrome. Nat Rev Urol 2015;12(10):560; with permission.)

of the morphologic and immunohistochemical features of BHD-associated lung cysts is needed in order to permit the pathologist to accurately distinguish BHD from emphysema.

Renal

Renal cancers of varying histology can be seen in patients with BHD. Pavlovich and colleagues[68] reviewed the histology from 130 surgically resected renal tumors resected from 30 patients with BHD. Hybrid oncocytic and chromophobe renal cell cancer was the most common histologic subtype, seen in 50% of the tumors, followed by chromophobe renal cell cancers (34%), clear cell renal cancers (9%), and less commonly, papillary cancers and other mixed subtypes.

Skin

The characteristic skin lesion in BHD is a benign hair follicle tumor, fibrofolliculoma. On histopathology, fibrofolliculomas appear as multiple anastomosing strands of 2 to 4 epithelial cells emanating from a central aberrant hair follicle, encapsulated by a thick connective tissue stroma (**Fig. 1**C, D).[69] A possible origin of fibrofolliculomas from the sebaceous gland mantle has been suggested, which could explain the preferential location of fibrofolliculomas in areas rich with sebaceous glands, such as the nose and perinasal skin.[69]

DIAGNOSTIC APPROACH

Patients with undiagnosed BHD who present with spontaneous pneumothorax are often misdiagnosed initially as having a primary spontaneous pneumothorax or emphysema, reflecting physician unfamiliarity with this rare disease. In order to avoid misdiagnosis, physicians need to consider BHD in patients presenting with a

personal or family history of pneumothorax, especially if skin lesions or renal tumors are present.[47,48] It is important to recognize, however, that there is wide phenotypic variability in the clinical presentation of BHD; absence of skin and renal findings does not exclude the diagnosis of BHD, especially in patients with a family history of pneumothoraces.[32–34] Other causes of familial spontaneous pneumothorax include Marfan syndrome, Ehlers-Danlos syndrome, homocystinuria, α1-antitrypsin deficiency, TSC-LAM, and cystic fibrosis.[70] Fortunately, most of these conditions have other characteristic clinical features to assist clinicians in making the correct diagnosis.[1]

A recently concluded analysis shows that performing an HRCT scan of the chest in patients presenting with a spontaneous pneumothorax is cost-effective to screen for the presence of BHD and other DCLDs.[71] The cyst characteristics of BHD are quite unique and can help differentiate BHD from other DCLDs with a high degree of certainty.[63] Confirmation of the diagnosis with skin biopsy or *FLCN* mutation analysis is recommended even if the HRCT is characteristic, however, because the diagnosis will commit patients to lifelong monitoring for renal neoplasms.[63]

Another scenario that should raise the suspicion for BHD is a patient presenting with early onset (age <50 years) multifocal or bilateral renal cancer or renal cancer of mixed chromophobe and oncocytic histology, especially if there is an accompanying family history of renal cancers.[21] Besides BHD, the combination of pulmonary cysts and renal tumors is also seen in patients with LAM. There are some key differences in the clinical features of BHD and LAM that can assist in distinguishing between the two disorders (**Table 2**).

Multiple diagnostic criteria exist in the literature for diagnosing BHD.[1,21,55] The authors suggest

Table 2
Summary of characteristic findings of lymphangioleiomyomatosis and Birt-Hogg-Dubé syndrome

Finding	LAM	BHD
Characteristic skin lesions	Angiofibromas in patients with TSC-LAM	Fibrofolliculomas and trichodiscomas
Characteristic renal tumors	Angiomyolipomas	Renal cancers of varying histology, with hybrid oncocytomas, and chromophobe cancers being the most common
Pulmonary cyst features on HRCT	Uniform, round cysts present in a diffuse distribution. May be associated with small nodules in patients with TSC-LAM (multifocal micronodular pneumocyte hyperplasia)	Basilar predominant round-lentiform shaped cysts, commonly seen in subpleural regions, and frequently abut the pulmonary vessels and interlobular septa
Sex predilection	Almost exclusively females; occasional males with TSC	Equal sex distribution
Mode of inheritance	Autosomal dominant in TSC-LAM	Autosomal dominant
Incidence of pneumothorax	60%–80%	24%–38%
Rate of recurrent pneumothorax	70%	75%

the following stepwise approach to confirm the diagnosis of BHD in patients with clinical and radiographic features suggestive of the disease:

1. Biopsy of skin lesions, if present: Care should be taken to avoid shallow sampling of the skin lesions. Punch biopsy, rather than shave biopsy, should be performed on these lesions.[38]
2. Genetic testing for *FLCN* mutations: Genetic testing not only confirms diagnosis but also allows for detection of at-risk asymptomatic family members. Detection of a genetic disease has insurability, employment, and psychosocial implications; thus, all patients should be referred for genetic counseling before genetic testing.[38]

MANAGEMENT

Following diagnosis, the presence and extent of skin, pulmonary, and renal involvement should be fully characterized. Ongoing management then focuses primarily on surveillance and treatment of renal cancers and prevention and treatment of pneumothoraces.

Management of Skin Lesions

The skin lesions in BHD, although benign, can occasionally be disfiguring, causing significant psychosocial burden.[55] Current treatment modalities for fibrofolliculomas include destructive techniques, such as ablative laser using an erbium-YAG or carbon dioxide laser, electrocoagulation,

and/or excision.[72] However, these treatment modalities are hampered by a high recurrence rate and the risk of complications, such as scarring, inflammation, hypopigmentation, and hyperpigmentation.[72] In a recent analysis, the use of topical rapamycin failed to provide any benefit in the treatment of fibrofolliculomas.[72] The authors recommend consultation with a dermatologist in order to allow patients to choose individual treatment options after discussing the potential risks and benefits.

Management of the Pulmonary Aspects of Birt-Hogg-Dubé Syndrome

Pneumothorax prevention and treatment are the main principles of pulmonary management in patients with BHD. As the risk of pneumothorax has been associated with the number of pulmonary cysts,[35] a baseline HRCT of the chest is suggested in all patients with BHD to better characterize the extent of the patients' pulmonary involvement and to facilitate patient education.[1,73]

Patients with BHD should be informed of their increased risk of developing a spontaneous pneumothorax and educated about the associated signs and symptoms. Smoking is a known risk factor for primary spontaneous pneumothorax; although the association between smoking and pneumothorax occurrence in BHD is unclear, smoking should be strongly discouraged.[74] Although no disease-specific data exist, patients with BHD should be advised against scuba diving as changes in ambient atmospheric pressure could predispose patients to develop pneumothoraces.[1,75] Similarly the lower atmospheric pressure in a pressurized cabin at cruising altitude when flying may result in gas expansion within pulmonary cysts and the development of a pneumothorax. However, studies in patients with LAM, in whom the cyst burden is generally higher, have suggested air travel is quite safe for these patients.[76–78] In general most patients with BHD should be able to undergo air travel safely; however, the authors suggest that patients should not board an airplane with unexplained chest pain or shortness of breath.[1]

Once a pneumothorax develops, the risk of recurrence is high; compared with primary spontaneous pneumothorax, a more aggressive approach to minimize recurrence is suggested. This approach is similar to patients with LAM presenting with pneumothorax, for whom chemical pleurodesis and surgery have been shown to be better than conservative therapy and associated with less morbidity.[79] Although management will vary depending on patients' preferences, consideration of pleurodesis is recommended with the first pneumothorax in all patients with BHD.

BHD-related cystic lung disease typically does not result in significant or progressive respiratory impairment, and reassurance regarding this fact plays a key role in patient management. The authors suggest performing baseline pulmonary function testing in all patients with pulmonary symptoms, significant cyst burden, or diagnostic uncertainty.

Management of the Renal Manifestations of Birt-Hogg-Dubé Syndrome

Renal cancer is the most life-threatening complication of BHD, and regular screening is essential in the long-term management of these patients in order to identify tumors at an early stage. However, the optimal mode, timing, and duration of surveillance remain unclear. CT and MRI are more sensitive than ultrasound in detecting smaller lesions.[80,81] However, the cumulative radiation dose from CT scanning can be prohibitive; thus, gadolinium-enhanced MRI is the preferred test for screening of renal cancers.[21,38,73]

There are no established guidelines related to the timing and duration of surveillance. Because renal cancer has been described in patients younger than 25 years, most experts suggest beginning screening around 20 years of age.[38,55,73] In the absence of any abnormality on initial screening, repeat imaging every 36 to 48 months is

reasonable and lifelong surveillance is recommended.[21,73] Once a renal mass is detected, subsequent imaging intervals are individualized based on the size and growth rate of tumors.[21,73]

Once a renal tumor reaches 3 cm in size, surgical resection using a nephron-sparing approach is recommended for definitive treatment. Other nephron-sparing techniques, such as cryoablation and radiofrequency ablation, may be appropriate depending on size, growth rate, location, comorbidities, and local expertise. In general, these techniques should be reserved for patients not deemed to be good surgical candidates.[21] Case reports suggest a possible role of mTOR inhibitors in management of renal cancer associated with BHD[82]; however, definitive clinical trials are needed before widespread use of these agents can be recommended. A phase II study evaluating the role of an mTOR inhibitor, everolimus, in patients with BHD-associated renal cancer is currently ongoing (ClinicalTrials.gov, NCT02504892).

SUMMARY

Significant advancements have been achieved in our understanding of the genetic and cellular pathways leading to the development of BHD. Although we have gained insight into the role of *FLCN* mutations in renal tumor formation, additional studies are needed to elucidate the exact mechanisms underlying pulmonary cyst formation in BHD. Biomarkers predicting an aggressive renal cancer subtype with a potential for metastases are needed for optimal patient management. Physicians need to maintain a high index of clinical suspicion for BHD, especially when evaluating patients with a spontaneous pneumothorax, in order to institute appropriate measures to prevent recurrent pneumothoraces and enable regular screening for renal cancers.

REFERENCES

1. Gupta N, Seyama K, McCormack FX. Pulmonary manifestations of Birt-Hogg-Dube syndrome. Fam Cancer 2013;12:387–96.
2. Hornstein OP, Knickenberg M. Perifollicular fibromatosis cutis with polyps of the colon–a cutaneointestinal syndrome sui generis. Arch Dermatol Res 1975;253:161–75.
3. Birt AR, Hogg GR, Dube WJ. Hereditary multiple fibrofolliculomas with trichodiscomas and acrochordons. Arch Dermatol 1977;113:1674–7.
4. Khoo SK, Bradley M, Wong FK, et al. Birt-Hogg-Dube syndrome: mapping of a novel hereditary neoplasia gene to chromosome 17p12-q11.2. Oncogene 2001;20:5239–42.

5. Schmidt LS, Warren MB, Nickerson ML, et al. Birt-Hogg-Dube syndrome, a genodermatosis associated with spontaneous pneumothorax and kidney neoplasia, maps to chromosome 17p11.2. Am J Hum Genet 2001;69:876–82.

6. Nickerson ML, Warren MB, Toro JR, et al. Mutations in a novel gene lead to kidney tumors, lung wall defects, and benign tumors of the hair follicle in patients with the Birt-Hogg-Dube syndrome. Cancer Cell 2002;2:157–64.

7. Schmidt LS, Nickerson ML, Warren MB, et al. Germline BHD-mutation spectrum and phenotype analysis of a large cohort of families with Birt-Hogg-Dube syndrome. Am J Hum Genet 2005;76:1023–33.

8. Lim DH, Rehal PK, Nahorski MS, et al. A new locus-specific database (LSDB) for mutations in the folliculin (FLCN) gene. Hum Mutat 2010;31:E1043–51.

9. Hasumi Y, Baba M, Ajima R, et al. Homozygous loss of BHD causes early embryonic lethality and kidney tumor development with activation of mTORC1 and mTORC2. Proc Natl Acad Sci U S A 2009;106:18722–7.

10. Okimoto K, Sakurai J, Kobayashi T, et al. A germ-line insertion in the Birt-Hogg-Dube (BHD) gene gives rise to the Nihon rat model of inherited renal cancer. Proc Natl Acad Sci U S A 2004;101:2023–7.

11. Chen J, Futami K, Petillo D, et al. Deficiency of FLCN in mouse kidney led to development of polycystic kidneys and renal neoplasia. PLoS One 2008;3:e3581.

12. Baba M, Furihata M, Hong SB, et al. Kidney-targeted Birt-Hogg-Dube gene inactivation in a mouse model: Erk1/2 and Akt-mTOR activation, cell hyperproliferation, and polycystic kidneys. J Natl Cancer Inst 2008;100:140–54.

13. Vocke CD, Yang Y, Pavlovich CP, et al. High frequency of somatic frameshift BHD gene mutations in Birt-Hogg-Dube-associated renal tumors. J Natl Cancer Inst 2005;97:931–5.

14. Hong SB, Oh H, Valera VA, et al. Tumor suppressor FLCN inhibits tumorigenesis of a FLCN-null renal cancer cell line and regulates expression of key molecules in TGF-beta signaling. Mol Cancer 2010;9:160.

15. Baba M, Hong SB, Sharma N, et al. Folliculin encoded by the BHD gene interacts with a binding protein, FNIP1, and AMPK, and is involved in AMPK and mTOR signaling. Proc Natl Acad Sci U S A 2006;103:15552–7.

16. Hasumi H, Baba M, Hong SB, et al. Identification and characterization of a novel folliculin-interacting protein FNIP2. Gene 2008;415:60–7.

17. Hasumi H, Baba M, Hasumi Y, et al. Folliculin-interacting proteins Fnip1 and Fnip2 play critical roles in kidney tumor suppression in cooperation with Flcn. Proc Natl Acad Sci U S A 2015;112:E1624–31.

18. van Slegtenhorst M, Khabibullin D, Hartman TR, et al. The Birt-Hogg-Dube and tuberous sclerosis complex homologs have opposing roles in amino acid homeostasis in Schizosaccharomyces pombe. J Biol Chem 2007;282:24583–90.

19. Hartman TR, Nicolas E, Klein-Szanto A, et al. The role of the Birt-Hogg-Dube protein in mTOR activation and renal tumorigenesis. Oncogene 2009;28:1594–604.

20. Hudon V, Sabourin S, Dydensborg AB, et al. Renal tumour suppressor function of the Birt-Hogg-Dube syndrome gene product folliculin. J Med Genet 2010;47:182–9.

21. Schmidt LS, Linehan WM. Molecular genetics and clinical features of Birt-Hogg-Dube syndrome. Nat Rev Urol 2015;12(10):558–69.

22. Tsun ZY, Bar-Peled L, Chantranupong L, et al. The folliculin tumor suppressor is a GAP for the RagC/D GTPases that signal amino acid levels to mTORC1. Mol Cell 2013;52:495–505.

23. Petit CS, Roczniak-Ferguson A, Ferguson SM. Recruitment of folliculin to lysosomes supports the amino acid-dependent activation of Rag GTPases. J Cell Biol 2013;202:1107–22.

24. Nookala RK, Langemeyer L, Pacitto A, et al. Crystal structure of folliculin reveals a hidDENN function in genetically inherited renal cancer. Open Biol 2012;2:120071.

25. Hong SB, Oh H, Valera VA, et al. Inactivation of the FLCN tumor suppressor gene induces TFE3 transcriptional activity by increasing its nuclear localization. PLoS One 2010;5:e15793.

26. Nahorski MS, Seabra L, Straatman-Iwanowska A, et al. Folliculin interacts with p0071 (plakophilin-4) and deficiency is associated with disordered RhoA signalling, epithelial polarization and cytokinesis. Hum Mol Genet 2012;21:5268–79.

27. Medvetz DA, Khabibullin D, Hariharan V, et al. Folliculin, the product of the Birt-Hogg-Dube tumor suppressor gene, interacts with the adherens junction protein p0071 to regulate cell-cell adhesion. PLoS One 2012;7:e47842.

28. Furuya M, Tanaka R, Koga S, et al. Pulmonary cysts of Birt-Hogg-Dube syndrome: a clinicopathologic and immunohistochemical study of 9 families. Am J Surg Pathol 2012;36:589–600.

29. Khabibullin D, Medvetz DA, Pinilla M, et al. Folliculin regulates cell-cell adhesion, AMPK, and mTORC1 in a cell-type-specific manner in lung-derived cells. Physiol Rep 2014;2 [pii: e12107].

30. Kumasaka T, Hayashi T, Mitani K, et al. Characterization of pulmonary cysts in Birt-Hogg-Dube syndrome: histopathological and morphometric analysis of 229 pulmonary cysts from 50 unrelated patients. Histopathology 2014;65:100–10.

31. Goncharova EA, Goncharov DA, James ML, et al. Folliculin controls lung alveolar enlargement and

epithelial cell survival through E-cadherin, LKB1, and AMPK. Cell Rep 2014;7:412–23.

32. Gunji Y, Akiyoshi T, Sato T, et al. Mutations of the Birt Hogg Dube gene in patients with multiple lung cysts and recurrent pneumothorax. J Med Genet 2007;44:588–93.

33. Graham RB, Nolasco M, Peterlin B, et al. Nonsense mutations in folliculin presenting as isolated familial spontaneous pneumothorax in adults. Am J Respir Crit Care Med 2005;172:39–44.

34. Painter JN, Tapanainen H, Somer M, et al. A 4-bp deletion in the Birt-Hogg-Dube gene (FLCN) causes dominantly inherited spontaneous pneumothorax. Am J Hum Genet 2005;76:522–7.

35. Toro JR, Pautler SE, Stewart L, et al. Lung cysts, spontaneous pneumothorax, and genetic associations in 89 families with Birt-Hogg-Dube syndrome. Am J Respir Crit Care Med 2007;175:1044–53.

36. Zbar B, Alvord WG, Glenn G, et al. Risk of renal and colonic neoplasms and spontaneous pneumothorax in the Birt-Hogg-Dube syndrome. Cancer Epidemiol Biomarkers Prev 2002;11:393–400.

37. Agarwal PP, Gross BH, Holloway BJ, et al. Thoracic CT findings in Birt-Hogg-Dube syndrome. AJR Am J Roentgenol 2011;196:349–52.

38. Gupta N, Vassallo R, Wikenheiser-Brokamp KA, et al. Diffuse cystic lung disease. Part II. Am J Respir Crit Care Med 2015;192:17–29.

39. Tomassetti S, Carloni A, Chilosi M, et al. Pulmonary features of Birt-Hogg-Dube syndrome: cystic lesions and pulmonary histiocytoma. Respir Med 2011;105:768–74.

40. Johannesma PC, van den Borne BE, Gille JJ, et al. Spontaneous pneumothorax as indicator for Birt-Hogg-Dube syndrome in paediatric patients. BMC Pediatr 2014;14:171.

41. Ayo DS, Aughenbaugh GL, Yi ES, et al. Cystic lung disease in Birt-Hogg-Dube syndrome. Chest 2007;132:679–84.

42. Johannesma PC, Houweling AC, van Waesberghe JH, et al. The pathogenesis of pneumothorax in Birt-Hogg-Dube syndrome: a hypothesis. Respirology 2014;19:1248–50.

43. Tobino K, Gunji Y, Kurihara M, et al. Characteristics of pulmonary cysts in Birt-Hogg-Dube syndrome: thin-section CT findings of the chest in 12 patients. Eur J Radiol 2011;77:403–9.

44. Houweling AC, Gijezen LM, Jonker MA, et al. Renal cancer and pneumothorax risk in Birt-Hogg-Dube syndrome; an analysis of 115 FLCN mutation carriers from 35 BHD families. Br J Cancer 2011;105:1912–9.

45. Toro JR, Wei MH, Glenn GM, et al. BHD mutations, clinical and molecular genetic investigations of Birt-Hogg-Dube syndrome: a new series of 50 families and a review of published reports. J Med Genet 2008;45:321–31.

46. Onuki T, Goto Y, Kuramochi M, et al. Radiologically indeterminate pulmonary cysts in Birt-Hogg-Dube syndrome. Ann Thorac Surg 2014;97:682–5.

47. Ren HZ, Zhu CC, Yang C, et al. Mutation analysis of the FLCN gene in Chinese patients with sporadic and familial isolated primary spontaneous pneumothorax. Clin Genet 2008;74:178–83.

48. Johannesma PC, Reinhard R, Kon Y, et al. Prevalence of Birt-Hogg-Dube syndrome in patients with apparently primary spontaneous pneumothorax. Eur Respir J 2015;45:1191–4.

49. Tobino K, Hirai T, Johkoh T, et al. Differentiation between Birt-Hogg-Dube syndrome and lymphangioleiomyomatosis: quantitative analysis of pulmonary cysts on computed tomography of the chest in 66 females. Eur J Radiol 2012;81:1340–6.

50. Nishida C, Yatera K, Yamasaki K, et al. Possible familial case of Birt-Hogg-Dube syndrome complicated with lung cancer: a possible link between these two disease entities. Respir Med 2015;109:923–5.

51. Furuya M, Nakatani Y. Birt-Hogg-Dube syndrome: clinicopathological features of the lung. J Clin Pathol 2013;66:178–86.

52. Roth JS, Rabinowitz AD, Benson M, et al. Bilateral renal cell carcinoma in the Birt-Hogg-Dube syndrome. J Am Acad Dermatol 1993;29:1055–6.

53. Toro JR, Glenn G, Duray P, et al. Birt-Hogg-Dube syndrome: a novel marker of kidney neoplasia. Arch Dermatol 1999;135:1195–202.

54. Pavlovich CP, Grubb RL 3rd, Hurley K, et al. Evaluation and management of renal tumors in the Birt-Hogg-Dube syndrome. J Urol 2005;173:1482–6.

55. Menko FH, van Steensel MA, Giraud S, et al. Birt-Hogg-Dube syndrome: diagnosis and management. Lancet Oncol 2009;10:1199–206.

56. Schulz T, Hartschuh W. Birt-Hogg-Dube syndrome and Hornstein-Knickenberg syndrome are the same. Different sectioning technique as the cause of different histology. J Cutan Pathol 1999;26:55–61.

57. Schaffer JV, Gohara MA, McNiff JM, et al. Multiple facial angiofibromas: a cutaneous manifestation of Birt-Hogg-Dube syndrome. J Am Acad Dermatol 2005;53:S108–11.

58. Nahorski MS, Lim DH, Martin L, et al. Investigation of the Birt-Hogg-Dube tumour suppressor gene (FLCN) in familial and sporadic colorectal cancer. J Med Genet 2010;47:385–90.

59. Chung JY, Ramos-Caro FA, Beers B, et al. Multiple lipomas, angiolipomas, and parathyroid adenomas in a patient with Birt-Hogg-Dube syndrome. Int J Dermatol 1996;35:365–7.

60. Maffe A, Toschi B, Circo G, et al. Constitutional FLCN mutations in patients with suspected Birt-Hogg-Dube syndrome ascertained for non-cutaneous manifestations. Clin Genet 2011;79:345–54.

61. Palmirotta R, Donati P, Savonarola A, et al. Birt-Hogg-Dube (BHD) syndrome: report of two novel germline mutations in the folliculin (FLCN) gene. Eur J Dermatol 2008;18:382–6.

62. Kilincer A, Ariyurek OM, Karabulut N. Cystic lung disease in Birt-Hogg-Dube syndrome: a case series of three patients. Eurasian J Med 2014;46:138–41.

63. Gupta N, Meraj R, Tanase D, et al. Accuracy of chest high-resolution computed tomography in diagnosing diffuse cystic lung diseases. Eur Respir J 2015;46(4):1196–9.

64. Gupta N, Vassallo R, Wikenheiser-Brokamp KA, et al. Diffuse cystic lung disease. Part I. Am J Respir Crit Care Med 2015;191:1354–66.

65. Choyke PL, Glenn GM, Walther MM, et al. Hereditary renal cancers. Radiology 2003;226:33–46.

66. Choyke PL. Imaging of hereditary renal cancer. Radiol Clin North Am 2003;41:1037–51.

67. Butnor KJ, Guinee DG Jr. Pleuropulmonary pathology of Birt-Hogg-Dube syndrome. Am J Surg Pathol 2006;30:395–9.

68. Pavlovich CP, Walther MM, Eyler RA, et al. Renal tumors in the Birt-Hogg-Dube syndrome. Am J Surg Pathol 2002;26:1542–52.

69. Vernooij M, Claessens T, Luijten M, et al. Birt-Hogg-Dube syndrome and the skin. Fam Cancer 2013;12:381–5.

70. Chiu HT, Garcia CK. Familial spontaneous pneumothorax. Curr Opin Pulm Med 2006;12:268–72.

71. Gupta N, Langenderfer D, McCormack FX, et al. HRCT screening for diffuse cystic lung diseases in patients presenting with spontaneous pneumothorax is cost-effective [abstract]. Am J Respir Crit Care Med 2016;104. A6261.

72. Gijezen LM, Vernooij M, Martens H, et al. Topical rapamycin as a treatment for fibrofolliculomas in Birt-Hogg-Dube syndrome: a double-blind placebo-controlled randomized split-face trial. PLoS One 2014;9:e99071.

73. Stamatakis L, Metwalli AR, Middelton LA, et al. Diagnosis and management of BHD-associated kidney cancer. Fam Cancer 2013;12:397–402.

74. Bense L, Eklund G, Wiman LG. Smoking and the increased risk of contracting spontaneous pneumothorax. Chest 1987;92:1009–12.

75. British Thoracic Society Fitness to Dive Group, Subgroup of the British Thoracic Society Standards of Care Committee. British Thoracic Society guidelines on respiratory aspects of fitness for diving. Thorax 2003;58:3–13.

76. Hu X, Cowl CT, Baqir M, et al. Air travel and pneumothorax. Chest 2014;145:688–94.

77. Pollock-BarZiv S, Cohen MM, Downey GP, et al. Air travel in women with lymphangioleiomyomatosis. Thorax 2007;62:176–80.

78. Taveira-DaSilva AM, Burstein D, Hathaway OM, et al. Pneumothorax after air travel in lymphangioleiomyomatosis, idiopathic pulmonary fibrosis, and sarcoidosis. Chest 2009;136:665–70.

79. Almoosa KF, Ryu JH, Mendez J, et al. Management of pneumothorax in lymphangioleiomyomatosis: effects on recurrence and lung transplantation complications. Chest 2006;129:1274–81.

80. Cohen HT, McGovern FJ. Renal-cell carcinoma. N Engl J Med 2005;353:2477–90.

81. Jamis-Dow CA, Choyke PL, Jennings SB, et al. Small (< or = 3-cm) renal masses: detection with CT versus US and pathologic correlation. Radiology 1996;198:785–8.

82. Nakamura M, Yao M, Sano F, et al. A case of metastatic renal cell carcinoma associated with Birt-Hogg-Dube syndrome treated with molecular-targeting agents. Hinyokika Kiyo 2013;59:503–6 [in Japanese].

α_1-Antitrypsin Deficiency

Umur Hatipoğlu, MD[a,*], James K. Stoller, MD, MS[b]

KEYWORDS

- α_1-Antitrypsin deficiency • Emphysema • Cirrhosis • Diagnostic testing • Targeted detection
- Augmentation therapy

KEY POINTS

- α_1-Antitrypsin deficiency (AATD) is common but under-recognized.
- Guidelines recommend testing all patients with fixed airflow obstruction.
- The weight of evidence supports the efficacy of intravenous augmentation therapy in slowing emphysema progression.

INTRODUCTION

In 1963, Carl-Bertil Laurell and Sten Eriksson[1] first described AATD based on their noting the absence of the α_1-protein band in serum protein electrophoreses from 5 patients. Three of them had emphysema at a young age (35–44 years) and a family history of emphysema was frequent.[1] The cardinal clinical features of AATD were thereby established: early-onset emphysema and a genetic predisposition both associated with a protein deficiency. In 1969, Sharp and colleagues[2] described cirrhosis in 10 children from 6 families who had severely decreased α_1-globulin and concomitant reductions in tryptic inhibitory capacity. In 1972, Berg and Eriksson[3] reported finding concomitant liver disease and emphysema in 12 of 13 autopsy specimens, suggesting that the disorders were linked to the same genetic defect. Only 53 years after these seminal findings, AATD has been established as one of the most common heritable conditions and provides fascinating insight into a class of clinical conditions called *serpinopathies*, in which defects in protein folding and synthesis confer clinical risk.[4]

This article presents a review of the genetics, pathophysiology, clinical manifestations, natural history, and treatment options for AATD, with an emphasis on lung disease.

GENETICS OF α_1-ANTITRYPSIN DEFICIENCY

AATD is inherited as an autosomal codominant condition. The gene responsible for producing α_1-antitrypsin (AAT) is SERPINA1, which is located on the long arm of chromosome 14 (14q31–32.3) and contains 6 introns, 4 coding (2, 3, 4, and 5) exons, and 3 noncoding (1a, 1b, and 1c) exons. More than 150 AAT allele variants have been described to date.

The protease inhibitor (PI) nomenclature has been devised to describe AAT variants according to their protein expression, which is designated the AAT phenotype. Accordingly, the variants are identified by their migration position in an isoelectric pH (4–5) gradient on gel electrophoresis from A for anodal variants to Z for slower migrating variants. For example, PI*MM, the most common and normal AAT type, describes normal individuals who are homozygous for expressing the M allele. In contrast, PI*ZZ describes individuals who are homozygous for the Z allele and who comprise the majority (95%) of those with clinical disease associated with AATD.

Disclosures: Dr U. Hatipoğlu has no relevant disclosures. Dr J.K. Stoller has served as a consultant to Grifols, CSL Behring, Baxalta, and Kamada. He serves on the Board of Directors of the Alpha-1 Foundation.
a Respiratory Institute, Cleveland Clinic Foundation, 9500 Euclid Avenue, Desk A-90, Cleveland, OH 44195, USA; b Education Institute, Cleveland Clinic Lerner School of Medicine, Cleveland Clinic, NA 22, Cleveland, OH 44195, USA
* Corresponding author.
E-mail address: hatipou@ccf.org

Clin Chest Med 37 (2016) 487–504
http://dx.doi.org/10.1016/j.ccm.2016.04.011
0272-5231/16/$ – see front matter © 2016 Elsevier Inc. All rights reserved.

chestmed.theclinics.com

In contrast to the phenotype, the AAT genotype refers to the specific allelic combination of an individual as demonstrated by allele-specific gene amplification tests or other gene sequencing techniques. For example, a PI*MM individual has a normal whole-gene nucleotide sequence. In contrast, an individual with the PI*ZZ genotype has a single nucleotide polymorphism at position 1096 (guanine to adenosine), which results in a single amino acid substitution (of lysine for glutamic acid at position 342), the latter detectable as the PI*ZZ phenotype if isoelectric focusing (IEF) were also performed.

For clinical purposes, AAT variants are categorized into 4 groups[5]:

1. Normal variants are characterized by normal serum AAT levels (20–53 μM, or approximately 80–220 mg/dL, by nephelometry) and normal AAT function.
2. Deficient variants are characterized by serum levels of AAT less than 20 μM and, for some alleles (eg, Z), concomitantly decreased functional activity of the AAT molecule.
3. Null variants are characterized by absent circulating AAT due to transcriptional or translational errors that interrupt protein synthesis. These variants have been classified PI*QO with specific descriptors, for example, PI*QO$_{cairo}$.
4. Dysfunctional variants are characterized by abnormal function of AAT, for example, with decreased binding to neutrophil elastase (as in the F variant) or with thrombin inhibitory activity (as in the Pittsburgh variant).[6]

EPIDEMIOLOGY OF α_1-ANTITRYPSIN DEFICIENCY

The prevalence of AATD has been estimated both by direct determination in population-based screening studies and by indirect estimates using genetic epidemiologic surveys. Population-based studies are conducted by screening an unselected group of individuals, that is, regardless of their pretest probability of having AATD. Alternately, case-finding or targeted detection is conducted when individuals who have clinical features that prompt suspicion of AATD (including family history) are tested.

The largest population-based screening study for AATD was conducted in Sweden in newborns between November 1972 and September 1974 and included 95% of all of the infants born in the country during that period.[7] Sveger detected 120 PI*ZZ and 2 PI*Z individuals, indicating a prevalence of severe deficiency of AAT of 1 per 1639

live births. In Oregon, O'Brien and colleagues[8] screened 107,038 newborns and identified 21 cases of homozygous-deficient genotypes (PI*ZZ or PI*Z Null) and 11 cases of variant genotypes (including PI*MZ, PI*SZ, and unspecified others), translating to a prevalence of 1/5097 of severe deficiency of AATD. Extrapolating the results of the Oregon study to the US population of approximately 322 million,[9] there are an estimated 63,000 Americans with severe deficiency of AAT, where severe deficiency is defined as having decreased serum levels of AAT that fall below a protective threshold value widely considered to be 11 μM (57 mg/dL by nephelometry).[10]

In a worldwide analysis of data from 514 cohorts (69 countries throughout 11 geographic regions of the world), de Serres[11] estimated the worldwide prevalence of PI*ZZ, PI*SZ, and PI*SS individuals as 3.4 million; when extrapolated to the world population in 2015 (7.3 billion vs 4.4 billion in 2002), the prevalence of AATD individuals is estimated at 5.64 million. There is significant variability in AATD prevalence among different ethnic groups. Although the highest gene frequency for the Z allele is recorded among individuals of Northern European descent,[7,12] AATD is uncommon in some Asian countries, such as China and Indonesia.[12] PI*Siiyama is the most common variant associated with AATD in Japan.[13] Severe AATD is uncommon among African Americans and Hispanic Americans living in the United States, comprising 0.5% and 7.8%, respectively, of the PI*ZZ genotype pool in the United States.[14]

In the context that AATD occurs universally and is common, ample evidence shows that AATD is under-recognized. Three lines of evidence suggest such under-recognition. First, direct surveys of practicing physicians indicate that a minority test for AATD. For example, Greulich and colleagues[15] surveyed 60 German and 30 Italian internists and found that only a third of the physicians reported performing AATD testing as part of their practice. In the same study, although 92% of 60 German pulmonologists surveyed reported screening for AATD, only 54% of 61 Italian pulmonologists performed AATD testing. Furthermore, when asked whether they test all chronic obstructive pulmonary disease (COPD) patients for AATD (in accordance with the guidelines from the American Thoracic Society and European Respiratory Society[5]), only 18% and 25% of German (N = 90) and Italian physicians (N = 65), respectively, responded affirmatively.

As a second line of evidence demonstrating under-recognition, epidemiologic studies consistently show that only a small minority of AATD individuals are recognized across a range of countries. For example, Tobin and colleagues[16] reported that only 4.5% (90/2000) of British AAT-deficient individuals had been identified. Similarly, in the United States, Silverman and colleagues[17] reported a detection rate of approximately 4% of the expected number of AAT-deficient individuals based on sampling blood specimens submitted to a St Louis blood bank. Even in Sweden, where AATD was first recognized and reported, Piitulainen and Tanash recently reported that only approximately 20% of all expected cases of AATD were reported to the Swedish national registry.[18] Recent data from the Canadian registry indicate that there are also significant regional disparities in rate of diagnosis, presumably due to lack of specialty referral centers and variation in public funding for augmentation therapy and genetic testing.[19]

The third line of evidence demonstrating under-recognition of AATD is that affected individuals frequently experience long delays, averaging 5 to 7 years, between the onset of initial symptoms and diagnosis and may see multiple health care providers before initial diagnosis.[15,20,21] These delay intervals have regrettably not changed over approximately 2 decades of observations.[21]

In summary, epidemiologic studies show that AATD is common but has been widely and persistently under-recognized. Because diagnosing AATD can affect a patient's clinical management (eg, lessen an individual's propensity for smoking,[7,8] affect occupational choices to limit dust exposure,[22] and create a management option to recommend augmentation therapy), cost-effective strategies to enhance detection of the many affected individuals are clearly needed.[23]

DIAGNOSIS OF α₁-ANTITRYPSIN DEFICIENCY

As suggested in official guidelines (**Table 1**),[5] laboratory testing for AATD begins with determining the serum level of AAT in individuals with risk factors. Acknowledging the different testing methods (eg, radial immunodiffusion, rocket immunoelectrophoresis, and, most recently, nephelometry) and consequent different reference ranges for AAT, the authors use serum AAT determination by nephelometry as an initial test. When serum levels are low (<100 mg/dL) or when pedigree analysis is needed to clarify familial patterns, phenotyping by IEF or, more commonly, genotyping (by polymerase chain reaction [PCR] assessment and/or gene sequencing) is used to detect an AAT protein variant. Phenotyping is performed by polyacrylamide gel IEF electrophoresis of serum in a gradient between pH 4 and pH 5. Although less costly than molecular genetic

testing, limitations of IEF include the difficulty in interpreting an atypical electrophoretic pattern, resulting from some rare AAT variants and the overlapping nature of some bands.

Genotyping (molecular genetic testing) is performed by analyzing genomic DNA that is extracted from circulating white blood cells or from mouth swabs for direct analysis. Molecular genetic testing usually begins by a targeted approach for the most frequent SERPINA1 pathogenic variants, the S and Z alleles, which account for 95% of clinical cases of AATD. Commercial dried blood spot kits and a free, confidential home-testing kit provided by the Alpha-1 Foundation (http://www.alpha-1foundation.org/alphas/?c=02-Get-Tested) enable simultaneous assessment of AAT serum levels and genotyping. Clinicians must bear in mind the limitation of PCR-based genotyping as it is currently widely practiced, that is, that only some alleles can be interrogated by PCR probes (Z, S commonly, and occasionally I and F). Thus, when these alleles are not found, the report can be misconstrued as indicating PI*MM when another undetected abnormal allele could be present.

If no explanation is found for a low-serum AAT after targeted mutation analysis or if the results of serum level, PCR-based genotyping, and/or the clinical picture are discordant, gene sequence analysis and/or deletion/duplication analysis may be undertaken. If there is suspicion of a specific allele, targeted sequencing can be performed. Increasingly, next-generation sequencing of the entire AAT gene is used to characterize AAT variants.

Serum levels of AAT may increase in certain circumstances, thereby confounding a diagnosis of AATD. The serum level of AAT rises up to 4-fold as an acute-phase reactant during episodes of acute inflammation, cancer, and liver disease in individuals without AATD. Similarly, increases may be seen in heterozygotes for 1 AAT variant, in those with mild AATD, in pregnancy and other high-estrogen states, and in persons receiving blood transfusions or intravenous augmentation therapy (ie, purified pooled human plasma AAT). In PI*ZZ individuals, however, the magnitude of the rise in serum AAT during acute stress is unlikely to be sufficient to mask the diagnosis of severe AATD.

Data from the Swiss Study on Air Pollution and Lung Disease in Adults (SAPALDIA) cohort have provided the first general population estimates for AAT serum ranges for the most common SERPINA1 variants.[24] In this study, a serum AAT level of 100 mg/dL represented an optimal threshold to differentiate between those

Table 1
Clinical indications for genetic testing

Indication	Genetic Testing	
	Recommended	Consider Testing
Pulmonary		
Symptomatic adult with emphysema, COPD, asthma with incompletely reversible airflow obstruction	X	
Asymptomatic with persistent obstruction and risk factors	X	
Symptomatic adult with emphysema, COPD, asthma with incompletely reversible airflow obstruction (in countries with prevalence < North America or Europe)		X
Adults with bronchiectasis without evident etiology		X
Adolescents with persistent airflow obstruction		X
Asymptomatic with persistent airflow obstruction and no risk factors		X
Extrapulmonary		
Unexplained liver disease	X	
Adult with necrotizing panniculitis	X	
Adult with c-ANCA–positive vasculitis		X
Sibling of adult with AATD	X	
Family history of COPD or liver disease not known to be caused by AATD		X
Distant relative of an individual with the PI*ZZ genotype		X
Offspring/parent of an individual the PI*ZZ genotype		X
Sibling, offspring, parent, or distant relative of a heterozygous individual (ie, with the PI*MZ genotype)		X
Carrier status assessment for reproduction planning		
Individual at high risk for AAT deficiency-related disease		X
Partner of individual with the PI*ZZ genotype or the PI*MZ genotype		X
Population screening		
In countries with AATD prevalence >1:1500, prevalent smoking, and adequate counseling services		X

From Stoller JK, Lacbawan FL, Aboussouan LS. Alpha-1 Antitrypsin Deficiency. 2006 Oct 27 [Updated 2014 May 1]. In: Pagon RA, Adam MP, Ardinger HH, et al., editors. GeneReviews® [Internet]. Seattle (WA): University of Washington, Seattle; 1993–2016; with permission.

genotypes with slightly increased emphysema risk (PI*SS and PI*MZ) versus not (PI*MM and PI*MS) (sensitivity 95.8% and specificity 94.8%). In a retrospective analysis of 72,229 consecutive samples referred for testing for AAT deficiency, the most common allele combinations were MM (80.4%), MS (7.6%), MZ (7.1%), ZZ (1.1%), and SZ (0.74%).[25] In that series, Bornhorst and colleagues[25] reported a 99.5% sensitivity and 96.5% specificity for detecting the PI*ZZ genotype using a serum AAT cutoff of 85 mg/dL. **Table 2** summarizes the relationship between genotype, serum level, and pulmonary risk. Based on early observations by Gadek and colleagues,[26] many clinicians regard a serum level of 57 mg/dL or 11 μM as the serum AAT protective threshold

value, that is, that value below which the risk of emphysema associated with AATD develops.

PATHOPHYSIOLOGY

AAT is a serine PI (serpin) with the chief function of neutralizing the proteolytic action of neutrophil elastase, an enzyme contained in the azurophilic granules of neutrophils. The name, *antitrypsin*, is historical and reflects the early observation that AAT can bind and inhibit the biological activity of the enzyme trypsin in vitro even though trypsin inhibition is unrelated to the biologic function of AAT in preventing emphysema. Other serpin proteins include $\alpha_1$antichymotrypsin, antithrombin III, C1 inhibitor, and neuroserpin. Also, conformational

Table 2
Relationship of α_1-antitrypsin protein variants to serum α_1-antitrypsin levels and emphysema risk in adults

α_1-Antitrypsin Protein Variants	Prevalence (%)			Serum α_1-Antitrypsin Levels		
	Worldwide	North America	Europe	True Level, µmol/L (Mean [5th–95th Percentile])	Commercial Standard, mg/dL (Median [5th–95th Percentile])	Emphysema Risk
MM	96.3	93.0	91.1	33 (20–53)	147 (102–254)	Background
MS	2.7	4.8	6.6	33 (18–52)	125 (86–218)	Background
MZ	0.8	2.1	1.9	25.4 (15–42)	90 (62–151)	Background[a]
SS	0.08	0.1	0.3	28 (20–48)	95 (43–154)	Background
SZ	0.02	0.1	0.1	16.5 (10–23)	62 (33–108)	20%–50%
ZZ	0.003	0.01	0.01	5.3 (3.4–7)	<29 (<29–52)	80%–100%
Null-Null	—	—	—	0	0	100%

[a] Smokers with the PI*MZ genotype may be at a higher risk of obstructive lung disease than PI*MM counterparts.[27,28]

From Stoller JK, Lacbawan FL, Aboussouan LS. Alpha-1 Antitrypsin Deficiency. 2006 Oct 27 [Updated 2014 May 1]. In: Pagon RA, Adam MP, Ardirger HH, et al., editors. GeneReviews® [Internet]. Seattle (WA): University of Washington, Seattle; 1993–2016; with permission.

disorders of serpins associated with their intracellular accumulation have been observed in several conditions which have been collectively named *serpinopathies*.

Fig. 1 shows the mousetrap-like mechanism by which AAT binds to and neutralizes neutrophil elastase. Serpinopathies are characterized by either a so-called toxic loss-of-function defect (ie, emphysema, angioedema, and thrombosis in the cases of AATD, C1 inhibitor, and antithrombin deficiency, respectively) or a toxic gain-of-function defect due to accumulation of abnormal protein (as in cirrhosis or dementia in the cases of AATD and neuroserpinopathy, respectively). In individuals with the PI*ZZ genotype, the single amino acid substitution of lysine for glutamic acid at position 342 causes a conformationally unstable Z-type AAT protein, which polymerizes within the endoplasmic reticulum of hepatocytes. Polymerization prevents protein secretion with only 15% of the Z-type AAT protein appearing in the serum.[29,30] The dual consequences are (1) accumulation of toxic Z-type AAT protein polymers in the liver (toxic gain of function) and (2) reduced serum antiproteolytic capacity (toxic loss of function). During periods of heightened neutrophilic inflammation in the lung, neutrophil elastase and other proteases can go unchecked, causing elastolysis and emphysema. In addition to a quantitative deficiency, Z-type AAT protein also has reduced affinity for neutrophil elastase.

Compounding the lack of a proteolytic screen, Z-type AATD predisposes to inflammation in several ways. Specifically, Alam and colleagues[31] demonstrated higher concentrations of pulmonary cytokines (tumor necrosis factor α, interleukin-6, and nuclear factor κB), inflammatory cells (neutrophils and macrophages), and increased endoplasmic reticulum stress in transgenic Z-type AAT mice lungs compared with M-type AAT counterparts. Furthermore, these investigators showed increases in intracellular Z protein AAT polymers, cytokine concentrations, and the endoplasmic reticulum stress response when Z AAT-transfected human pulmonary epithelial cells were incubated with cigarette smoke extract. An inhibitor of polymerization, an antioxidant (*N*-acetylcysteine), and an inhibitor of endoplasmic reticulum stress response all significantly mitigated the inflammatory response associated with cigarette smoke extract. Taken together, these findings indicate multiple mechanisms that predispose to emphysema in

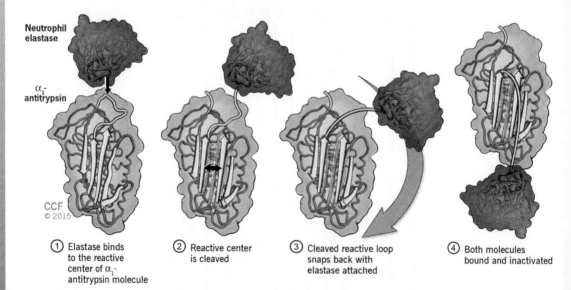

Neutrophil elastase

α_1-antitrypsin

CCF
© 2015

① Elastase binds to the reactive center of α_1-antitrypsin molecule

② Reactive center is cleaved

③ Cleaved reactive loop snaps back with elastase attached

④ Both molecules bound and inactivated

Fig. 1. The binding of AAT protein to neutrophil elastase and subsequent neutralization of neutrophil elastase. The reactive center of the AAT molecule, a methionine amino acid side chain, is cleaved on binding of the neutrophil elastase. Akin to a mousetrap, the cleaved reactive loop snaps back with the bound neutrophil elastase to the contralateral pole of the AAT molecule, inactivating the enzyme by squeezing it. (Images based on original models created using Molecular Maya [https://clarafi.com/tools/mmaya/] and PDB: 1ATU [Ryu SE, Choi HJ. The Native Strains in the Hydrophobic Core and Flexible Reactive Loop of a Serine Protease Inhibitor: Crystal Structure of an Uncleaved Alpha 1-antitrypsin at 2.7 A. Structure 1996;4:1181–92]; and PDB: 5AOC [vonNussbaum F, Li VMJ, Allerheiligen S, et al. Crystal structure of human neutrophil elastase in complex with a dihydropyrimidone inhibitor.])

PI*ZZ AATD. Environmental factors, such as cigarette smoke, are significant instigators of such inflammation and subsequent lung injury.

PULMONARY MANIFESTATIONS OF α_1-ANTITRYPSIN DEFICIENCY

AATD has been clearly associated with COPD, including emphysema, chronic bronchitis, and bronchiectasis. Findings from the National Heart, Lung, and Blood Institute (NHLBI) registry show that individuals with severe deficiency of AATD manifest the same symptoms as do patients with usual, or AAT-replete, COPD.[32] These symptoms (in order of decreasing frequency) include dyspnea (84%), wheezing with upper respiratory infections (76%), wheezing with dyspnea (51%), increased cough and phlegm (50%), usual phlegm (46%), and usual cough (40%).

The high prevalence of wheezing among AATD individuals and the observation, as with usual COPD, that a component of reversible airflow obstruction (defined as a 12% and 200-mL rise in the forced expiratory volume in the first second of expiration [FEV_1] postbronchodilator) is common among AATD individuals (ie, 61% prevalence with 3 serial spirometries) supports testing those patients with irreversible airflow obstruction who carry the clinical impression of asthma.

In the face of the similarity between symptoms of AATD and usual COPD, some features may help distinguish those with AATD. For example, although the signs and symptoms of emphysema frequently first become apparent in the seventh decade in patients with AAT-replete or usual COPD, patients with AATD commonly first manifest symptoms in the fourth or fifth decade of life. In the NHLBI registry of 1129 individuals with severe AATD, the average age of subjects was 46 years and most experienced dyspnea.[32] In earlier series, the mean age of presentation was reported between 32 and 41 years of age.[16,33,34] In a follow-up study of 35-year-old PI*ZZ individuals who were diagnosed at birth, early CT evidence of emphysema was evident only in smokers.[35]

Another distinctive clinical feature of AATD regards the anatomic distribution of emphysema in the lung. In AATD, emphysema more commonly involves the lower lung zones (so-called basilar-predominant hyperlucency) than in usual COPD, where apical involvement predominates. Parr and colleagues[36] observed that 64% of 120 PI*ZZ individuals had lower lobe–predominant emphysema on chest CT; the remainder had upper lobe–predominant emphysema, emphasizing the importance of testing all COPD patients for AATD, lest those with more typical COPD features escape diagnosis.

As with usual COPD, the pulmonary function test features of patients with AATD include fixed airflow obstruction (often with a component of reversible airflow obstruction as noted in Ref.[32]) and reduced diffusion capacity.

How individuals are detected (or ascertained) relates to their clinical features and prognosis. For example, in the NHLBI registry, individuals with normal lung function (postbronchodilator FEV_1 >80% and diffusing capacity of lung for carbon monoxide $\geq$80%) were more likely to have been ascertained as so-called nonindex cases (ie, those detected because they were family members of probands) compared with those with abnormal lung function (79% vs 12%).

NATURAL HISTORY OF α_1-ANTITRYPSIN DEFICIENCY–RELATED LUNG DISEASE

Individuals with severe AATD experience accelerated decline of lung function on average. Among 927 subjects of the NHLBI registry[37] who had greater than or equal to 2 FEV_1 measurements at least 1 year apart, mean rates of FEV_1 decline were 67 mL/y, 54 mL/y, and 109 mL/y, respectively, in never-smokers, former smokers, and current smokers. In the Swedish national AATD registry,[38] a cohort of 608 adult PI*ZZ patients followed over a median of 5.5 years had mean rates of FEV_1 decline of 47 mL/y, 41 mL/y, and 70 mL/y in never-smokers, exsmokers, and current smokers, respectively. Rates of FEV_1 decline vary by Global Initiative for Chronic Obstructive Lung Disease (GOLD) strata in AATD, with those with GOLD 2 and GOLD 3 COPD experiencing the fastest rates of decline (90.1 ± 19.7 mL/y and 51.9 ± 7.6 mL/y, respectively).[39] In addition to smoking, factors associated with faster decline of lung function in AATD include baseline functional capacity, exacerbation frequency, reversible airway disease, and low body mass index.[39] As with symptoms, the method of ascertaining AATD affects the natural history. In a retrospective observational study of 591 subjects with severe AATD from the British ADAPT (Antitrypsin Deficiency and Program for Treatment) database,[40] index cases had earlier impairment in pulmonary function, poorer health-related quality-of-life scores, and more emphysema on CT scan of the chest compared with nonindex cases. The study also clarified the temporal progression of pulmonary manifestations of AATD in never-smoking, nonindex cases (**Fig. 2**).

Smoking status also conditions prognosis and interacts with ascertainment method in AATD. Specifically, Tanash and colleagues[41] reported

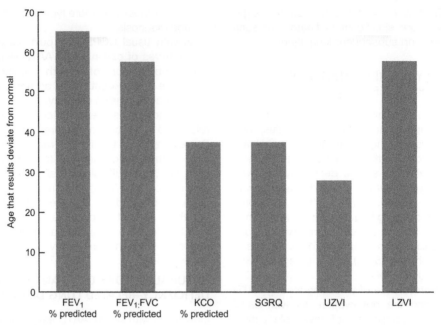

Fig. 2. Age at which pulmonary function, quality-of-life, and radiological parameters deviated from normal among never-smoking nonindex subjects. After splitting the cohort into 5-year age strata, measurements that were less than 80% of predicted (pulmonary function values) or greater than 1.96 standard errors above the mean data derived from the normal population (quality-of-life and radiological parameters) were deemed abnormal. The earliest age group in which the proportion of subjects with abnormal values was consistently greater than 50% was taken as "the age at which results deviated from normal." The order of onset of signs and symptoms (from early onset to later) is upper lung zone emphysema, impairment of diffusion capacity (predicted transfer factor), abnormal health-related quality of life, lower zone emphysema on CT, decreased FEV_1/FVC ratio, and, lastly, decreased FEV_1 % predicted. Decreased FEV_1 lagged behind CT presentation by approximately 28 years. KCO, carbon monoxide transfer factor corrected for alveolar volume; LZVI, lower zone voxel index; SGRQ, St. George's Respiratory Questionnaire; UZVI, upper zone voxel index. (*Adapted from* Holme J, Stockley JA, Stockley RA. Age related development of respiratory abnormalities in non-index α-1 antitrypsin deficient studies. Respir Med 2013;107(3):391.)

that never-smoking PI*ZZ individuals identified as nonindex individuals with no symptoms had normal life spans compared with the Swedish general population (odds ratio [OR] of death 0.7). In contrast, those presenting with lung or liver symptoms both experienced impaired prognoses (ie, standardized mortality ratios >1).

Environmental factors also modify the decline in lung function in patients with AATD. In a cross-sectional study of 128 PI*ZZ individuals, occupational exposures to dust, fume, smoke, and gas were independently associated with worse lung function and the presence of respiratory symptoms.[22] Wood and colleagues[42] reported associations between particulate matter exposure and faster decline in FEV_1 as well as ozone exposure and faster decline in gas transfer among 220 PI*ZZ subjects in the UK national registry for AATD. Furthermore, a 4-year longitudinal cohort study among New York City firefighters who had inhalational exposure to particulate material after the World Trade Center collapse demonstrated

faster declines in FEV_1 in subjects with moderate (PI*MZ, PI*SZ; n = 4) and mild (PI*MS, PI*SS; n = 7) AATD compared with normal subjects (PI*MM; n = 79).[43]

The main cause of death in individuals with severe deficiency of AAT is also conditioned by the method of ascertainment. In the NHLBI registry where 84% of subjects were former smokers, emphysema accounted for 72% of deaths and cirrhosis for 12%.[37] In the Swedish national registry, respiratory disease accounted for 58% of all deaths followed by liver disease in 12%.[44] Among never-smokers, however, emphysema accounted for 45% of deaths and liver disease accounted for 28% of deaths, consistent with the notion that never-smokers may escape the early ravages of emphysema but potentially succumb to later onset of cirrhosis and its sequelae.

Recent studies suggest that a subset of PI*MZ heterozygote smokers also may be susceptible to developing COPD. Molloy and colleagues[45] reported a family-based study in which 89 nonindex

PI*MZ subjects were compared with 99 PI*MM subjects related to the same 51 index probands with COPD. In aggregate, PI*MZ heterozygotes were found to have lower postbronchodilator FEV_1, FEV_1/forced vital capacity (FVC) ratio, and FEF 25-75% compared with PI*MM subjects. The adjusted OR for a spirometric diagnosis of COPD in ever-smoking PI*MZ heterozygotes was 10.65 (95% CI, 2.17–52.29). There was no increased risk, however, for COPD among never-smoking individuals with PI*MZ (OR 0.24; 95% CI, 0.01–5.21). Also, a recent report that combined a Norwegian case-control study (n = 1669) with a family-based International COPD Genetics Network study (n = 2707) also suggests that the PI*MZ genotype is associated with slightly higher risk of airflow obstruction as measured by FEV_1/FVC ratio, although no significant difference was demonstrated for FEV_1.[46] Furthermore, PI*MZ subjects who had low tobacco smoke exposure (<20 pack years) had more severe emphysema, as determined by the percent of lung voxels with low attenuation area ($\leq$ 950 HU) on chest CT compared with PI*MM subjects in both cohorts.

Radiographic evidence of bronchiectasis is frequent among individuals with PI*ZZ AATD, occurring in 95% of chest CT scans.[47] In that same series by Parr and colleagues,[47] clinical bronchiectasis was less frequent (27%). At the same time, Cuvelier and colleagues[48] reported that in a series of consecutive patients with bronchiectasis, AATD was no more prevalent than among normal subjects. On this basis, official guidelines suggest testing for AATD among patients with bronchiectasis when other causes of bronchiectasis (eg, hypogammaglobulinemia and cystic fibrosis) have been excluded (see **Table 1**).[5]

LIVER DISEASE IN α_1-ANTITRYPSIN DEFICIENCY

Sharp and colleagues[2] first reported both the association between AATD and liver disease in 10 children from 6 different kindreds and the characteristic periodic acid–Schiff/diastase-resistant globules, which were later found to be polymerized Z-AAT protein within hepatocytes. Liver involvement in AATD includes hepatitis, cirrhosis, and hepatoma and is caused by intrahepatocyte AAT polymerization with subsequent interruption of protein secretion. The 4 alleles reported to be associated with AAT polymerization are Z, Mmalton, King's, and Siiyama.[49] Null genotypes are not associated with liver disease because no AAT protein is produced.

The natural history of liver disease in AATD has been clarified by longitudinal studies of individuals identified with AATD at birth. In the Swedish newborn screening cohort, 22 of the 122 PI*Z newborns (18%) displayed liver function abnormalities that included obstructive jaundice and abnormal liver enzymes.[7] Four deaths during infancy were attributed to cirrhosis (2), aplastic anemia (n = 1, whose postmortem examination confirmed cirrhosis), and an accidental death with the postmortem showing early liver fibrosis. Cholestasis afflicted 11% of newborns with AATD and was transient.

Estimates suggest that 2% to 3% of PI*ZZ children develop liver cirrhosis during childhood.[50] Liver symptoms manifest in early adulthood but may develop later; a postmortem study of 94 deceased PI*ZZ individuals in the Swedish cohort showed evidence of cirrhosis in 37% of cases.[27,28] The older age of individuals with cirrhosis compared with individuals without cirrhosis (65.5 vs 53.6 years of age) supports the idea that those who escape emphysema in earlier years may develop liver disease later in life.[28]

In the absence of specific therapy for liver disease other than liver transplantation – at least currently – the prognosis of individuals with cirrhosis associated with AATD is generally poor, with an estimated mean survival of approximately 2 years.[28]

Although the evidence is mixed,[51] conventional wisdom has been that AATD confers an increased risk of liver cancer – both hepatocellular carcinoma and cholangiocarcinoma. Liver cancer has developed independent of the presence of cirrhosis and in also heterozygous PI*Z AAT individuals.[52]

Surveillance for liver disease in patients with AATD is recommended,[5] although the optimal assessment strategy is unclear. Dawwas and colleagues[53] evaluated the role of blood tests (liver function profiles and complete blood cell counts) as well as hepatic ultrasound in identifying liver disease in a series of 57 PI*ZZ individuals with established lung disease. The absence of abnormal liver echogenicity on hepatic ultrasound had 100% negative predictive value for liver disease. An elevated ALT (>70 U/L) and low platelets ($\leq$174,000/mm^3) showed 95% and 100% specificity for severe liver fibrosis or cirrhosis, respectively. On this basis, Dawwas and colleagues recommend periodic liver function tests, a complete blood cell count, and hepatic ultrasound to detect advanced liver disease in individuals with PI*ZZ AATD and lung disease. Although some studies have found liver function tests to have limited utility in detecting liver disease in AATD,[54] official guidelines recommend regular assessment of simple liver function tests in elderly individuals with AAT deficiency who lack liver symptoms.[5]

VASCULITIS IN α_1-ANTITRYPSIN DEFICIENCY

The association between antiproteinase 3 (PR3) antibody–positive vasculitis (usually c–antineutrophil cytoplasmic autoantibody [ANCA] positive) and AATD was reported more than 20 years ago.[55,56] Among patients with c-ANCA–positive vasculitis, prevalence estimates for the Z allele are between 5.6% and 17.6%, exceeding the frequency among normal individuals by 3-fold to 9-fold.[57] Furthermore, having a Z allele may be associated with a poor prognosis in c-ANCA–positive vasculitis. Among patients with PR3-ANCA–positive vasculitis, the mortality rate was increased in heterozygotes for the Z-allele compared with non-PI*Z carriers (39% vs 16%, respectively).[58] Moreover, Mota and colleagues[59] reported a 24% reduction in specific AAT activity among 27 patients with granulomatosis with polyangiitis compared with 63 controls, despite no significant difference in serum AAT concentrations, leading to speculation that increased oxidation or enzymatic degradation accounts for the reduced AAT enzymatic activity.

The association between c-ANCA–positive vasculitis and AATD has prompted the recommendation that testing for AATD should be considered in all adults with c-ANCA–positive vasculitis[5] (see **Table 1**). Simultaneous determination of the phenotype or genotype along with the serum AAT level is usually required in testing GPA patients for AATD because the acute-phase reactivity of AAT can cause serum AAT levels to rise during the acute inflammation of vasculitis.[57,58]

PANNICULITIS AND OTHER PROPOSED DISEASE ASSOCIATIONS WITH α_1-ANTITRYPSIN DEFICIENCY

Panniculitis refers to inflammation of the subcutaneous adipose tissue[60,61] and was first reported in association with AATD by Warter and colleagues.[60] Panniculitis is a rare clinical feature of AATD with fewer than 100 individuals with AATD-associated panniculitis reported in the literature. In the NHLBI registry, only 1 of 1129 study subjects reported panniculitis.[32] Several AAT genotypes have been associated with panniculitis, including PI*ZZ, PI*SZ, PI*SS, and PI*MS. Clinically, panniculitis manifests as painful, hot, red, tender nodules, characteristically in areas of trauma (eg, thighs and/or buttocks). Ulceration, fluid drainage, and histologic evidence of both elastic tissue damage and necrosis are more prevalent in AATD-associated panniculitis than in other types.[62,63] Traumatic injuries are reported in one-third of patients as a precipitating event.[63] Although the prognosis is mostly determined by the presence of other AATD-related organ complications like cirrhosis or emphysema, AATD-associated panniculitis may cause debilitating disfigurement (eg, breast necrosis). Because panniculitis is thought to be a consequence of unopposed proteolysis in the subcutaneous tissue, several reports have described favorable responses to infusing purified pooled human plasma AAT (ie, augmentation therapy).[64,65]

TREATMENT OF α_1-ANTITRYPSIN DEFICIENCY

In general, treatment of COPD due to AATD resembles treatment of usual COPD, with smoking cessation, long-acting bronchodilators, preventive vaccinations, pulmonary rehabilitation, supplemental oxygen if indicated, and lung transplantation for advanced disease.[66–68] The role of lung volume reduction surgery (LVRS) does differ in AATD, because the sparse available experience has shown a shorter duration and smaller magnitude of effect of LVRS in AATD compared with individuals with AAT-replete COPD.[69] Currently, specific therapy for AATD-associated lung disease is called augmentation therapy.

Augmentation Therapy

Augmentation therapy is the intravenous infusion of purified pooled human plasma AAT with a biochemical goal to raise and maintain serum AAT levels above the serum protective threshold and a clinical goal to slow the progression of emphysema and enhance the duration and quality of life. Four preparations of purified AAT have received Food and Drug Administration approval based on satisfying biochemical criteria for efficacy, that is, that regular infusions raise serum levels above the protective threshold values, that such levels remain above the protective threshold for most of the dosing interval, and that the infused AAT retains its functional activity to neutralize neutrophil elastase activity.

In examining the evidence for clinical efficacy of augmentation therapy (**Table 3**), large observational studies[37,70–72] are generally concordant in showing that augmentation therapy recipients experienced a slower rate of FEV_1 decline than nonrecipients. In the NHLBI registry, the greatest benefit in slowing FEV_1 rate of decline was observed in individuals with moderate degrees of airflow obstruction, that is, values of FEV_1 between 35% and 65% predicted.[37] In a before–after study by Wencker and colleagues,[71] the greatest effect of augmentation therapy in changing FEV_1 slope was observed in individuals with a rapid FEV_1 decline before augmentation therapy was initiated (ie, FEV_1 decline 256 mL/y before therapy vs 53 mL/y during therapy).

Table 3
Clinical efficacy studies of augmentation therapy

First Author (Reference), Year	Design	Infusion Interval	Main Results
Stone et al,[73] 1995	Observational cohort	Monthly	Urine desmosine level fell while on treatment
Seersholm et al,[70] 1997	Observational cohort, concurrent controls	Weekly	In patients with FEV_1 31%–65% predicted, augmentation slowed the decline of FEV_1 by 21 mL/y ($P = .04$).
NHLBI registry,[37] 1998	Observational cohort, concurrent controls	51% Weekly 25% Biweekly 22% Monthly	In patients with FEV_1 35%–49% predicted, augmentation slowed the decline of FEV_1 by 27 mL/y ($P = .03$). In the whole group, the risk ratio of death was 0.64 compared with nonrecipients ($P = .02$).
Dirksen et al,[74] 1999	Randomized controlled trial	Every 28 d	Loss of lung tissue (by CT densitometry) was 1.5 g/L/y with augmentation and 2.6 g/L/y with placebo ($P = .07$). FEV_1 decline was not significantly reduced.
Gottlieb et al,[75] 2000	Descriptive	Weekly	Augmentation did not reduce elastin degradation rate.
Lieberman,[76] 2000	Observational (Web-based survey)	56% Weekly 36% Biweekly	7% Monthly The number of lung infections per year decreased from 3 to 5 preaugmentation to 0–1 postaugmentation.
Wencker et al,[71] 2001	Observational (before–after)	Weekly	Rates of FEV_1 decline preaugmentation and postaugmentation were 49.2 vs 34.2 mL/y, respectively ($P = .019$).
Stockley et al,[77] 2002	Descriptive	Weekly	Augmentation reduced sputum leukotriene B4.
Dirksen et al,[78] 2009	Randomized controlled trial	Weekly	Using the first and last CT scans with covariates adjustment, loss of lung tissue was 2.9 g/L with augmentation therapy vs 4.1 g/L in placebo ($P<.05$).
Tonelli et al,[72] 2009	Observational	Weekly	In augmentation therapy recipients, rate of FEV_1 change was +10.6 + 21.4 mL/y vs −39.96 + 12.1 mL/y in nonrecipients ($P = .05$).
Schmid et al,[79] 2012	Descriptive	Weekly	Augmentation reduced serum IL-8 levels.
Barros-Tizón[80] 2012	Observational (retrospective)	6.3% Weekly 17.3% Biweekly 76.4% Every 3 wk	Augmentation reduced exacerbation rate in the population with exacerbation history (2.0 ± 1.6 vs 1.4 ± 2.7 per year).
Ma et al,[81] 2013	Observational with controls (retrospective)	Not available	Augmentation (inhaled and intravenous) was associated with significant reduction in elastin degradation, although not to control levels.
Chapman et al,[82] 2015	Randomized controlled trial	Weekly	Augmentation led to reduction in the annual rate of loss in lung density measured at TLC (-1.45 ± 0.23 g/L vs -2.19 ± 0.25 g/L).

Adapted from Stoller JK, Aboussouan LS. A review of α-1 antitrypsin deficiency. Am J Respir Crit Care Med 2012;185(3):253; with permission.

Three randomized, placebo-controlled trials of augmentation therapy have been conducted[74,78,82] and, although none is definitive in the authors' view, the aggregate evidence shows that augmentation therapy can slow emphysema progression as measured by declines in CT lung density. None of the randomized trials shows that augmentation therapy is associated with slowing FEV_1 decline or reduction in overall exacerbation frequency, although some post hoc analyses suggest a lessening of exacerbation severity.[78]

On the basis of the available evidence, the American Thoracic Society/European Respiratory Society recommendations regarding augmentation therapy are as follows: "Recognizing that supportive evidence of efficacy comes from concordant observational studies but not from a randomized controlled clinical trial, the Task Force recommends intravenous augmentation therapy for individuals with established airflow obstruction from AAT deficiency. Evidence that augmentation therapy confers benefit (eg, slowed rate of FEV_1 decline and decreased mortality) is stronger for individuals with moderate airflow obstruction (eg, FEV_1 35%–60% predicted) than for those with severe airflow obstruction. Augmentation therapy is not currently recommended for individuals without emphysema, and benefits in individuals with severe (eg, $FEV_1 \leq 35\%$ predicted) or mild (eg, $FEV_1 \geq 50\%$–60% predicted) airflow obstruction are less clear." Although multiple dosing regimens have been examined,[83,84] the only Food and Drug Administration–approved regimen for augmentation therapy currently is 60 mg/kg once weekly. Dose-ranging studies to examine the possible benefits of higher doses (120 mg/kg/wk) are under way.[85]

Augmentation therapy is not recommended for PI*MZ heterozygotes who may have COPD,[86] based on the absence of any supportive evidence of efficacy for heterozygotes and the biologic unlikelihood of benefit for such individuals; PI*MZ heterozygotes rarely have serum levels below the serum protective threshold value of 11 μM. For PI*SZ heterozygotes, approximately 10% of such individuals may have serum levels below 11 μM.[87] Therefore, despite the absence of studies specifically addressing the issue, symptomatic PI*SZ individuals with COPD may be candidates for augmentation therapy.

Augmentation therapy is well tolerated and safe. Wencker and colleagues[88] reported the experience of 443 augmentation therapy recipients, of whom 65 experienced a total of 124 adverse events. The most common adverse reactions were fever/chills (17 patients), urticaria (18 patients), nausea and vomiting (21 patients), and fatigue (7 patients). No deaths were observed. In the NHLBI registry, among 747 augmentation therapy recipients, 174 subjects reported 720 adverse events, the most common of which were dyspnea (47%) and dizziness/fainting (17%). The overall incidence of adverse events was very low (approximately 0.02 events per patient-month). Augmentation therapy recipients experienced on average less than 2 adverse events over 5 years of continuous therapy. Hepatitis, HIV, or prion disease transmission has not been linked to intravenous augmentation therapy to date.

Available studies of the cost-effectiveness of augmentation therapy have shown that it fails to satisfy conventional criteria for a cost-effective intervention (<$50,000/quality-adjusted life-year). All augmentation therapy drugs are expensive (approximately $100,000/y or more in the United States). In the study by Gildea and colleagues,[89] augmentation therapy given until FEV_1 fell below 35% predicted had an incremental cost-effectiveness ratio of $207,841/quality-adjusted life-year. At the same time, until an alternative, effective treatment becomes available, augmentation therapy remains the only specific therapy available for AATD-associated COPD and has been recommended in specific contexts.[5,90]

Lung Transplantation

AATD accounts for approximately 5% of all lung transplantations performed in the United States. According to the registry of the International Society for Heart and Lung Transplantation, AATD-COPD patients who received lung transplantation (n = 2187) had better long-term survival compared with those with usual COPD (n = 9616) (survival half-life 6.1 vs 5.2 years; $P = .01$).[91] The registry data suggested bilateral lung transplant recipients fared better than single lung recipients. Outcomes of lung transplantation vary considerably, however, across individual centers, likely reflecting local variation in candidate selection and practice. For example, reports from Washington University Medical Center in St. Louis,[92] the Copenhagen National Lung Transplant Group,[93] and Zurich University Hospital[94] reported no difference in 5-year survival rates between AATD-COPD and usual COPD recipients. In contrast, the Toronto group reported that AATD patients had lower 10-year survival (23% vs 43%) compared with usual COPD patients.[95] A recent study from the 2 national lung transplantation centers in Sweden[96] documented a median survival time for AATD-COPD patients of 12 years compared with only 6 years for usual COPD patients. This difference persisted after adjustment for age, smoking status, body mass index, oxygen use, exercise capacity, donor age, cytomegalovirus mismatch, and transplant type.

The question of whether lung transplantation confers a survival advantage over the natural history of the disease has been addressed in preliminary fashion in a case-control study by Tanash and colleagues.[97] These investigators matched 83 severe AATD-COPD patients who underwent lung transplantation with 70 control cases (AATD-COPD patients who did not undergo transplantation selected from the Swedish national AATD registry). The estimated median survival time was 11 years in transplant recipients versus 5 years in controls. Banga and colleagues[98] recently reported the natural history of lung function after lung transplantation for patients with usual (231 patients) versus AATD-COPD (45 patients) at the Cleveland Clinic. Although the overall rate of decline in FEV_1 slope and survival did not differ between the 2 groups, a trend toward worse early post–lung transplantation survival was observed in the AATD group. Also, though unexplained, the rate of FEV_1 decline among AATD patients who received double lung transplantation was faster than among single lung recipients.

Lung Volume Reduction

Results of the National Emphysema Treatment Trial[69] have clearly shown that in carefully selected subsets, LVRS for COPD can confer significant physiologic, functional, and survival benefits. Data regarding the efficacy of LVRS for individuals with AATD are more limited and generally less favorable in that the magnitude and duration of FEV_1 improvement following LVRS in AATD individuals was smaller. For example, in analyzing the AATD subset within NETT, Stoller and colleagues[99] compared outcomes in the 10 AATD individuals with 554 AAT-replete subjects. As shown in **Fig. 3**, the magnitude and duration of FEV_1 improvement was more modest in the AATD subjects. Similar observations from other small series of AATD LVRS recipients[100–103] support the limited utility of LVRS in AATD. Although clinical practice varies markedly, most clinicians do not recommend LVRS for individuals with AATD, with some advocating LVRS as a bridge to lung transplantation.[104] Guidelines from the American Thoracic Society/European

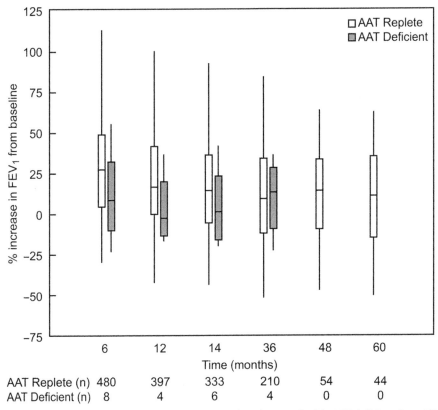

	6	12	14	36	48	60
AAT Replete (n)	480	397	333	210	54	44
AAT Deficient (n)	8	4	6	4	0	0

Fig. 3. Comparison of improvement in FEV_1 among AAT replete (n = 554) with AAT-deficient (n = 10) subjects in the NETT (National Emphysema Treatment Trial) cohort. The magnitude and duration of FEV_1 improvement was more modest in the AATD subjects. None of the AAT-deficient subjects were in the upper lobe–predominant, low exercise capacity subset of patients who derive the greatest benefit from LVRS. (*From* Stoller JK, Gildea TR, Ries AL, et al. Lung volume reduction surgery in patients with emphysema and alpha-1 antitrypsin deficiency. Ann Thorac Surg 2007;83(1):247; with permission.)

Respiratory Society regarding LVRS state: "The scant evidence regarding the efficacy of LVRS (with possible resection of lower lobes) in individuals with AAT deficiency suggests that improvement in dyspnea, lung function, and functional status is possible. However, well studied, robust selection criteria for ideal candidates remain elusive and the duration of LVRS benefit appears shorter than individuals with AAT-replete COPD."

Given the promise of reversibility and lower postprocedure morbidity and mortality, endoscopic lung volume reduction by inserting 1-way endobronchial valves has been studied in a small number of AATD individuals.[105,106] For example, Tuohy and colleagues[105] reported experience with placing a second-generation endobronchial 1-way valve, the Zephyr (Emphasys, Redwood City, California) in 6 patients with severe symptomatic AATD-COPD and reported a median 330 mL improvement in FEV_1 as well as improvement in the body mass index, airflow obstruction, dyspnea, and exercise capacity (BODE) index to less than 7 in 2 of the 6 subjects. Procedure-related complications (pneumothorax, expectoration of valve, and frequent infective exacerbations) were reported in 4 of the 6 patients. Similarly, in a series of 15 consecutive patients with AATD-COPD who underwent endobronchial placement of Zephyr valves for severe emphysema, Hillerdal and colleagues[106] reported an average FEV_1 improvement of 397 mL compared with baseline. This improvement was sustained in the 6 patients who were followed for 2 years, in 3 patients for 3 years, and in 3 patients for 4 years. Because an intact fissure line on the CT scan was an inclusion criterion for the study, Hillerdal and colleagues[106] speculated that the sustained improvement was related to preserved fissures and the absence of collateral ventilation.

FUTURE DIRECTIONS

Many promising lines of research are under way regarding new treatment strategies for AATD, regarding both pulmonary and hepatic manifestations. These include gene therapy by delivering (through various approaches) recombinant adeno-associated virus carrying the human AAT gene,[107,108] inhibiting intrahepatic polymerization of AAT,[109,110] promoting hepatic secretion of AAT,[111,112] prolonging the serum half-life of AAT by pegylation,[113] inhalation of AAT, interfering with mutant (and native) AAT production by small interfering RNA, enhancing intrahepatic degradation of mutant AAT by stimulating autophagy (eg, by carbamazepine[114] or rapamycin[115]), and varying the delivered dose of intravenous

augmentation therapy. A recent dose escalation trial of recombinant adeno-associated virus expressing normal human AAT in 9 PI*ZZ AAT–deficient subjects showed that the highest dose produced levels less than 7% of the protective threshold value of 11 μM.[116] Because AAT expression was limited by vector dosage (ie, the highest dose required 100 intramuscular injections), improvements in vector delivery are necessary to attain adequate AAT expression. Approaches currently under investigation include isolated limb perfusion and intrapleural instillation of the vector.[117] Delivery of AAT by inhalation is also currently being studied (https://clinicaltrials.gov/ct2/show/study/NCT01217671) and offers the prospect of lower cost and enhanced convenience.[118] Human studies have established complete inhibition of neutrophil elastase activity and marked reduction in elastin degradation[81] in bronchoalveolar lavage fluid after inhaled AAT treatment.

In summary, in the 54 years since AATD was first described, impressive strides in understanding the pathobiology and clinical course of AATD have been made. At the same time, continuing challenges include how to detect all affected individuals and how to better slow emphysema progression and liver disease in affected individuals. Emerging management options show great promise in improving outcomes of patients with AATD.

REFERENCES

1. Laurell CB, Eriksson S. The electrophoretic alpha-1 globulin pattern of serum in alpha-1 antitrypsin deficiency. Scand J Clin Lab Invest 1963;(15):132–40.
2. Sharp HL, Bridges RA, Krivit W, et al. Cirrhosis associated with alpha-1 antitrypsin deficiency: a previously unrecognized inherited disorder. J Lab Clin Med 1969;73(6):934–9.
3. Berg NO, Eriksson S. Liver disease in adults with alpha-1 antitrypsin deficiency. N Engl J Med 1972;287(25):1264–7.
4. Carrell RW, Lomas DA. Alpha-1 antitrypsin deficiency–a model for conformational diseases. N Engl J Med 2002;346(1):45–53.
5. American Thoracic Society, European Respiratory Society. American Thoracic Society/European respiratory Society Statement: Standards for the diagnosis and management of individuals with alpha-1 antitrypsin deficiency. Am J Respir Crit Care Med 2003;168(7):818–900.
6. Owen MC, Brennan SO, Lewis JH, et al. Mutation of antitrypsin to antithrombin. Alpha-1 antitrypsin Pittsburgh (358 met leads to arg), a fatal bleeding disorder. N Engl J Med 1983;309(12):694–8.

7. Sveger T. Liver disease in alpha-1 antitrypsin deficiency detected by screening of 200,000 infants. N Engl J Med 1976;294(24):1316–21.

8. O'Brien ML, Buist NR, Murphey WH. Neonatal screening for alpha-1 antitrypsin deficiency. J Pediatr 1978;92(6):1006–10.

9. United States Census Bureau. US and world population clock. Available at: http://www.census.gov/popclock. Accessed August 26, 2015.

10. Guidelines for the approach to the patient with severe hereditary alpha-1-antitrypsin deficiency. American Thoracic Society. Am Rev Respir Dis 1989;140(5):1494–7.

11. de Serres FJ. Worldwide racial and ethnic distribution of alpha-1 antitrypsin deficiency: summary of an analysis of published genetic epidemiologic surveys. Chest 2002;122(5):1818–29.

12. de Serres FJ, Blanco I. Prevalence of alpha-1 antitrypsin deficiency alleles PI*S and PI*Z worldwide and effective screening for each of the five phenotypic classes PI*MS, PI*MZ, PI*SS, PI*SZ, and PI*ZZ: a comprehensive review. Ther Adv Respir Dis 2012;6(5):277–95.

13. Seyama K, Nukiwa T, Takabe K, et al. Siiyama (serine 53 (TCC) to phenylalanine 53 (TTC)). A new alpha-1 antitrypsin-deficient variant with mutation on a predicted conserved residue of the serpin backbone. J Biol Chem 1991;266(19):12627–32.

14. de Serres FJ, Blanco I, Fernandez-Bustillo E. Ethnic differences in alpha1 antitrypsin deficiency in the United States of America. Ther Adv Respir Dis 2010;4(2):63–70.

15. Greulich T, Ottaviani S, Bals R, et al. Alpha-1antitrypsin deficiency - diagnostic testing and disease awareness in Germany and Italy. Respir Med 2013;107(9):1400–8.

16. Tobin MJ, Cook PJ, Hutchison DC. Alpha-1 antitrypsin deficiency: the clinical and physiological features of pulmonary emphysema in subjects homozygous for Pi type Z. A survey by the British Thoracic Association. Br J Dis Chest 1983;77(1):14–27.

17. Silverman EK, Miletich JP, Pierce JA, et al. Alpha-1 antitrypsin deficiency. high prevalence in the St. Louis area determined by direct population screening. Am Rev Respir Dis 1989;140(4):961–6.

18. Piitulainen E, Tanash HA. The clinical profile of subjects included in the Swedish national register on individuals with severe alpha-1 antitrypsin deficiency. COPD 2015;12(Suppl 1):36–41.

19. Bradi AC, Audisho N, Casey DK, et al. Alpha-1 antitrypsin deficiency in Canada: regional disparities in diagnosis and management. COPD 2015;12(Suppl 1):15–21.

20. Stoller JK, Smith P, Yang P, et al. Physical and social impact of alpha-1 antitrypsin deficiency: results of a survey. Cleve Clin J Med 1994;61(6):461–7.

21. Stoller JK, Sandhaus RA, Turino G, et al. Delay in diagnosis of alpha-1 antitrypsin deficiency: a continuing problem. Chest 2005;128(4):1989–94.

22. Mayer AS, Stoller JK, Bucher Bartelson B, et al. Occupational exposure risks in individuals with PI*Z alpha-1 antitrypsin deficiency. Am J Respir Crit Care Med 2000;162(2 Pt 1):553–8.

23. Stoller JK, Brantly M. The challenge of detecting alpha-1 antitrypsin deficiency. COPD 2013;10(Suppl 1):26–34.

24. Ferrarotti I, Thun GA, Zorzetto M, et al. Serum levels and genotype distribution of alpha-1 antitrypsin in the general population. Thorax 2012;67(8):669–74.

25. Bornhorst JA, Greene DN, Ashwood ER, et al. Alpha-1 antitrypsin phenotypes and associated serum protein concentrations in a large clinical population. Chest 2013;143(4):1000–8.

26. Gadek JE, Klein HG, Holland PV, et al. Replacement therapy of alpha-1 antitrypsin deficiency. Reversal of protease-antiprotease imbalance within the alveolar structures of PiZ subjects. J Clin Invest 1981;68(5):1158–65.

27. Eriksson S, Carlson J, Velez R. Risk of cirrhosis and primary liver cancer in alpha-1 antitrypsin deficiency. N Engl J Med 1986;314(12):736–9.

28. Eriksson S. Alpha-1 antitrypsin deficiency and liver cirrhosis in adults. An analysis of 35 Swedish autopsied cases. Acta Med Scand 1987;221(5):461–7.

29. Lomas DA, Mahadeva R. Alpha-1 antitrypsin polymerization and the serpinopathies: pathobiology and prospects for therapy. J Clin Invest 2002;110(11):1585–90.

30. Sivasothy P, Dafforn TR, Gettins PG, et al. Pathogenic alpha-1 antitrypsin polymers are formed by reactive loop-beta-sheet A linkage. J Biol Chem 2000;275(43):33663–8.

31. Alam S, Li Z, Atkinson C, et al. Z alpha-1 antitrypsin confers a proinflammatory phenotype that contributes to chronic obstructive pulmonary disease. Am J Respir Crit Care Med 2014;189(8):909–31.

32. McElvaney NG, Stoller JK, Buist AS, et al. Baseline characteristics of enrollees in the national heart, lung and blood institute registry of alpha-1 antitrypsin deficiency. Alpha-1 antitrypsin deficiency registry study group. Chest 1997;111(2):394–403.

33. Janus ED, Phillips NT, Carrell RW. Smoking, lung function, and alpha-1 antitrypsin deficiency. Lancet 1985;1(8421):152–4.

34. Rawlings W Jr, Kreiss P, Levy D, et al. Clinical, epidemiologic, and pulmonary function studies in alpha-1 antitrypsin-deficient subjects of Pi Z type. Am Rev Respir Dis 1976;114(5):945–53.

35. Piitulainen E, Montero LC, Nystedt-Duzakin M, et al. Lung function and CT densitometry in subjects with alpha-1 antitrypsin deficiency and healthy controls at 35 years of age. COPD 2015;12(2):162–7.

36. Parr DG, Stoel BC, Stolk J, et al. Pattern of emphysema distribution in alpha-1 antitrypsin deficiency influences lung function impairment. Am J Respir Crit Care Med 2004;170(11):1172–8.

37. The Alpha-1 Antitrypsin Deficiency Registry Study Group. Survival and FEV_1 decline in individuals with severe deficiency of α_1-antitrypsin. Am J Respir Crit Care Med 1998;158(1):49–59.

38. Piitulainen E, Eriksson S. Decline in FEV1 related to smoking status in individuals with severe alpha-1 antitrypsin deficiency (PiZZ). Eur Respir J 1999; 13(2):247–51.

39. Dawkins PA, Dawkins CL, Wood AM, et al. Rate of progression of lung function impairment in alpha-1 antitrypsin deficiency. Eur Respir J 2009;33(6):1338–44.

40. Holme J, Stockley JA, Stockley RA. Age related development of respiratory abnormalities in non-index alpha-1 antitrypsin deficient studies. Respir Med 2013;107(3):387–93.

41. Tanash HA, Nilsson PM, Nilsson JA, et al. Clinical course and prognosis of never-smokers with severe alpha-1 antitrypsin deficiency (PiZZ). Thorax 2008;63(12):1091–5.

42. Wood AM, Harrison RM, Semple S, et al. Outdoor air pollution is associated with rapid decline of lung function in alpha-1 antitrypsin deficiency. Occup Environ Med 2010;67(8):556–61.

43. Banauch GI, Brantly M, Izbicki G, et al. Accelerated spirometric decline in New York City firefighters with alpha-1 antitrypsin deficiency. Chest 2010;138(5):1116–24.

44. Tanash HA, Nilsson PM, Nilsson JA, et al. Survival in severe alpha-1 antitrypsin deficiency (PiZZ). Respir Res 2010;11:44.

45. Molloy K, Hersh CP, Morris VB, et al. Clarification of the risk of chronic obstructive pulmonary disease in alpha-1 antitrypsin deficiency PiMZ heterozygotes. Am J Respir Crit Care Med 2014;189(4):419–27.

46. Sorheim IC, Bakke P, Gulsvik A, et al. Alpha-1) antitrypsin protease inhibitor MZ heterozygosity is associated with airflow obstruction in two large cohorts. Chest 2010;138(5):1125–32.

47. Parr DG, Guest PG, Reynolds JH, et al. Prevalence and impact of bronchiectasis in alpha1-antitrypsin deficiency. Am J Respir Crit Care Med 2007; 176(12):1215–21.

48. Cuvelier A, Muir JF, Hellot MF, et al. Distribution of alpha(1)-antitrypsin alleles in patients with bronchiectasis. Chest 2000;117(2):415–9.

49. Teckman JH, Qu D, Perlmutter DH. Molecular pathogenesis of liver disease in alpha-1antitrypsin deficiency. Hepatology 1996;24(6):1504–16.

50. Sveger T. The natural history of liver disease in alpha-1 antitrypsin deficient children. Acta Paediatr Scand 1988;77(6):847–51.

51. Antoury C, Lopez R, Zein N, et al. Alpha-1 antitrypsin deficiency and the risk of hepatocellular carcinoma in end-stage liver disease. World J Hepatol 2015;7(10):1427–32.

52. Zhou H, Ortiz-Pallardo ME, Ko Y, et al. Is heterozygous alpha-1 antitrypsin deficiency type PiZ a risk factor for primary liver carcinoma? Cancer 2000; 88(12):2668–76.

53. Dawwas MF, Davies SE, Griffiths WJ, et al. Prevalence and risk factors for liver involvement in individuals with PiZZ-related lung disease. Am J Respir Crit Care Med 2013;187(5):502–8.

54. Clark VC, Dhanasekaran R, Brantly M, et al. Liver test results do not identify liver disease in adults with alpha—1 antitrypsin deficiency. Clin Gastroenterol Hepatol 2012;10(11):1278–83.

55. Esnault VL, Testa A, Audrain M, et al. Alpha-1 antitrypsin genetic polymorphism in ANCA-positive systemic vasculitis. Kidney Int 1993;43(6):1329–32.

56. O'Donoghue DJ, Guickian M, Blundell G, et al. Alpha-1 proteinase inhibitor and pulmonary haemorrhage in systemic vasculitis. Adv Exp Med Biol 1993;336:331–5.

57. Mahr AD, Edberg JC, Stone JH, et al. Alpha—1 antitrypsin deficiency-related alleles Z and S and the risk of Wegener's granulomatosis. Arthritis Rheum 2010;62(12):3760–7.

58. Segelmark M, Elzouki AN, Wieslander J, et al. The PiZ gene of alpha-1 antitrypsin as a determinant of outcome in PR3-ANCA-positive vasculitis. Kidney Int 1995;48(3):844–50.

59. Mota A, Sahebghadam Lotfi A, Jamshidi AR, et al. Alpha-1 antitrypsin activity is markedly decreased in Wegener's granulomatosis. Rheumatol Int 2014; 34(4):553–8.

60. Warter J, Storck D, Grosshans E, et al. Weber-Christian syndrome associated with an alpha-1 antitrypsin deficiency. Familial investigation. Ann Med Interne (Paris) 1972;123(10):877–82.

61. Geraminejad P, DeBloom JR 2nd, Walling HW, et al. Alpha-1 antitrypsin associated panniculitis: the MS variant. J Am Acad Dermatol 2004;51(4):645–55.

62. Smith KC, Pittelkow MR, Su WP. Panniculitis associated with severe alpha-1 antitrypsin deficiency. Treatment and review of the literature. Arch Dermatol 1987;123(12):1655–61.

63. Smith KC, Su WP, Pittelkow MR, et al. Clinical and pathologic correlations in 96 patients with panniculitis, including 15 patients with deficient levels of alpha-1 antitrypsin. J Am Acad Dermatol 1989; 21(6):1192–6.

64. Chowdhury MM, Williams EJ, Morris JS, et al. Severe panniculitis caused by homozygous ZZ alpha-1 antitrypsin deficiency treated successfully with human purified enzyme (prolastin). Br J Dermatol 2002;147(6):1258–61.

65. O'Riordan K, Blei A, Rao MS, et al. Alpha-1 antitrypsin deficiency-associated panniculitis: Resolution with intravenous alpha-1 antitrypsin

administration and liver transplantation. Transplantation 1997;63(3):480–2.

66. Stoller JK. Clinical practice. acute exacerbations of chronic obstructive pulmonary disease. N Engl J Med 2002;346(13):988–94.

67. Sutherland ER, Cherniack RM. Management of chronic obstructive pulmonary disease. N Engl J Med 2004;350(26):2689–97

68. Decramer M, Janssens W, Miravitlles M. Chronic obstructive pulmonary disease. Lancet 2012; 379(9823):1341–51.

69. Fishman A, Martinez F, Naunheim K, et al. A randomized trial comparing lung-volume-reduction surgery with medical therapy for severe emphysema. N Engl J Med 2003;348(21):2059–73.

70. Seersholm N, Wencker M, Banik N, et al. Does alpha-1 antitrypsin augmentation therapy slow the annual decline in FEV1 in patients with severe hereditary alpha-1 antitrypsin deficiency? Wissenschaftliche Arbeitsgemeinschaft zur Therapie von Lungenerkrankungen (WATL) Alpha1-AT Study Group. Eur Respir J 1997;10(10):2260–3.

71. Wencker M, Fuhrmann B, Banik N, et al. Wissenschaftliche Arbeitsgemeinschaft zur Therapie von Lungenerkrankungen. Longitudinal follow-up of patients with alpha-1 protease inhibitor deficiency before and during therapy with IV alpha-1 protease inhibitor. Chest 2001;119(3):737–44.

72. Tonelli AR, Rouhani F, Li N, et al. Alpha-1 antitrypsin augmentation therapy in deficient individuals enrolled in the Alpha-1 Foundation DNA and Tissue Bank. Int J Chron Obstruct Pulmon Dis 2009;4:443–52.

73. Stone PJ, Morris TA 3rd, Franzblau C, et al. Preliminary evidence that augmentation therapy diminishes degradation of cross-linked elastin in alpha-1 antitrypsin-deficient humans. Respiration 1995;62(2):76–9.

74. Dirksen A, Dijkman JH, Madsen F, et al. A randomized clinical trial of Alpha—1 antitrypsin augmentation therapy. Am J Respir Crit Care Med 1999;160(5 Pt 1):1468–72.

75. Gottlieb DJ, Luisetti M, Stone PJ, et al. Short-term supplementation therapy does not affect elastin degradation in severe alpha(1)-antitrypsin deficiency. The American-Italian AATD Study Group. Am J Respir Crit Care Med 2000;162(6):2069–72.

76. Lieberman J. Augmentation therapy reduces frequency of lung infections in antitrypsin deficiency: a new hypothesis with supporting data. Chest 2000;118(5):1480–5.

77. Stockley RA, Bayley DL, Unsal I, et al. The effect of augmentation therapy on bronchial inflammation in alpha-1 antitrypsin deficiency. Am J Respir Crit Care Med 2002;165(11):1494–8.

78. Dirksen A, Piitulainen E, Parr DG, et al. Exploring the role of CT densitometry: a randomised study of augmentation therapy in alpha-1 antitrypsin deficiency. Eur Respir J 2009;33(6):1345–53.

79. Schmid ST, Koepke J, Dresel M, et al. The effects of weekly augmentation therapy in patients with PiZZ alpha-1 antitrypsin deficiency. Int J Chron Obstruct Pulmon Dis 2012;7:687–96.

80. Barros-Tizón JC, Torres ML, Blanco I, et al. Investigators of the rEXA study group. Reduction of severe exacerbations and hospitalization-derived costs in alpha-1-antitrypsin-deficient patients treated with alpha-1 antitrypsin augmentation therapy. Ther Adv Respir Dis 2012;6(2):67–78.

81. Ma S, Lin YY, He J, et al. Alpha-1 antitrypsin augmentation therapy and biomarkers of elastin degradation. COPD 2013;10(4):473–81.

82. Chapman KR, Burdon JG, Piitulainen E, et al. Intravenous augmentation treatment and lung density in severe alpha-1 antitrypsin deficiency (RAPID): a randomised, double-blind, placebo-controlled trial. Lancet 2015;386(9991):360–8.

83. Hubbard RC, Crystal RG. Alpha-1 antitrypsin augmentation therapy for alpha-1 antitrypsin deficiency. Am J Med 1988;84(6A):52–62.

84. Barker AF, Iwata-Morgan I, Oveson L, et al. Pharmacokinetic study of alpha-1antitrypsin infusion in alpha1-antitrypsin deficiency. Chest 1997;112(3):607–13.

85. Campos MA, Kueppers F, Stocks JM, et al. Safety and pharmacokinetics of 120 mg/kg versus 60 mg/kg weekly intravenous infusions of alpha-1 proteinase inhibitor in alpha-1 antitrypsin deficiency: a multicenter, randomized, double-blind, crossover study (SPARK). COPD 2013;10(6):687–95.

86. Sandhaus RA, Turino G, Stocks J, et al. Alpha-1 antitrypsin augmentation therapy for PI*MZ heterozygotes: a cautionary note. Chest 2008;134(4):831–4.

87. Turino GM, Barker AF, Brantly ML, et al. Clinical features of individuals with PI*SZ phenotype of alpha-1 antitrypsin deficiency. Alpha-1 Antitrypsin Deficiency Registry Study Group. Am J Respir Crit Care Med 1996;154(6 Pt 1):1718–25.

88. Wencker M, Banik N, Buhl R, et al. Long-term treatment of alpha-1antitrypsin deficiency-related pulmonary emphysema with human alpha-1 antitrypsin. Wissenschaftliche Arbeitsgemeinschaft zur Therapie von Lungenerkrankungen (WATL) Alpha1-AT Study Group. Eur Respir J 1998;11(2):428–33.

89. Gildea TR, Shermock KM, Singer ME, et al. Cost-effectiveness analysis of augmentation therapy for severe alpha-1 antitrypsin deficiency. Am J Respir Crit Care Med 2003;167(10):1387–92.

90. Marciniuk DD, Hernandez P, Balter M, et al. Alpha-1 antitrypsin deficiency targeted testing and augmentation therapy: a Canadian Thoracic Society clinical practice guideline. Can Respir J 2012;19(2):109–16.

91. Christie JD, Edwards LB, Kucheryavaya AY, et al. The registry of the International Society for Heart

and Lung Transplantation: twenty-eighth adult lung and heart-lung transplant report–2011. J Heart Lung Transplant 2011;30(10):1104–22.

92. Cassivi SD, Meyers BF, Battafarano RJ, et al. Thirteen-year experience in lung transplantation for emphysema. Ann Thorac Surg 2002;74(5):1663–9 [discussion: 1669–70].

93. Burton CM, Milman N, Carlsen J, et al. The Copenhagen National Lung Transplant Group: survival after single lung, double lung, and heart-lung transplantation. J Heart Lung Transplant 2005;24(11):1834–43.

94. Inci I, Schuurmans M, Ehrsam J, et al. Lung transplantation for emphysema: impact of age on short- and long-term survival. Eur J Cardiothorac Surg 2015;48(6):906–9.

95. de Perrot M, Chaparro C, McRae K, et al. Twenty-year experience of lung transplantation at a single center: Influence of recipient diagnosis on long-term survival. J Thorac Cardiovasc Surg 2004;127(5):1493–501.

96. Tanash HA, Riise GC, Ekstrom MP, et al. Survival benefit of lung transplantation for chronic obstructive pulmonary disease in Sweden. Ann Thorac Surg 2014;98(6):1930–5.

97. Tanash HA, Riise GC, Hansson L, et al. Survival benefit of lung transplantation in individuals with severe alpha1-anti-trypsin deficiency (PiZZ) and emphysema. J Heart Lung Transplant 2011; 30(12):1342–7.

98. Banga A, Gildea T, Rajeswaran J, et al. The natural history of lung function after lung transplantation for alpha—1 antitrypsin deficiency. Am J Respir Crit Care Med 2014;190(3):274–81.

99. Stoller JK, Gildea TR, Ries AL, et al. National Emphysema Treatment Trial Research Group. Lung volume reduction surgery in patients with emphysema and alpha-1 antitrypsin deficiency. Ann Thorac Surg 2007;83(1):241–51.

100. Cassina PC, Teschler H, Konietzko N, et al. Two-year results after lung volume reduction surgery in alpha-1 antitrypsin deficiency versus smoker's emphysema. Eur Respir J 1998;12(5):1028–32.

101. Gelb AF, McKenna RJ, Brenner M, et al. Lung function after bilateral lower lobe lung volume reduction surgery for alpha-1 antitrypsin emphysema. Eur Respir J 1999;14(4):928–33.

102. Tutic M, Bloch KE, Lardinois D, et al. Long-term results after lung volume reduction surgery in patients with alpha-1 antitrypsin deficiency. J Thorac Cardiovasc Surg 2004;128(3):408–13.

103. Dauriat G, Mal H, Jebrak G, et al. Functional results of unilateral lung volume reduction surgery in alpha-1 antitrypsin deficient patients. Int J Chron Obstruct Pulmon Dis 2006;1(2):201–6.

104. Donahue JM, Cassivi SD. Lung volume reduction surgery for patients with alpha-1 antitrypsin deficiency emphysema. Thorac Surg Clin 2009;19(2): 201–8.

105. Tuohy MM, Remund KF, Hilfiker R, et al. Endobronchial valve deployment in severe alpha-1 antitrypsin deficiency emphysema: a case series. Clin Respir J 2013;7(1):45–52.

106. Hillerdal G, Mindus S. One- to four-year follow-up of endobronchial lung volume reduction in alpha-1 antitrypsin deficiency patients: a case series. Respiration 2014;88(4):320–8.

107. Brantly ML, Chulay JD, Wang L, et al. Sustained transgene expression despite T lymphocyte responses in a clinical trial of rAAV1-AAT gene therapy. Proc Natl Acad Sci U S A 2009;106(38): 16363–8.

108. Flotte TR. Adeno-associated virus-based gene therapy for inherited disorders. Pediatr Res 2005; 58(6):1143–7.

109. Parfrey H, Dafforn TR, Belorgey D, et al. Inhibiting polymerization: new therapeutic strategies for Z alpha-1 antitrypsin-related emphysema. Am J Respir Cell Mol Biol 2004;31(2):133–9.

110. Zhou A, Stein PE, Huntington JA, et al. How small peptides block and reverse serpin polymerisation. J Mol Biol 2004;342(3):931–41.

111. Burrows JA, Willis LK, Perlmutter DH. Chemical chaperones mediate increased secretion of mutant alpha-1 antitrypsin (alpha-1 AT) Z: a potential pharmacological strategy for prevention of liver injury and emphysema in alpha-1 AT deficiency. Proc Natl Acad Sci U S A 2000;97(4): 1796–801.

112. Marcus NY, Perlmutter DH. Glucosidase and mannosidase inhibitors mediate increased secretion of mutant alpha-1 antitrypsin Z. J Biol Chem 2000; 275(3):1987–92.

113. Cantin AM, Woods DE, Cloutier D, et al. Polyethylene glycol conjugation at Cys232 prolongs the half-life of alpha-1 proteinase inhibitor. Am J Respir Cell Mol Biol 2002;27(6):659–65.

114. Hidvegi T, Ewing M, Hale P, et al. An autophagy-enhancing drug promotes degradation of mutant alpha-1 antitrypsin Z and reduces hepatic fibrosis. Science 2010;329(5988):229–32.

115. Kaushal S, Annamali M, Blomenkamp K, et al. Rapamycin reduces intrahepatic alpha-1 antitrypsin mutant Z protein polymers and liver injury in a mouse model. Exp Biol Med (Maywood) 2010; 235(6):700–9.

116. Flotte TR, Trapnell BC, Humphries M, et al. Phase 2 clinical trial of a recombinant adeno-associated viral vector expressing alpha-1 antitrypsin: interim results. Hum Gene Ther 2011;22(10):1239–47.

117. Loring HS, Flotte TR. Current status of gene therapy for alpha-1 antitrypsin deficiency. Expert Opin Biol Ther 2015;15(3):329–36.

118. Monk R, Graves M, Williams P, et al. Inhaled alpha-1 antitrypsin: Gauging patient interest in a new treatment. COPD 2013;10(4):411–5.

Hermansky-Pudlak Syndrome

Souheil El-Chemaly, MD, MPH[a], Lisa R. Young, MD[b,c],*

KEYWORDS

- Pulmonary fibrosis • Interstitial lung disease • Albinism
- Biogenesis of lysosome-related organelle complex • Adaptor protein 3
- Hermansky-Pudlak syndrome

KEY POINTS

- Hermansky-Pudlak syndrome (HPS) is an autosomal recessive disorder that is associated with oculocutaneous albinism, bleeding diatheses, granulomatous colitis, and highly penetrant pulmonary fibrosis in some subtypes, including HPS-1, HPS-2, and HPS-4.
- HPS pulmonary fibrosis shows many of the clinical, radiologic, and histologic features found in idiopathic pulmonary fibrosis (IPF), but occurs at a younger age.
- The extent of albinism in HPS is variable, and it may not be readily appreciated in patients with presumed IPF unless carefully assessed.
- HPS gene products are ubiquitously expressed and assemble into hetero-oligomeric complexes called BLOCs (biogenesis of lysosome-related organelle complexes), which are critical in trafficking to lysosomelike organelles, such as melanosomes, platelet dense granules, and lamellar bodies.
- Although HPS is a rare disease worldwide, it is common in Puerto Rico, where 1 in 1800 individuals are affected because of a founder mutation.

INTRODUCTION

Hermansky-Pudlak syndrome (HPS) is an autosomal recessive disorder associated with highly penetrant pulmonary fibrosis in young adults with subtypes HPS-1, HPS-2, and HPS-4. Other clinical features of HPS include oculocutaneous albinism (OCA) and bleeding diathesis, enabling identification of at-risk individuals before the onset of lung disease. This article summarizes current knowledge about the clinical features and natural history of HPS, provides current recommendations for diagnosis and management of HPS, and highlights recent progress in elucidating disease pathogenesis and ongoing work in this field.

EPIDEMIOLOGY

HPS is a very rare autosomal recessive disease with 10 known subtypes.[1] HPS has been described in many regions of the world and in different ethnic backgrounds, including Western

Disclosure: The authors have nothing to disclose.
Funding: NIH/NHLBI R01 HL119503, NIH/NCATS/NHLBI U54 HL127672 (L.R. Young). The Rare Lung Diseases Consortium is part of the Rare Diseases Clinical Research Network, an initiative of the Office of Rare Diseases Research (ORDR), National Center for Advancing Translational Sciences (NCATS), with funding through collaboration between NCATS and the National Heart, Lung, and Blood Institute. S. El-Chemaly receives research grant funding from the ATS Foundation/American Lung Association.
[a] Division of Pulmonary and Critical Care Medicine, Brigham and Women's Hospital, Harvard Medical School, 75 Francis Street, Boston, MA 02115, USA; [b] Division of Pulmonary Medicine, Department of Pediatrics, Vanderbilt University School of Medicine, 2200 Children's Way, Doctor's Office Tower 11215, Nashville, TN 37232, USA; [c] Division of Allergy, Pulmonary, and Critical Care, Department of Medicine, Vanderbilt University School of Medicine, 1161 21st Avenue South, B-1220 Medical Center North, Nashville, TN 37232, USA
* Corresponding author. Division of Pulmonary Medicine, Vanderbilt University Medical Center, 2200 Children's Way, Doctor's Office Tower 11215, Nashville, TN 37232.
E-mail address: lisa.young@vanderbilt.edu

Clin Chest Med 37 (2016) 505–511
http://dx.doi.org/10.1016/j.ccm.2016.04.012
0272-5231/16/$ – see front matter © 2016 Elsevier Inc. All rights reserved.

Europe, the Indian subcontinent, Japan, China, the Middle East, and non–Puerto Rican Hispanic people.[2–7] To date, more than 1200 individuals with HPS have registered with The HPS Network, Inc, a volunteer self-help, not-for-profit support group for people and families dealing with HPS that was founded in 1992 (Appell D, RN, personal communication, 2016.). The true frequency of the disease and of the different subtypes is not known. In northwest Puerto Rico, 1 in 21 persons is a carrier of the founder mutation (16-base pair [bp] duplication in exon 15 of HPS1[8]) and 1 in 1800 persons has HPS-1.[9] Because of another founder mutation (3904-bp deletion in HPS3), 1 in 4000 people in central Puerto Rico is affected with HPS-3.[10,11] Multiple other HPS1 mutations have been identified and HPS-1 is also the most common subtype of HPS in non–Puerto Ricans.[1] A few case reports describe patients affected by the other HPS subtypes, especially HPS-3 in individuals with Ashkenazi Jewish background.[12]

PATHOGENESIS

The 10 reported genetically distinct subtypes of HPS (denoted HPS-1 to HPS-10) share the common features of OCA and a platelet storage pool deficiency.[2,13–15] HPS gene products are ubiquitously expressed and assemble into hetero-oligomeric complexes called BLOCs (biogenesis of lysosome-related organelle complexes), which are critical in trafficking to lysosome like organelles, such as melanosomes and platelet dense granules.[16] The HPS1 gene product is a component of BLOC3, and HPS1 mutations cause highly penetrant pulmonary fibrosis. In contrast, the HPS3 gene product is part of BLOC2, a different trafficking complex; pulmonary fibrosis has not been observed in patients with HPS-3. The best characterized of the HPS gene products is HPS2, which in mice and humans is the β3A subunit of the adapter protein-3 (AP-3) complex (named independently of the BLOCs).[17] AP-3 is a ubiquitously expressed hetero-oligomer that functions in organelle biogenesis and early endosomal protein trafficking. In HPS-2, mutations in the β3A subunit of AP-3 result in instability and ubiquitin-mediated degradation of the entire AP-3 complex.

There is a growing body of work focusing on the cell biology of HPS. Patients with HPS have macrophage-mediated inflammation preceding the onset of pulmonary fibrosis. Studies show that bronchoalveolar lavage (BAL) fluid from patients with HPS contains increased numbers of BAL macrophages and that these macrophages are constitutively activated, elaborating excess cytokines and chemokines.[18] One study suggests abnormalities in fibroblasts, with increased expression of galectin-3, a β-galactosidase–binding lectin with profibrotic effects.[19] Further, patients with HPS with pulmonary fibrosis (HPSPF) have been found to have increased numbers of circulating C-X-C chemokine receptor type 4 (CXCR-4) positive fibrocytes compared with subjects with HPS without lung disease or healthy control subjects.[20]

Limited availability of human lung tissue has prompted substantial HPS research in murine models. In mice, as in humans, there is considerable locus heterogeneity for HPS-like syndromes. Most of the HPS mouse models are naturally occurring and maintained as congenic mutants on the C57BL/6J inbred strain. HPS mice reliably model important features of the human disease, including hypopigmentation, deficiency of platelet dense granules, and genotype-specific constitutive alveolar macrophage activation and susceptibility to profibrotic stimuli. Although spontaneous fibrosis does not occur in naturally occurring HPS mice, HPS-1 and HPS-2 models have an exaggerated fibrotic response to fibrotic stimuli, including silica[21] and bleomycin.[22–24] Spontaneous lung fibrosis has been reported in a HPS-1/HPS-2 double-mutant model.[25]

Macrophage-mediated inflammation is also present in HPS mouse models.[26,27] However, murine bone marrow transplant studies have shown that macrophage abnormalities and fibrotic susceptibility are caused by epithelial dysfunction, not intrinsic macrophage defects.[22] Additional studies implicate alveolar epithelial cell apoptosis,[25] interleukin-13Rα2 localization and signaling,[24] and autophagy[28] as potential mechanisms. The mechanisms underlying how HPS trafficking defects result in alveolar epithelial cell dysfunction and resultant pulmonary fibrosis remain incompletely understood.

DIAGNOSIS
Clinical Features

To satisfy criteria for diagnosis, all patients with HPS, regardless of subtype, must have (1) tyrosinase-positive OCA, and (2) a bleeding disorder caused by platelet dysfunction that ranges from mild to severe.[3] OCA is characterized by hypopigmentation of the hair and skin. Retinal hypopigmentation is characterized by reduced iris and retinal pigment associated with a severe reduction in visual acuity and the presence of horizontal nystagmus.[13,29] Tyrosinase-positive OCA implies that eumelanin or brown/black pigment is absent from hair, eyes, and skin, whereas pheomelanin or yellow/orange pigment is present and builds up with age.[30] Importantly, the degree of albinism is variable and can be subtle in patients with HPS, potentially masked by the use of hair-coloring products.

In the absence of overt OCA, HPS could be confused with idiopathic pulmonary fibrosis (IPF), nonspecific interstitial pneumonia, or pulmonary fibrosis from a variety of other causes. The differential diagnosis of HPS also includes Chédiak-Higashi syndrome (CHS), a recessive disorder that shares the features of mild albinism and bleeding. CHS is also associated with innate immunodeficiency, often with recurrent infections and an accelerated lymphoproliferative phase.

Diagnostic Testing

Platelet electron microscopy
The bleeding disorder in HPS stems from the absence of dense bodies (delta granules) in platelets despite the presence of normal numbers of platelets. Platelet storage granules (alpha and delta granules) release their contents (ATP, ADP, serotonin) to attract other platelets after the initiation of the platelet aggregation cascade. Historically, the bleeding time was used to test for platelet aggregation defects, but this test has been shown to be unreliable and is not recommended.[29] The most accurate diagnostic test remains the study of freshly isolated platelets with electron microscopy to establish the complete (or near-complete) absence of delta granules.[31] Platelet transmission electron microscopic study is currently available only in selected laboratories (www.mayomedicallaboratories.com).

Genetic testing
Genetic testing is recommended to determine the specific disease subtype in individuals with HPS because there are important phenotypic differences between subtypes that have critical implications for follow-up and prognosis. As suggested by Gahl and colleagues,[1] if available, one strategy could be to test a multigene panel containing the 10 genes now identified to cause HPS. Alternatively, a testing strategy focusing on the ethnic background or the specific phenotypic presentation of patients with OCA and a bleeding disorder would be appropriate (**Fig. 1**).

- *HPS1* should be investigated in patients from northwest Puerto Rico and those who are severely affected and present with interstitial lung disease (ILD).
- *HPS3* testing is particularly indicated in patients from central Puerto Rico or with Ashkenazi Jewish ancestry.
- *HPS2* should be tested in patients with neutropenia or infections.
- *HPS4* should be tested in severely affected patients and those with ILD.

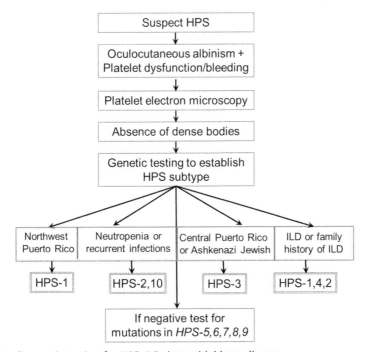

Fig. 1. Approach to diagnostic testing for HPS. ILD, interstitial lung disease.

- Other HPS subtypes can be pursued in patients with a milder phenotype or in whom testing for *HPS1-4* is negative.

Diagnosis of Interstitial Lung Disease

High-resolution computed tomography of the chest

Patients with HPS-1 universally develop pulmonary fibrosis. The frequency of HPSPF in HPS-4 and HPS-2 is not known. Patients generally develop ILD in the third decade of life,[32] but some reports indicate the presence of symptomatic lung disease in late adolescence.[29] The diagnosis of ILD is established with a high-resolution computed tomography (HRCT) scan of the chest. Characteristic HRCT findings are increased reticular opacities, thickened interlobular septa, and ground-glass infiltrates in addition to fibrotic changes, including traction bronchiectasis and honeycombing (**Fig. 2**).[33] These imaging findings evolve over time. With advanced disease there is universal development of reticular changes and traction bronchiectasis, with ~60% of patients developing honeycombing and ground-glass infiltrates.[33] The severity of changes on HRCT has been shown to correlate with decline in lung function and mortality.[33] Intriguingly, when patients were grouped by the severity of their disease by pulmonary function tests (PFTs) (no disease, mild changes, moderate changes, and severe changes) and HRCT findings, the average age was similar among all groups, highlighting the heterogeneity of lung function decline in HPSPF, even among individuals with the same HPS mutations.[32] The timing of the first screening HRCT should likely be in late adolescence based on reports of the earliest onset of ILD.[29]

Importantly, lung biopsy is not recommended for ILD diagnosis in individuals with HPS, because the risk of bleeding is considerable and the high pretest likelihood that fibrotic changes are caused by HPS obviate a surgical lung biopsy in this setting. However, examination of the lung tissue from patients with HPSPF when available has revealed changes that are similar to the usual interstitial pneumonia pattern characteristic of IPF. Additional characteristic changes are foamy swelling of alveolar macrophages and epithelial cells.[7,34–36]

NATURAL HISTORY AND PROGNOSIS

Data regarding the rate of lung function decline and prognosis in HPS are derived from studies conducted at the National Institutes of Health (NIH).[37,38] The natural history of pulmonary fibrosis in HPS has been reported as variable but universally progressive, with mortality commonly occurring in the fourth to fifth decades of life. However, the age of death has ranged from 26 to 74 years. Gahl and colleagues[37] reported a biphasic distribution of lung function and rate of decline. A first peak was seen in young adults (20–25 years old) with a steady decline in forced vital capacity (FVC) percentage predicted from 88% to 63% by the age of 36 to 40 years. For those patients with normal FVC (mean 89% predicted) at 45 years of age, a subsequent steady decline to 67% predicted was observed by the age of 56 to 60 years.[37] When outcomes were analyzed independent of age for subjects starting with mild to moderate disease (FVC >50% predicted), average annual decline in FVC and carbon monoxide diffusion in the lung (DLco) were -2.8 ± 5.0 (% predicted) and -2.0 ± 4.5 (% predicted), respectively.[38] However, additional data indicate that some patients experience a much more rapid decline.[37,38]

Similarly, a recent study examining the role of circulating fibrocytes as biomarkers of disease progression in HPSPF enrolled 40 subjects with HPS-1, 37 of whom had ILD and an average FVC of 71% predicted (60–80 interquartile range). Over the average study follow-up period of more than 600 days, average lung function was stable. However, individual patients experienced

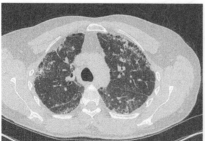 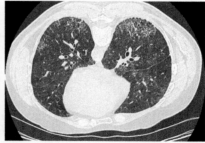

Fig. 2. Examples of chest CT imaging findings in 2 individuals with HPS1.

lung function decline.[20] A threshold level of CXCR-4-positive circulating fibrocytes was associated with increased risk of death during a median follow-up duration of 6.1 years.[20] However, fibrocyte levels were not predictive of lung function decline (FVC or DLco) in this cohort. In summary, beyond an accelerated decline in lung function (500 mL/y) that has been reported to be associated with death from HPSPF,[37] there are no clinically available biomarkers to predict disease progression in HPS.

CLINICAL MANAGEMENT
Management of Pulmonary Disease

Patients with HPS-1, HPS-4 and HPS-2 subtypes at risk for pulmonary fibrosis should have a thorough lung examination, an early HRCT scan, and serial PFTs to determine their own rate of lung function decline.

Pirfenidone in Hermansky-Pudlak Syndrome with Pulmonary Fibrosis

Although there are no known specific therapies for HPSPF, patients with HPSPF were the first to enroll in clinical trials with pirfenidone in the United States.[37,38] There have been 2 placebo-controlled trials of pirfenidone in HPSPF conducted at the NIH Clinical Center. The first trial enrolled 23 subjects with HPSPF with mildly to severely decreased lung function (FVC 40%–75% predicted), with 1:1 randomization to placebo or pirfenidone (800 mg 3 times a day). Analysis by the repeated measures model showed that pirfenidone-treated patients lost lung function as assessed by FVC at a rate that was 5% of predicted (approximately 400 mL) per year slower than placebo-treated patients, with post-hoc analysis showing greater benefit to patients with an initial FVC of at least 50% of predicted. After 44 months, based on assessment of efficacy, the trial was stopped on the recommendation of the Data Safety and Monitoring Board, although US Food and Drug Administration approval for pirfenidone was not granted based on the trial data.

Therefore, based on the results of the first pirfenidone trial, a second controlled trial was conducted in which patients with mild to moderate disease were randomized to pirfenidone versus placebo in a 2:1 ratio. An interim analysis, performed 12 months after 30 of the targeted 39 patients were enrolled, showed that subjects in the group treated with pirfenidone (801 mg 3 times a day) had a rate of decline in FVC that was 0.7% predicted per month less than that in the placebo group. However, because FVC in the placebo group declined at a much slower rate (2.5% per year) than expected, the trial was stopped for futility, because showing a difference between groups had become a statistical impossibility.[37] In these studies, pirfenidone was safe and well tolerated in patients with HPSPF.

Lung Transplantation

Patients with HPSPF (ie, HPS-1, HPS-4, and HPS-2) should be referred for lung transplant evaluation early in the disease process. Successful lung transplant has been performed in HPS-1 despite the risks of bleeding.[39] Careful evaluation for bleeding and other potential complications while on the waiting list and after transplant are of critical importance and early referral to a lung transplant center mitigates some of the potential barriers to transplant.

Additional Recommendations for Pulmonary Management

Similar to other patients with pulmonary disease, patients with HPSPF should receive yearly influenza immunizations. Pneumococcal polysaccharide vaccinations (PPSV23) should be offered to all patients with HPS with ILD or at risk for ILD, and pneumococcal conjugate vaccine (PCV13) to those more than 65 years of age. Patients should also be referred to pulmonary rehabilitation programs as needed and in preparation for lung transplant evaluation and listing.

Management of Extrapulmonary Complications

Skin and eye protection
Patients with albinism are at increased risk for skin cancers such as squamous and basal cell carcinomas, as well as melanoma. Protection from the sun from a young age, as well as yearly screening examinations by a dermatologist, are indicated.

Bleeding complications
Patients with HPS are counseled to wear medical alert bracelets. Medications such as aspirin, ibuprofen, and warfarin are generally avoided because of bleeding complications. Platelet transfusions may be required in the setting of trauma, severe bleeding episodes, or surgical procedures, with recommendation for use of a single donor when possible to reduce cumulative antibody sensitization over time. Desmopressin may also be used to prevent bleeding complications.

Inflammatory bowel disease
Involvement of the gastrointestinal tract by a granulomatous colitis has been described in patients

with HPS-1, HPS-4, and HPS-6.[40–43] The disease resembles Crohn's disease clinically and pathologically, and most often involves the colon to a greater extent than other regions of the gastrointestinal tract. In a study of 122 subjects with HPS, 8% were found to have colitis, and, among those who presented with gastrointestinal symptoms, 33% were diagnosed with colitis.[42] Treatment of HPS-related colitis mirrors that of the treatment of Crohn's disease with antiinflammatory drugs, immunosuppressants, and infliximab.[41,42] Because of the universal presence of platelet dysfunction, the role of aminosalicylates is controversial. Surgery should be a last resort, for intractable cases.[29]

FUTURE DIRECTIONS

Natural history studies and investigations into the molecular basis of HPS are ongoing at the NIH Clinical Center (NCT00001456). A longitudinal study of HPS pulmonary fibrosis (NCT02368340) is being conducted by the Rare Lung Diseases Consortium, which is part of the Rare Diseases Clinical Research Network, an initiative of the Office of Rare Diseases Research (ORDR), National Center for Advancing Translational Sciences (NCATS), with funding through collaboration between NCATS and the National Heart, Lung, and Blood Institute. Additional efforts are needed to further characterize the molecular and cellular pathogenesis of HPS pulmonary fibrosis, to define the overlap between HPS pathogenesis and IPF, to identify biomarkers, and to develop targeted therapies for this serious disease.

SUMMARY

HPS is an autosomal recessive disorder that is associated with OCA, bleeding diatheses, granulomatous colitis, and highly penetrant pulmonary fibrosis in some subtypes, including HPS-1, HPS-2, and HPS-4. HPS pulmonary fibrosis shows many of the clinical, radiologic, and histologic features found in IPF, but occurs at a younger age. Improved understanding of the pathogenesis of HPS holds great promise for development of molecularly targeted therapies for this rare disease and may have implications for other fibrotic lung disorders.

REFERENCES

1. Gahl WA, Huizing M. Hermansky-Pudlak syndrome. In: Pagon RA, Adam MP, Ardinger HH, et al, editors. GeneReviews®. Seattle (WA): University of Washington; 1993.

2. Cullinane AR, Curry JA, Carmona-Rivera C, et al. A BLOC-1 mutation screen reveals that PLDN is mutated in Hermansky-Pudlak syndrome type 9. Am J Hum Genet 2011;88:778–87.

3. Cullinane AR, Curry JA, Golas G, et al. A BLOC-1 mutation screen reveals a novel BLOC1S3 mutation in Hermansky-Pudlak syndrome type 8. Pigment Cell Melanoma Res 2012;25:584–91.

4. Badolato R, Prandini A, Caracciolo S, et al. Exome sequencing reveals a pallidin mutation in a Hermansky-Pudlak-like primary immunodeficiency syndrome. Blood 2012;119:3185–7.

5. Jones ML, Murden SL, Brooks C, et al. Disruption of AP3B1 by a chromosome 5 inversion: a new disease mechanism in Hermansky-Pudlak syndrome type 2. BMC Med Genet 2013;14:42.

6. Carmona-Rivera C, Golas G, Hess RA, et al. Clinical, molecular, and cellular features of non-Puerto Rican Hermansky-Pudlak syndrome patients of Hispanic descent. J Invest Dermatol 2011;131:2394–400.

7. Kanazu M, Arai T, Sugimoto C, et al. An intractable case of Hermansky-Pudlak syndrome. Intern Med 2014;53:2629–34.

8. Oh J, Bailin T, Fukai K, et al. Positional cloning of a gene for Hermansky-Pudlak syndrome, a disorder of cytoplasmic organelles. Nat Genet 1996; 14:300–6.

9. Witkop CJ, Almadovar C, Pineiro B, et al. Hermansky-Pudlak syndrome (HPS). An epidemiologic study. Ophthalmic Paediatr Genet 1990;11:245–50.

10. Anikster Y, Huizing M, White J, et al. Mutation of a new gene causes a unique form of Hermansky-Pudlak syndrome in a genetic isolate of central Puerto Rico. Nat Genet 2001;28:376–80.

11. Santiago Borrero PJ, Rodriguez-Perez Y, Renta JY, et al. Genetic testing for oculocutaneous albinism type 1 and 2 and Hermansky-Pudlak syndrome type 1 and 3 mutations in Puerto Rico. J Invest Dermatol 2006;126:85–90.

12. Huizing M, Anikster Y, Fitzpatrick DL, et al. Hermansky-Pudlak syndrome type 3 in Ashkenazi Jews and other non-Puerto Rican patients with hypopigmentation and platelet storage-pool deficiency. Am J Hum Genet 2001;69:1022–32.

13. Gahl WA, Brantly M, Kaiser-Kupfer MI, et al. Genetic defects and clinical characteristics of patients with a form of oculocutaneous albinism (Hermansky-Pudlak syndrome). N Engl J Med 1998;338:1258–64.

14. Gochuico BR, Huizing M, Golas GA, et al. Interstitial lung disease and pulmonary fibrosis in Hermansky-Pudlak syndrome type 2, an adaptor protein-3 complex disease. Mol Med 2012;18:56–64.

15. Ammann S, Schulz A, Krageloh-Mann I, et al. Mutations in AP3D1 associated with immunodeficiency and seizures define a new type of Hermansky-Pudlak syndrome. Blood 2016;127(8):997–1006.

16. Di Pietro SM, Dell'Angelica EC. The cell biology of Hermansky-Pudlak syndrome: recent advances. Traffic 2005;6:525–33.

17. Dell'Angelica EC. AP-3-dependent trafficking and disease: the first decade. Curr Opin Cell Biol 2009; 21:552–9.

18. Rouhani FN, Brantly ML, Markello TC, et al. Alveolar macrophage dysregulation in Hermansky-Pudlak syndrome type 1. Am J Respir Crit Care Med 2009;180:1114–21.

19. Cullinane AR, Yeager C, Dorward H, et al. Dysregulation of galectin-3. Implications for Hermansky-Pudlak syndrome pulmonary fibrosis. Am J Respir Cell Mol Biol 2014;50:605–13.

20. Trimble A, Gochuico BR, Markello TC, et al. Circulating fibrocytes as biomarker of prognosis in Hermansky-Pudlak syndrome. Am J Respir Crit Care Med 2014;190:1395–401.

21. Yoshioka Y, Kumasaka T, Ishidoh K, et al. Inflammatory response and cathepsins in silica-exposed Hermansky-Pudlak syndrome model pale ear mice. Pathol Int 2004;54:322–31.

22. Young LR, Gulleman PM, Bridges JP, et al. The alveolar epithelium determines susceptibility to lung fibrosis in Hermansky-Pudlak syndrome. Am J Respir Crit Care Med 2012;186:1014–24.

23. Young LR, Pasula R, Gulleman PM, et al. Susceptibility of Hermansky-Pudlak mice to bleomycin-induced type II cell apoptosis and fibrosis. Am J Respir Cell Mol Biol 2007;37:67–74.

24. Zhou Y, He CH, Herzog EL, et al. Chitinase 3-like-1 and its receptors in Hermansky-Pudlak syndrome-associated lung disease. J Clin Invest 2015;125: 3178–92.

25. Mahavadi P, Korfei M, Henneke I, et al. Epithelial stress and apoptosis underlie Hermansky-Pudlak syndrome-associated interstitial pneumonia. Am J Respir Crit Care Med 2010;182:207–19.

26. Atochina-Vasserman EN, Bates SR, Zhang P, et al. Early alveolar epithelial dysfunction promotes lung inflammation in a mouse model of Hermansky-Pudlak syndrome. Am J Respir Crit Care Med 2011;184:449–58.

27. Young LR, Borchers MT, Allen HL, et al. Lung-restricted macrophage activation in the pearl mouse model of Hermansky-Pudlak syndrome. J Immunol 2006;176:4361–8.

28. Ahuja S, Knudsen L, Chillappagari S, et al. MAP1LC3B overexpression protects against Hermansky-Pudlak syndrome type - 1 induced defective autophagy in vitro. Am J Physiol Lung Cell Mol Physiol 2015. [Epub ahead of print].

29. Seward SL Jr, Gahl WA. Hermansky-Pudlak syndrome: health care throughout life. Pediatrics 2013; 132:153–60.

30. Ramsay M, Colman MA, Stevens G, et al. The tyrosinase-positive oculocutaneous albinism locus maps to chromosome 15q11.2-q12. Am J Hum Genet 1992;51:879–84.

31. Witkop CJ, Krumwiede M, Sedano H, et al. Reliability of absent platelet dense bodies as a diagnostic criterion for Hermansky-Pudlak syndrome. Am J Hematol 1987;26:305–11.

32. Brantly M, Avila NA, Shotelersuk V, et al. Pulmonary function and high-resolution CT findings in patients with an inherited form of pulmonary fibrosis, Hermansky-Pudlak syndrome, due to mutations in HPS-1. Chest 2000;117:129–36.

33. Avila NA, Brantly M, Premkumar A, et al. Hermansky-Pudlak syndrome: radiography and CT of the chest compared with pulmonary function tests and genetic studies. AJR Am J Roentgenol 2002;179: 887–92.

34. Thomas de Montpreville V, Mussot S, Dulmet E, et al. [Pulmonary fibrosis in Hermansky-Pudlak syndrome is not fully usual]. Ann Pathol 2006;26:445–9.

35. El-Chemaly S, Malide D, Yao J, et al. Glucose transporter-1 distribution in fibrotic lung disease: association with [(1)(8)F]-2-fluoro-2-deoxyglucose-PET scan uptake, inflammation, and neovascularization. Chest 2013;143:1685–91.

36. Kelil T, Shen J, O'Neill AC, et al. Hermansky-Pudlak syndrome complicated by pulmonary fibrosis: radiologic-pathologic correlation and review of pulmonary complications. J Clin Imaging Sci 2014;4:59.

37. Gahl WA, Brantly M, Troendle J, et al. Effect of pirfenidone on the pulmonary fibrosis of Hermansky-Pudlak syndrome. Mol Genet Metab 2002;76:234–42.

38. O'Brien K, Troendle J, Gochuico BR, et al. Pirfenidone for the treatment of Hermansky-Pudlak syndrome pulmonary fibrosis. Mol Genet Metab 2011; 103:128–34.

39. Lederer DJ, Kawut SM, Sonett JR, et al. Successful bilateral lung transplantation for pulmonary fibrosis associated with the Hermansky-Pudlak syndrome. J Heart Lung Transplant 2005;24:1697–9.

40. Schinella RA, Greco MA, Cobert BL, et al. Hermansky-Pudlak syndrome with granulomatous colitis. Ann Intern Med 1980;92:20–3.

41. Hazzan D, Seward S, Stock H, et al. Crohn's-like colitis, enterocolitis and perianal disease in Hermansky-Pudlak syndrome. Colorectal Dis 2006; 8:539–43.

42. Hussain N, Quezado M, Huizing M, et al. Intestinal disease in Hermansky-Pudlak syndrome: occurrence of colitis and relation to genotype. Clin Gastroenterol Hepatol 2006;4:73–80.

43. Uhlig HH. Monogenic diseases associated with intestinal inflammation: implications for the understanding of inflammatory bowel disease. Gut 2013; 62:1795–805.

Hereditary Hemorrhagic Telangiectasia

Joseph G. Parambil, MD

KEYWORDS

- Hereditary hemorrhagic telangiectasia • Arteriovenous malformation • Telangiectasia

KEY POINTS

- Hereditary hemorrhagic telangiectasia (HHT) is an autosomal-dominant angiodysplasia that has an estimated prevalence of 1 in 5000 individuals.
- The most common pulmonary manifestation is arteriovenous malformation (AVM), present in 50% of patients. Complications of pulmonary AVMs include hemoptysis, hemothorax, stroke, and cerebral abscess.
- Pulmonary hypertension can also complicate HHT, due either to high output heart failure from hepatic vascular malformations or to pulmonary arteriopathy.
- Vascular anomalies can also develop in the nasal mucosa, brain, spinal cord, liver, and gastrointestinal tract, necessitating a variety of screening and diagnostic procedures to detect, and mandating a multidisciplinary approach to care.

INTRODUCTION

Hereditary hemorrhagic telangiectasia (HHT) is an autosomal-dominant disorder that leads to the formation of dysplastic blood vessels in mucocutaneous surfaces.[1,2] Dysplastic telangiectasias and arteriovenous malformations (AVMs) can frequently develop within internal organs as well, such as the lungs, brain, liver, and gastrointestinal (GI) tract.[2,3] HHT has an estimated prevalence of 1 in 5000 individuals with no racial predilection and displays an age-dependent penetrance with the diagnosis not suspected until adolescence or later in most patients.[4]

The management of HHT focuses on reducing chronic bleeding along with screening and targeted interventions for internal organ involvement, which can often be silent.[5] Chronic bleeding is mainly from the nose and GI tract, with associated iron-deficiency anemia seen in nearly 30% of patients, requiring iron and/or blood transfusions in order to keep up with continued losses.[5,6]

Today, HHT remains underdiagnosed and underrecognized by practitioners as well as families, leading to life-threatening strokes and hemorrhage in both children and adults. Because of the frequent presence of pulmonary manifestations, this review summarizes the currently available evidence on HHT for the pulmonologist who may often be the first practitioner to encounter these patients.

GENETICS

Thus far, 5 putative HHT disease-causing genes have been located, but genetic screening is clinically available for only 3 of these: *ENG* encoding endoglin (HHT type 1); *ACVRL1* encoding ALK-1 (HHT type 2); and *MADH4* encoding SMAD4 (combined syndrome of HHT and juvenile polyposis syndrome that predisposes patients to both HHT and juvenile polyps of the GI tract, especially the colon and stomach, with a high risk of malignant transformation).[7-9] The 2 remaining unidentified

Disclosures and Source of Funding: None.
Conflict-of-Interest Statement: There are no conflicts of interest in this article.
Department of Medicine, Respiratory Institute, Cleveland Clinic, A-90, 9500 Euclid Avenue, Cleveland, OH 44195, USA
E-mail address: parambj@ccf.org

Clin Chest Med 37 (2016) 513–521
http://dx.doi.org/10.1016/j.ccm.2016.04.013
0272-5231/16/$ – see front matter Published by Elsevier Inc.

HHT-causing genes are on chromosomes 5 and 7.[2] The 3 known genes in HHT encode for proteins involved in transforming growth factor-β (TGF-β) superfamily signaling[10] and are predominantly expressed on endothelial cells.[8,9] This has led to propositions that aberrant endothelial cell reparative responses to TGF-β may be the pathobiological abnormality responsible for dysregulated angiogenesis and disease manifestation.[10,11]

Despite this available genetic information, controversy over disease pathogenesis still exists because of the nonuniform and selective involvement of specific vascular beds. Also, there is significant variability in clinical manifestations, even within family members harboring identical mutations.[2] This has led to suggestions that additional factors, such as modifier genes or environmental factors, may influence the formation of these dysplastic vessels.[12] To support this, Park and colleagues[13] showed in ALK-1-deficient mice that wounding as a second hit triggers an abnormal vascular response to injury necessary for dysregulated angiogenesis, especially in the presence of pro-angiogenic stimuli such as vascular endothelial growth factor (VEGF).[14] This may explain why angiodysplasia tends to occur frequently in the nose, sun-exposed skin, and mouth, which are in constant contact with the external environment and are subject to chronic injury and/or inflammation that may induce a similar wounding-response reaction. This also supports the clinical benefits noted from use of antiangiogenic agents (bevacizumab [anti-VEGF antibody]) in treating certain manifestations of HHT.[15–17]

DIAGNOSIS

HHT is a clinical diagnosis, and the Curaçao criteria are the mainstay of diagnosis.[18] Definite HHT is diagnosed in the presence of 3 or more features, including (1) spontaneous, recurrent nosebleeds; (2) mucocutaneous telangiectasias at multiple characteristic sites such as fingertips, lips, oral mucosa, and/or tongue; (3) visceral involvement with GI telangiectasia and pulmonary, hepatic, cerebral, and/or spinal AVMs; and (4) family history of an affected first-degree relative. If only 2 criteria are present, then HHT is possible, and HHT is unlikely if one or less criterion is present. Because of the age-related penetrance of HHT, there is risk of missing this clinical diagnosis in children and young adults, who might not have epistaxis or visible telangiectasias and yet have HHT and harbor silent life-threatening internal organ lesions. Herein lies one of the cardinal benefits of genetic testing.[19]

The intent of genetic testing in HHT is to facilitate diagnosis in unaffected relatives (often children and young adults) who cannot be excluded clinically and in patients with possible HHT in whom a positive genetic test would be confirmatory, and to clarify the specific mutation in a family. Currently available genetic techniques carry a mutation detection rate of approximately 85%.[20] Because there is considerable overlap in clinical manifestations, even within family members harboring identical mutations, the presence of a specific genotype should not influence screening for visceral involvement,[6] except in the setting of a SMAD4 mutation that would necessitate institution of GI screening for malignancy.[21] The inability to detect a causative mutation in a family does not exclude the disease because mutations may not found in about 15% of patients.

PULMONARY INVOLVEMENT
Pulmonary Arteriovenous Malformations

Pulmonary arteriovenous malformations (PAVMs) are present in approximately 50% of patients with HHT. Conversely, HHT is the underlying cause in nearly 80% of patients found to have PAVMs.[22] PAVMs often remain undiagnosed and are frequently asymptomatic, but can present clinically with hypoxemia due to right-to-left shunting, digital clubbing and cyanosis, and/or an audible thoracic bruit, but these features are present in less than 10% of patients.[22,23] PAVMs can also be associated with massive hemoptysis or hemothorax because of spontaneous rupture, or with transient ischemic attack (TIA), stroke, or cerebral abscess as a consequence of aseptic or septic emboli.[24] TIA and stroke are thought to result from paradoxic embolization of asymptomatic venous thrombus through the PAVMs or, alternatively, the thrombus could potentially originate in situ within the PAVM.[23,24] Cerebral abscess results from paradoxic embolization of bacterial biofilms that often arise from an oral source; this risk appears to be highest following dental procedures.[23] Multiple PAVMs have been associated with a higher risk of stroke, whereas male sex and hypoxemia appear to increase the risk of cerebral abscess.[22] Risk of these complications as well as PAVM growth appears to be greater during pregnancy, most likely due to gravidity-related increase in cardiac output (CO) and/or hormone-induced changes in PAVM wall stability.[25]

The detection of silent lesions before the development of these above-mentioned life-threatening complications supports the premise for screening all HHT patients for PAVMs. Different imaging modalities, physiologic quantification of intrapulmonary shunt fraction with either arterial blood gas analysis or radionuclide perfusion lung scanning, and transthoracic contrast echocardiography (TTCE) have been evaluated as potential screening tests.[22,26] Of these, TTCE with agitated saline to evaluate delayed contrast visualization after 3 to 8 cardiac cycles in the left atrium has been demonstrated to have the best combination of a high sensitivity of greater than 90% and low risk and is the current screening test of choice.[27] This test has its limitations, however, because its high sensitivity can result in an increased false positive rate due to detection of shunting through normal intrapulmonary arteriovenous anastomoses that can be open in approximately 20% of normal individuals at rest.[28] The high sensitivity can also result in overdetection of clinically unimportant microscopic PAVMs. To address these concerns, a TTCE grading system has been described, with an increasing grade predicting an elevated probability of radiographically present PAVMs. However, this grading system is operator-dependent and has not yet been validated.[29] If PAVM is indeed suspected on initial screening, then multidetector-row helical computed tomography (CT) scan of the chest is used to confirm the presence, location, size, and number of malformations, as well as to assess the diameter of the feeding afferent vessels (**Fig. 1**).[30] On CT, PAVMs are usually multiple and more often in the lower lobes. In approximately 5% of cases, they are diffuse and innumerable and pose as problematic because of difficulties in treating them.[23,30] Most PAVMs in HHT are simple fistulas, with feeding arteries arising from one segment in 80% of cases, while in the remainder these are complex with multiple feeding vessels arising from several segments.[23]

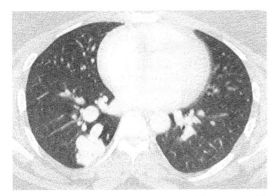

Fig. 1. CT chest scan from a 34-year-old woman with recurrent epistaxis, exertional dyspnea, and an audible thoracic bruit demonstrating a large lobulated AVM in the right lower lobe. She underwent subsequent genetic testing with the presence of a missense ENG mutation.

Transcatheter vaso-occlusive embolotherapy with detachable stainless steel coils is the treatment of choice for PAVMs. This technique has demonstrated excellent procedural success and long-term efficacy in both adults and children and has also been safely used during pregnancy.[31] Hence, there no longer appears to be a role for resective surgery in PAVM management. Occasionally, detachable balloons or Amplatzer occluders can also be used, especially to treat PAVMs with very large feeding arteries.[32] A feeding artery 3 mm or greater is currently the threshold for initiating treatment, because most complications from untreated lesions have been described in patients with a feeding artery of at least that size or larger.[24] Smaller ones could be treated as well, especially if deemed to be symptomatic and/or technically feasible.[31]

The most common short-term complication of embolotherapy is pleuritic chest pain that is most often self-limited. On long-term (>5 years) follow-up, clinical complications occurred very rarely, but reperfusion of treated lesions occurred in 15%, and growth of untreated small PAVMs occurred in 18% of patients.[31] Early and long-term follow-up is hence essential to detect lesions that may need additional therapy, because nearly half of patients undergoing embolotherapy have small detectable residual PAVMs. This can be achieved with a follow-up CT chest scan at 6 to 12 months to ensure involution of the treated aneurysmal sac, and subsequent screening scans every 3 to 5 years to detect reperfusion and/or growth of residual PAVMs. TTCE has not been useful to screen after embolotherapy, because it remains positive in greater than 90% of patients after vaso-occlusion.[23]

Certain precautions are recommended for all HHT patients with PAVMs, regardless of feeding vessel size or history of embolotherapy. Antibiotic prophylaxis for bacteremic, especially dental, procedures is recommended to prevent cerebral abscess.[6] In addition, cautious attention to avoid air bubbles in all intravenous (IV) lines or the use of IV air filters is recommended to prevent central nervous system (CNS) complications from air embolism. For the same reason, patients are advised to avoid scuba diving.

Bronchial Telangiectasias

Endobronchial telangiectasias causing hemoptysis have been described in HHT.[33] They are often multiple, and the appearance and distribution of the lesions are indistinguishable from those seen in scleroderma or isolated bronchial telangiectasia.[33] Management of symptomatic endobronchial telangiectasias comes from isolated case reports and includes the successful bronchoscopic use of electrocoagulation and laser photocoagulation.[34]

Pulmonary Hypertension

Two distinct clinical phenotypes of pulmonary hypertension (PH) have been described in HHT. Most commonly, PH occurs in association with hepatic vascular malformations (VMs), with high-output heart failure (HOHF).[26] Here there is elevation in mean pulmonary artery (mPA) pressure, with associated elevation in pulmonary capillary wedge pressure (PCWP), high CO, and low pulmonary vascular resistance (PVR). Rarely, patients develop a true fibroproliferative arteriopathy with pulmonary artery hypertension (PAH) that is characterized hemodynamically by elevated mPA pressures, normal PCWP, normal/reduced CO, and increased PVR.[35]

In HOHF, PH results from high pulmonary blood flow and left heart failure that accompanies the high output state from shunting through hepatic VMs.[36] These patients are often symptomatic with dyspnea, palpitations, and peripheral edema. HOHF results from shunting of blood between hepatic arteries and hepatic veins and contrast-enhanced CT or MRI of the liver invariably identifies these VMs.[37] HOHF tends to occur more frequently in women and presents late, often in the sixth or seventh decade of life.[36]

Physical examination of patients with HOHF usually reveals a triad of a wide pulse pressure with a low diastolic pressure and bounding pulses, a systolic ejection murmur at the left sternal border from tricuspid regurgitation, and a pulsatile liver with an audible hepatic bruit. Transthoracic echocardiography is useful in assessing patients with suspected HOHF.[26] The most common findings are normal left ventricular size and systolic function with left atrial enlargement. The right ventricle (RV) varies according to the severity and duration of disease with the RV appearing normal early in the disease, but enlarging and becoming dysfunctional later on in the disease course.

Right heart catheterization (RHC) is the gold standard for diagnosing PH, and the typical findings, besides an elevated mPA pressure, include a high CO, an elevated PCWP, and a low PVR. Oxygen saturation studies often reveal a large step-up between the inferior vena cava and right atrium, reflecting significant hepatic artery to vein shunting with resultant oxygen content of hepatic venous blood approaching that of arterial blood.[38]

The treatment of HOHF is directed at managing volume overload, anemia, and atrial fibrillation.[38] Diuretics are the mainstay of treatment to reduce the pulmonary venous congestion. Correction of anemia with iron and/or blood transfusions to maintain a hemoglobin concentration greater than 10 gm/dL is essential to reduce cardiac work and therefore the high output state. Atrial fibrillation is common in these patients because of left atrial stretching, and an aggressive approach toward rhythm control with cardioversion and/or use of antiarrhythmic medications should be considered.[38] Liver transplantation has been reserved for patients with refractory HOHF, despite the above medical therapies, with good success in reducing CO and alleviating symptoms.[39] However, because of the surgical risks of hemorrhage and need for long-term immunosuppression after liver transplantation, alternative treatments have been pursued. Recently, the short-term benefits of antiangiogenic therapy with anti-VEGF antibodies (bevacizumab) have proven to be effective in improving HOHF by reducing the size of hepatic VMs,[16] but the long-term risks and benefits of this approach and of other antiangiogenic therapies still need to be defined.

PAH is a rare complication of HHT.[35] Although mutations and polymorphisms in another member of the TGF-β superfamily, the *BMPR2* gene, are identified in a significant proportion of patients with heritable PAH and in some cases of idiopathic PAH, this has been found only in isolated care reports of patients with HHT-related PAH.[40] However, mutations in ALK-1 (*ACVRL1*) have been implicated in these patients, while mutations in *ENG* are rarely identified.[41] Interestingly, localization of *ACVRL1* mutations specifically within exons 8 and 10 appear to be common in HHT-related PAH.[41] Intimal hyperplasia with plexiform lesions, medial hypertrophy, and in situ thrombosis characterize the histopathology of HHT-related PAH, which is indistinguishable from the fibroproliferative arteriopathy seen in idiopathic PAH.[42]

RHC in these patients reveals a hemodynamic profile similar to that found in patients with idiopathic PAH, with an elevated mPA pressure, a normal PCWP, a low CO, and an elevated PVR. Patients with HHT-related PAH also follow a natural history of progressive right heart failure, albeit with a worse prognosis compared with their idiopathic PAH counterparts.[43] This worse prognosis may be due to the uniqueness of their genetic mutations, or alternatively to the additive stress to the failing RV from chronic anemia with associated hypovolemia demanding an increased workload on the heart and/or from reduced myocardial oxygen delivery.

The benefits of pulmonary arterial vasodilators, including prostanoids, endothelin-receptor antagonists, and phosphodiesterase inhibitors, in idiopathic PAH have been extrapolated as a rationale for using these agents in HHT-related PAH, especially given the similarities in histopathology, hemodynamics, and natural history.[43] However, there are no systematic studies, besides isolated case reports, specifically evaluating outcomes of these medications in patients with HHT-related PAH.[40] Evidence to support the efficacy of these expensive therapies in HHT-related PAH requires further studies to evaluate changes in hemodynamics, functional capacity, and quality-of-life measures.

Judicious administration of these pulmonary vasodilators in HHT is warranted because they can also dilate systemic dysplastic vessels and exaggerate epistaxis and GI bleeding, with consequent undue strain on a failing RV.[35] Also, patients with concurrent PAVMs and PAH warrant special consideration.[38] Because PAVMs decompress the resistive load on the RV, embolizing these malformations can lead to an acute increase in RV afterload and precipitate right heart failure. Concomitant measurement of hemodynamics during temporary occlusion of the PAVM before coil deployment allows for determination of whether embolotherapy can be safely performed without any deleterious consequences to the RV.

NASAL INVOLVEMENT

Recurrent spontaneous epistaxis is the most common symptom of HHT, and it manifests in approximately 50% of patients by age 20, and 96% develop this by age 40.[44,45] Because its occurrence and duration are quite variable, the Epistaxis Severity Score was created to objectively assess severity, thereby allowing care providers to tailor optimal treatment plans for HHT patients.[46] The goals of epistaxis management focus on reducing chronic nasal bleeding, management of anemia, and treatment of acute episodes.

Reduction of chronic bleeding focuses on maintaining nasal mucosal integrity, and this is attempted through various interventions, but mainly with saline humidification.[44] Various topical medications, including lubricants (saline gel, sesame/rose-geranium oil), hormones (estriol), antifibrinolytics (tranexamic acid), and antibiotics (mupirocin), have been tried with variable success. There are insufficient data on long-term control with these agents, precluding recommendation of one agent over another.[44] Various invasive procedures have

been developed to further reduce epistaxis in cases inadequately palliated with medical therapy and include different endonasal techniques using various laser therapies, electrical and chemical cautery, replacement of nasal mucosa by skin or buccal mucosa (septal dermoplasty), and surgical closure of the nostrils (Young procedure).[44,45] Recent reports on submucosal endonasal injections of different substances (sclerosants, like sodium tetradecyl sulfate, and antiangiogenic agents, like bevacizumab) have documented efficacy in mitigating chronic epistaxis.[15] The long-term management of chronic epistaxis still needs to be optimized, and the incomplete efficacy of currently available therapies has propelled ongoing studies on different medical treatments that may diminish chronic blood loss.

Anemia management is still a key element in chronic epistaxis, and iron replacement and even blood transfusions may be necessary to maintain blood counts and to keep up with continued losses.[6] Treatments for acute epistaxis include compressive techniques; use of expansive, resorbable wicks, sponges, and gels; and insertion of minimally traumatic, well-lubricated, or low-pressure pneumatic packing devices.[44] In acute epistaxis refractory to the above measures, there appears to be a role for nasal artery embolization with excellent immediate success.[47]

CENTRAL NERVOUS SYSTEM INVOLVEMENT

A variety of vascular abnormalities with different morphologies have been described in the CNS in HHT, including cerebral arteriovenous malformations (CAVMs) (Fig. 2), arteriovenous fistulas (AVFs), telangiectasias, cavernous malformations, developmental venous anomalies (DVAs), and vein of Galen malformations.[48] Of these, CAVMs, AVFs, and telangiectasias are most commonly involved. AVFs of the brain and spinal cord occur mainly in children under 5 years of age, while CAVMs and telangiectasias occur later in life.[48,49]

Cerebral or spinal AVMs are typically discovered following spontaneous rupture and subsequent bleeding, with malformations developing before the age of 5 years more likely to present in this fashion.[49,50] Also, CAVMs and AVFs appear to have a more aggressive behavior, while cavernous malformations, telangiectasias, and DVAs appear to have a more benign course.[48] When these various vascular anomalies involve the brain, clinical manifestations include cerebral hemorrhage, seizures, headaches, HOHF (especially from high-flow AVFs), hydrocephalus, and cognitive deficits.[48,49] Symptoms of spinal involvement are just as varied and include back pain, sciatica,

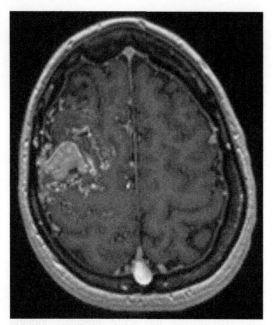

Fig. 2. MRI brain scan from a 23-year-old woman with a known ENG mutation presenting with slurred speech and numbness and weakness of her left arm showing a large right frontal lobe AVM.

paraparesis or tetraparesis, and bowel and bladder disturbances.[48]

The rationale for screening for CNS lesions is to detect a treatable lesion before the development of a life-threatening or disabling event.[50] MRI is considered the screening test of choice for CNS involvement, and the addition of contrast enhancement (gadolinium for patients >2 years) and/or inclusion of gradient echo sequences to detect blood products increases its sensitivity.[6] Once identified, cerebral angiography is considered the gold-standard intervention to define the type of CNS VM.[48]

Once a VM has been defined, obliteration is generally required to effectively eliminate the future risk of hemorrhage. Obliteration can be achieved with a variety of treatment strategies, including transcatheter vaso-occlusive embolization, microsurgery, stereotactic radiation, or combinations of these.[51] Although treatment may provide a significant reduction in spontaneous rupture, procedural risks, although uncommon, are not inconsequential, especially stroke.[51] Therefore, given the rarity of these malformations, the varied natural course based on lesion morphology, and the associated risks of treatment, HHT patients should be individually managed at experienced neurovascular centers with significant expertise in all treatment modalities.

GASTROINTESTINAL INVOLVEMENT

Telangiectasias can be found anywhere in the GI tract, but the stomach and small bowel are mainly affected in approximately 80% of patients.[52] Despite this high frequency, only 25% of patients will develop symptomatic GI bleeding, which usually does not present until the fifth or sixth decades of life and tends to mainly afflict women.[52] Gastric and duodenal telangiectasias are the main sources of bleeding, and the associated morbidity is proportional to the severity of resultant anemia.[52] Given the location of the lesions, esophagogastroduodenoscopy (EGD) is considered the initial diagnostic step for evaluating GI bleeding, and its utility is mainly in the assessment of anemia and/or iron-deficiency that is clinically unexplained by epistaxis.[53] If EGD is unrevealing for active hemorrhage, then small-bowel video-capsule endoscopy can be considered for noninvasive visualization of the entire small bowel, because jejunal telangiectasias could be contributory.

The management of GI bleeding involves treatment of anemia and iron deficiency, and therapies to reduce chronic bleeding, including medical and endoscopic interventions.[54] Medical treatments have included hormonal therapies (estrogen/progesterone, danacrine), antifibrinolytics (tranexamic acid, aminocaproic acid), immunomodulators (thalidomide, interferon, sirolimus), and angiogenesis inhibitors (bevacizumab).[17,54] Endoscopic treatments include argon-plasma coagulation and Nd:YAG laser delivered via EGD and/or push enteroscopy.[53] These treatments are based on retrospective case series and isolated case reports, and there is insufficient evidence to recommend any therapy over another. These options should be considered when iron replacement is insufficient in controlling anemia.

HEPATIC INVOLVEMENT

Hepatic VMs and telangiectasias have been observed to varying extents in the nearly 80% of patients with HHT, but only approximately 8% of these patients will develop symptomatic disease.[36] Clinical manifestations are determined by the predominant type of intrahepatic shunt: HOHF, ischemic cholangiopathy, and mesenteric ischemia are associated with hepatic artery–hepatic vein shunts; portal hypertension with hepatic artery–portal vein shunts; and hepatic encephalopathy with portal vein–hepatic vein shunts.[36] Of these various complications, HOHF is the most frequent.[37]

Several different imaging modalities have been studied to help screen and diagnose hepatic

VMs in HHT.[37] These imaging modalities include Doppler ultrasonography (US), triphasic spiral CT, contrast-enhanced MRI, and invasive angiography. Even though the reference standard for diagnosing hepatic VMs is invasive selective angiography, the various noninvasive scanning approaches have largely supplanted this approach. Doppler US is currently considered sufficiently accurate as a first-line screening modality of the liver in HHT.[37] The advantages of CT and MRI over Doppler US include the ability to describe the morphology of the liver lesions similar to invasive angiography as well as to directly visualize the anatomic type of intrahepatic shunt (**Fig. 3**).

Most patients with hepatic VMs in HHT are asymptomatic. Treatment is only recommended for symptomatic patients and depends on the type of complication. The treatment of HOHF was described earlier, whereas portal hypertension is treated as recommended for cirrhotic patients.[36] Accumulating evidence from case reports and small series has demonstrated significant benefits from antiangiogenic therapy with bevacizumab for hepatic VMs, especially in the setting of ischemic cholangiopathy and HOHF.[16,55] Patients who do not respond to medical therapy may be considered for liver transplantation, although the associated mortality and morbidity in HHT remain a limiting factor.[39]

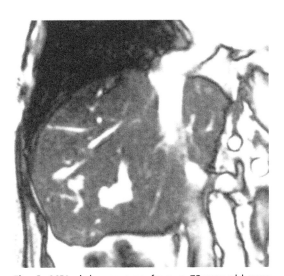

Fig. 3. MRI abdomen scan from a 73-year-old man with definite HHT and a known ALK-1 mutation demonstrating multiple tortuous vascular channels throughout the liver with dilated portal veins and early filling of the hepatic veins, suggesting shunting from the portal to the hepatic veins. He presented with progressive confusion and had asterixis on examination consistent with hepatic encephalopathy.

SUMMARY

Research in the areas of translational genetics and angiogenesis regulation is yielding significant insights into the pathogenesis of HHT. In addition, development of safer and less-invasive management and screening protocols is improving the care of patients with HHT. Most notably, encouraging pathobiological data suggest a promising role for antiangiogenic medical therapy in disease management, and further evidence-based studies on the efficacy and safety of these agents are being conducted. Despite these advances, a major problem remains the significant underrecognition of this condition by afflicted patients and families, and by professional caregivers. Fortunately, the work of patient-oriented foundations as well as dedicated HHT centers is helping to address this.

REFERENCES

1. Kjeldsen AD, Vase P, Green A. Hereditary hemorrhagic telangiectasia: a population-based study of prevalence and mortality in Danish patients. J Intern Med 1999;245:31–9.
2. Abdalla SA, Letarte M. Hereditary hemorrhagic telangiectasia: current views on genetics and mechanisms of disease. J Med Genet 2006;43:97–110.
3. Porteous ME, Burn J, Proctor SJ. Hereditary hemorrhagic telangiectasia: a clinical analysis. J Med Genet 1992;29:527–30.
4. Plauchu H, de Chadarevian JP, Bideau A, et al. Age-related clinical profile of hereditary hemorrhagic telangiectasia in an epidemiologically recruited population. Am J Med Genet 1989;32:291–7.
5. Parambil JG. Hereditary hemorrhagic telangiectasia: update on screening, diagnosis, and management. Clin Pulm Med 2014;21:269–74.
6. Faughnan ME, Palda VA, Garcia-Tsao G, et al. International guidelines for the diagnosis and management of hereditary hemorrhagic telangiectasia. J Med Genet 2011;48:73–87.
7. McAllister KA, Grogg KM, Johnson DW, et al. Endoglin, a TGF-beta binding protein of endothelial cells, is the gene for hereditary hemorrhagic telangiectasia type 1. Nat Genet 1994;8:345–51.
8. Johnson DW, Berg JN, Baldwin MA, et al. Mutations in the activin receptor-like kinase 1 gene in hereditary hemorrhagic telangiectasia type 2. Nat Genet 1996;13:189–95.
9. Gallione CJ, Repetto GM, Legius E, et al. A combined syndrome of juvenile polyposis and hereditary hemorrhagic telangiectasia associated with mutations in MADH4 (SMAD4). Lancet 2004;363:852–9.
10. Mahmoud M, Upton PD, Arthur HM. Angiogenesis regulation by TGFβ signaling: clues from an

inherited vascular disease. Biochem Soc Trans 2011;39:1659–66.

11. Bobik A. Transforming growth factor-βs and vascular disorders. Arterioscler Thromb Vasc Biol 2006;26:1712–20.

12. Bourdeau A, Faughnan ME, McDonald ML, et al. Potential role of modifier genes influencing transforming growth factor-beta1 levels in the development of vascular defects in endoglin heterozygous mice with hereditary hemorrhagic telangiectasia. Am J Pathol 2001;158:2011–20.

13. Park SO, Wankhede M, Lee YJ, et al. Real-time imaging of de novo arteriovenous malformation in a mouse model of hereditary hemorrhagic telangiectasia. J Clin Invest 2009;119:3487–96.

14. Chen W, Guo Y, Walker EJ, et al. Reduced mural cell coverage and impaired vessel integrity after angiogenic stimulation in the Alk1-deficient brain. Arterioscler Thromb Vasc Biol 2013;33:305–10.

15. Karnezis TT, Davidson TM. Treatment of hereditary hemorrhagic telangiectasia with submucosal and topical bevacizumab therapy. Laryngoscope 2012;122:495–7.

16. Dupuis-Girod S, Ginon I, Saurin JC, et al. Bevacizumab in patients with hereditary hemorrhagic telangiectasia and severe hepatic vascular malformations and high cardiac output. JAMA 2012;307:948–55.

17. Lupu A, Stefanescu C, Treton X, et al. Bevacizumab as rescue treatment for severe recurrent gastrointestinal bleeding in hereditary hemorrhagic telangiectasia. J Clin Gastroenterol 2013;47:256–7.

18. Shovlin CL, Guttmacher AE, Buscarini E, et al. Diagnostic criteria for hereditary hemorrhagic telangiectasia (Rendu–Osler–Weber syndrome). Am J Med Genet 2000;91:66–7.

19. Giordano P, Nigro A, Lenato GM, et al. Screening for children from families with Rendu-Osler-Weber disease: from geneticist to clinician. J Thromb Haemost 2006;4:1237–45.

20. Prigoda NL, Savas S, Abdalla SA, et al. Hereditary hemorrhagic telangiectasia: mutation detection, test sensitivity and novel mutations. J Med Genet 2006;43:722–8.

21. O'Malley M, LaGuardia L, Kalady MF, et al. The prevalence of hereditary hemorrhagic telangiectasia in juvenile polyposis syndrome. Dis Colon Rectum 2012;55:886–92.

22. Cottin V, Chinet T, Lavole A, et al. Pulmonary arteriovenous malformations in hereditary hemorrhagic telangiectasia: a series of 126 patients. Medicine 2007;86:1–17.

23. Gossage JR, Kanj G. Pulmonary arteriovenous malformations. A state of the art review. Am J Respir Crit Care Med 1998;158:643–61.

24. Swanson KL, Prakash UB, Stanson AW. Pulmonary arteriovenous fistulas: Mayo Clinic experience, 1982-1997. Mayo Clin Proc 1999;74:671–80.

25. Shovlin CL, Winstock AR, Peters AM, et al. Medical complications of pregnancy in hereditary hemorrhagic telangiectasia. QJM 1995;88:879–87.

26. Montejo Baranda M, Perez M, De Andres J, et al. High output congestive heart failure as first manifestation of Osler-Weber-Rendu disease. Angiology 1984;35:568–76.

27. Barzilai B, Waggoner AD, Spessert C, et al. Two-dimensional contrast echocardiography in the detection and follow-up of congenital pulmonary arteriovenous malformations. Am J Cardiol 1991;68:1507–10.

28. Lovering AT, Riemer RK, Thébaud B. Intrapulmonary arteriovenous anastomoses. Physiological, pathophysiological, or both? Ann Am Thorac Soc 2013;10:504–8.

29. Zukotynski K, Chan RP, Chow CM, et al. Contrast echocardiography grading predicts pulmonary arteriovenous malformations on CT. Chest 2007;132:18–23.

30. Remy J, Remy-Jardin M, Giraud F, et al. Angioarchitecture of pulmonary arteriovenous malformations: clinical utility of three- dimensional helical CT. Radiology 1994;191:657–64.

31. White RI Jr, Lynch-Nyhan A, Terry P, et al. Pulmonary arteriovenous malformations: techniques and long-term outcome of embolotherapy. Radiology 1988;169:663–9.

32. Lee DW, White RI Jr, Egglin TK, et al. Embolotherapy of large pulmonary arteriovenous malformations: long-term results. Ann Thorac Surg 1997;64:930–9.

33. Lincoln MJ, Shigeoka JW. Pulmonary telangiectasia without hypoxemia. Chest 1988;93:1097–8.

34. Tremblay A, Marquette CH. Endobronchial electrocautery and argon plasma coagulation: a practical approach. Can Respir J 2004;11:305–10.

35. Abdalla SA, Gallione CJ, Barst RJ, et al. Primary pulmonary hypertension in families with hereditary hemorrhagic telangiectasia. Eur Respir J 2004;23:373–7.

36. Garcia-Tsao G, Korzenik JR, Young L, et al. Liver disease in patients with hereditary hemorrhagic telangiectasia. N Engl J Med 2000;343:931–6.

37. Memeo M, Scardapane A, De Blasi R, et al. Diagnostic imaging in the study of visceral involvement of hereditary hemorrhagic telangiectasia. Radiol Med 2008;113:547–66.

38. Faughnan ME, Granton JT, Young LH. The pulmonary vascular complications of hereditary hemorrhagic telangiectasia. Eur Respir J 2009;33:1186–94.

39. Lerut J, Orlando G, Adam R, et al, European Liver Transplant Association. Liver transplantation for hereditary hemorrhagic telangiectasia: report of the European Liver Transplant Registry. Ann Surg 2006;244:854–62.

40. Rigelsky CM, Jennings C, Lehtonen R, et al. BMPR2 mutation in a patient with pulmonary arterial

hypertension and suspected hereditary hemorrhagic telangiectasia. Am J Med Genet 2008;146A: 2551–6.

41. Trembath RC, Thomson JR, Machado RD, et al. Clinical and molecular genetic features of pulmonary hypertension in patients with hereditary hemorrhagic telangiectasia. N Engl J Med 2001;345:325–34.

42. Meyrick B, Reid L. Pulmonary hypertension. Anatomic and physiologic correlates. Clin Chest Med 1983;4:199–217.

43. Girerd B, Montani D, Coulet F, et al. Clinical outcomes of pulmonary arterial hypertension in patients carrying an ACVRL1 (ALK1) mutation. Am J Respir Crit Care Med 2010;18:851–61.

44. Sautter NB, Smith TL. Hereditary hemorrhagic telangiectasia-related epistaxis: innovations in understanding and management. Int Forum Allergy Rhinol 2012;2:422–31.

45. Hitchings AE, Lennox PA, Lund VJ, et al. The effect of treatment for epistaxis secondary to hereditary hemorrhagic telangiectasia. Am J Rhinol 2005;19: 75–8.

46. Hoag JB, Terry P, Mitchell S, et al. An epistaxis severity score for hereditary hemorrhagic telangiectasia. Laryngoscope 2010;120:838–43.

47. Andersen PJ, Kjeldsen AD, Nepper-Rasmussen J. Selective embolization in the treatment of intractable epistaxis. Acta Otolaryngol 2005;125:293–7.

48. Krings T, Ozanne A, Chang SM, et al. Neurovascular phenotypes in hereditary hemorrhagic telangiectasia patients according to age. Review of 50 consecutive patients aged 1 day-60 years. Neuroradiology 2005; 47:711–20.

49. Cullen S, Alvarez H, Rodesch G, et al. Spinal arteriovenous shunts presenting before 2 years of age: analysis of 13 cases. Childs Nerv Syst 2006;22: 1103–10.

50. Willemse RB, Mager JJ, Westermann CJ, et al. Bleeding risk of cerebrovascular malformations in hereditary hemorrhagic telangiectasia. J Neurosurg 2000;92:779–84.

51. Haw CS, terBrugge K, Willinsky R, et al. Complications of embolization of arteriovenous malformations of the brain. J Neurosurg 2006;104:226–32.

52. Vase P, Grove O. Gastrointestinal lesions in hereditary hemorrhagic telangiectasia. Gastroenterology 1986;91:1079–83.

53. Proctor DD, Henderson KJ, Dziura JD, et al. Enteroscopic evaluation of the gastrointestinal tract in symptomatic patients with hereditary hemorrhagic telangiectasia. J Clin Gastroenterol 2005;39:115–9.

54. Zarrabeitia R, Albiñana V, Salcedo M, et al. A review on clinical management and pharmacological therapy on hereditary hemorrhagic telangiectasia (HHT). Curr Vasc Pharmacol 2010;8:473–81.

55. Vlachou PA, Colak E, Koculym A, et al. Improvement of ischemic cholangiopathy in three patients with hereditary hemorrhagic telangiectasia following treatment with bevacizumab. J Hepatol 2013;59:186–9.

Pulmonary Capillary Hemangiomatosis and Pulmonary Veno-occlusive Disease

Neal F. Chaisson, MD[a], Mark W. Dodson, MD, PhD[b,c],
Charles Gregory Elliott, MD[b,c],*

KEYWORDS

- Pulmonary veno-occlusive disease • Pulmonary capillary hemangiomatosis
- Pulmonary hypertension • Genetics • Pulmonary disorder

KEY POINTS

- Pulmonary veno-occlusive disease (PVOD) and pulmonary capillary hemangiomatosis (PCH) are rare pulmonary vascular disorders that must be differentiated from other causes of pulmonary hypertension.
- Distinguishing PVOD or PCH from other causes of pulmonary hypertension can be challenging for clinicians, radiologists, and pathologists.
- Recognition of PVOD or PCH is important because vasodilators used to evaluate and treat pulmonary arterial hypertension can cause acute pulmonary edema in PVOD or PCH.
- The recent discovery that mutations in *EIF2AK4* cause autosomal recessive inheritance of PVOD and PCH is a major advance for diagnosis, management, and understanding of these disorders.

INTRODUCTION

Over the past 20 years, physicians have developed increased awareness of pulmonary arterial hypertension (PAH), a disease in which pulmonary arteriolar remodeling leads to increased pulmonary vascular resistance, right heart failure, and death.

It is important for physicians who diagnose and treat PAH to be familiar with pulmonary veno-occlusive disease (PVOD) and pulmonary capillary hemangiomatosis (PCH). Both entities are similar to PAH, but their distinct characteristics can lead to dramatic worsening of symptoms or death when pulmonary vasodilators are given. This article provides an overview of PVOD and PCH to aid physicians who may encounter these rare, but important, pulmonary vascular disorders.

PULMONARY VENO-OCCLUSIVE DISEASE
History

In 1934 Hora[1] described occlusion of the small pulmonary veins of a 48-year-old man with

Disclosure: Advisory Panel, Actelion Pharmaceuticals (N.F. Chaisson). Steering Committee iNO, Bellerophon, Steering Committee CTEPH Registry (Bayer), Steering Committee United States Pulmonary Hypertension Scientific Registry (Actelion) (C.G. Elliott).
[a] Respiratory Institute, Cleveland Clinic, Lerner College of Medicine of Case Western Reserve University, 9500 Euclid Avenue, A-90, Cleveland, OH 44195, USA; [b] Pulmonary Division, University of Utah, 24 North 1900 East Wintrobe Building, Room 701, Salt Lake City, UT 84132, USA; [c] Department of Medicine, Intermountain Medical Center, 5121 South Cottonwood Street, Suite 307, Murray, UT 84107, USA
* Corresponding author. Department of Medicine, Intermountain Medical Center, 5121 South Cottonwood Street, Suite 307, Murray, UT 84107.
E-mail address: greg.elliott@imail.org

Clin Chest Med 37 (2016) 523–534
http://dx.doi.org/10.1016/j.ccm.2016.04.014
0272-5231/16/$ – see front matter © 2016 Elsevier Inc. All rights reserved.

progressive dyspnea, cyanosis, and pulmonary edema. Questions persisted as to whether this disorder was a postmortem artifact until 1966 when Heath and colleagues[2] described similar histologic findings in a living patient and introduced the term PVOD.

Pathology

The characteristic appearance of PVOD is of disorganized smooth muscle hypertrophy and collagen matrix deposition within small pulmonary veins and venules, leading to occlusion of the lumen and arterialization of vessel walls (**Fig. 1A**).[3] Intravascular thrombosis and fibrinous recanalization are common.[4] Extravascular changes, including interlobular septal thickening, dilated pulmonary lymph nodes, and pulmonary lymphatic vessels, and pulmonary edema also occur (**Table 1**).[3,5–7] Upstream capillaries appear engorged and loop-like (**Fig. 1B**).[4] Pulmonary arterial changes, including medial hypertrophy and eccentric intimal fibrosis,[6] also occur and can mimic PAH (**Fig. 1C**). However, plexiform arteriopathy (**Fig. 2**) differentiates PAH from PVOD.[8]

Epidemiology

The incidence and prevalence of PVOD remain unclear. Although some estimates suggest the prevalence is between 0.3 and 1.4 cases per million persons, several factors, including the need for pathologic diagnosis, disease misclassification, and lack of large studies, prevent better estimation.[9]

PVOD has been reported in patients aged 1 week to almost 70 years,[4,5,9,10] with most cases occurring in adults 30 to 50 years old. However, the heritable form of PVOD may present at a younger age than cases with sporadic disease, suggesting a potential bimodal distribution that reflects different pathogenesis, but a common end

disorder.[11] Because the understanding of PVOD is largely limited to case reports and small case series, heterogeneity also exists regarding gender preference. Most studies suggest no gender preference, whereas at least 1 case series suggests that PVOD may show male predominance.[4,5,9,10,12] What is clear is that PVOD does not show a female predominance as is seen in idiopathic PAH (IPAH).

Risk Factors

The list of conditions associated with PVOD includes connective tissue diseases (CTDs), malignancy, prior exposure to chemotherapy (especially alkylating agents and some antitumor antibiotics), stem cell transplant, and exposure to organic solvents[13–16] (**Box 1**). It is suggested that up to 15% of reported PVOD cases may be attributable to prior chemotherapy[14,15] and a recent case control study suggested an association of PVOD with organic solvents, especially trichloroethylene.[16]

Genetic Factors

Reports of siblings with PVOD suggested an autosomal recessive heritable predisposition to PVOD,[17–19] in contrast with the autosomal dominant inheritance pattern seen in familial PAH.[20] Following the discovery of *BMPR2* mutations and their association with familial PAH, *BMPR2* mutations were identified in isolated PVOD cases, but without clear heritable features.[21–24]

In 2014, Eyries and colleagues[11] reported *EIF2AK4* mutations in 5 sporadic PVOD cases and identified this as the cause of autosomal recessive inheritance among 13 families. *EIF2AK4* regulates angiogenesis and is found in the smooth muscle of pulmonary vessels, lung macrophages, and interstitial tissue,[11,25] suggesting that

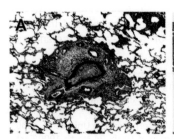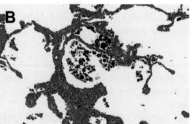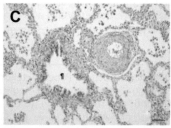

Fig. 1. (*A*) Preseptal pulmonary vein with occlusive lesion characteristic of PVOD (Movat stain, original magnification ×40). (*B*) Engorgement of alveolar capillaries and hemosiderin deposition in macrophages accompanying PVOD (hematoxylin and eosin, original magnification ×100). (*C*) Pulmonary arteriole adjacent to bronchiole (*paragraph mark*) shows medial hypertrophy and intimal fibrosis (hematoxylin and eosin, scale bar equals 200 μm). These lesions may accompany PVOD and PCH. ([*A*, *B*] *Courtesy of* Carol Farver, MD, Department of Anatomic Pathology, Cleveland Clinic, Cleveland, OH; and [*C*] *From* Montani D, Price LC, Dorfmuller P, et al. Pulmonary veno-occlusive disease. Eur Respir J 2009;33:191; with permission.)

Table 1
Common pathologic features of PAH, PVOD, and PCH

	PAH	PVOD	PCH
Pulmonary veins/venules involved	No	Yes	Yes, secondary to capillary invasion
Pulmonary vein/venule thromboses	No	Yes	Yes
Pulmonary capillaries involved	No	Yes, dilated, congested, looplike appearance	Yes, well-circumscribed proliferation of capillaries
Pulmonary arterioles involved	Yes	Yes, secondary to passive congestion	Yes, secondary to passive congestion
Arterial plexiform lesions	Yes	No	No
Pulmonary edema	No	Yes	Yes
Interlobular septal thickening	No	Yes	Yes
Engorged pulmonary lymphatic vessels	No	Yes	Yes
Pulmonary lymphadenopathy	No	Yes	Yes
Alveolar hemorrhage	No	Yes	Yes

mutations in this gene play a significant role in PVOD pathogenesis.

Clinical Features

PVOD can be difficult to differentiate from PAH because patients with both entities usually present with symptoms that reflect right ventricular (RV) dysfunction. Almost all patients report exertional dyspnea and fatigue.[4,10,26] Other symptoms include substernal chest pain, lightheadedness, hoarseness (cardiovocal or Ortner syndrome), productive or nonproductive cough, and lower extremity edema.[9,10,26]

Physical examination features may include a loud P2, a murmur located at the left lower sternal border, and right parasternal heave.[4,10] Other features include jugular venous distention, hepatomegaly, ascites, and peripheral edema.[4,10,26]

Clubbing occurs in many patients with PVOD and has been suggested as a feature that should prompt consideration of PVOD in patients otherwise suspected of having PAH.[9,10] Presence of crackles is variable and may reflect more advanced disease.[9,10]

Imaging

Chest imaging often provides clues that suggest PVOD. On chest radiograph (CXR), Kerley B lines

Box 1
Conditions with reported association to PVOD

- Myelodysplastic syndrome
- Lung cancer
- Hodgkin lymphoma
- Stem cell transplant
- Prior chemotherapy, especially alkylating agents
- Radiation exposure
- Tobacco
- Congenital heart disease
- Scleroderma and other CTDs
- Sarcoidosis
- Hashimoto thyroiditis
- Pulmonary Langerhans cell granulomatosis
- Antiphospholipid antibody syndrome
- Fenfluramine use
- Oral contraceptive use
- Human immunodeficiency virus

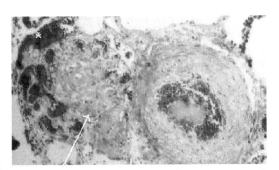

Fig. 2. Plexiform lesion (*arrow*) adjacent to a preacinar artery with dilation lesion (*asterisk*). Plexiform lesions are not seen in PVOD or PCH (smooth muscle actin stain, original magnification ×60). (*From* Pietra GG, Capron F, Stewart S, et al. Pathologic assessment of vasculopathies in pulmonary hypertension. J Am Coll Cardiol 2004;43:28S; with permission.)

and basilar ground-glass opacities are common.[27] High-resolution computed tomography of the chest (HRCT) is more likely to detect PVOD than CXR. Characteristic HRCT findings include a triad of centrilobular nodules and ground-glass opacities, thickened interlobular septa, and enlarged (short diameter, >1 cm) mediastinal lymph nodes (**Fig. 3**).[28] Recent evidence suggests that in patients with features of PAH, presence of 2 or more of these features on HRCT is highly predictive of PVOD.[24,29]

Current guidelines recommend perfusion lung scans to screen for chronic thromboembolic pulmonary hypertension (PH).[30] Unlike HRCT, these scans are not useful in distinguishing PVOD from PAH. Most patients with PVOD or PAH have normal lung perfusion scans or patterns that suggest a low probability of pulmonary emboli.[31] However, clinicians should be aware of reports that describe patients with PVOD with high-probability perfusion lung scan patterns without pulmonary artery occlusion on pulmonary angiography.[32]

Laboratory Studies

Most patients with PVOD have normal or nearly normal spirometry with severely decreased lung diffusion capacity for carbon monoxide (DLco).[24,33] Reductions of DLco tend to be more severe for patients with PVOD than for patients with IPAH[24,33]; and evidence suggests that normal spirometry coupled with a markedly reduced DLco may help to identify patients with PVOD.[30]

Although surgical lung biopsy may be difficult to perform in patients suspected of PVOD, evaluation of sputum cytology may provide a helpful alternative.[24,34,35] Venous obstruction in PVOD causes increased transcapillary pressures and can lead to occult pulmonary hemorrhage. Investigators have reported a higher percentage of hemosiderin-laden macrophages in patients with PVOD than in patients with IPAH[34,35] and have suggested that bronchoalveolar lavage or sputum cytology can differentiate PVOD from IPAH with high sensitivity and specificity.

Hemodynamics

Current methods of hemodynamic analysis cannot differentiate PVOD from PAH because both diseases show increased pulmonary artery pressures and pulmonary vascular resistance with normal pulmonary artery wedge pressures. This phenomenon reflects the fact that the wedged pulmonary artery catheter measures pressures in larger pulmonary veins and does not measure pressures in small pulmonary veins or capillaries. Current guidelines[30] do not recommend vasoreactivity testing for patients suspected of PVOD because of increased risk of developing pulmonary edema during testing and rare benefit from calcium channel blocker therapy.[24,30]

Prognosis and Therapy

Morbidity and mortality in PVOD is substantial, with a mean survival from symptom onset of 24.4 ± 22.2 months.[24] In pediatric populations, disease progression may be faster.[4] Therapeutic options are limited and lung transplant remains the only viable cure.[30,36] However, many patients die in the process of waiting or are too debilitated for transplant at the time of referral. A recent analysis suggested that patients with PVOD are twice as likely to die waiting for transplant as those with IPAH, despite similar wait times.[37]

There is consensus that pulmonary vasodilator therapy is tolerated poorly in patients with PVOD compared with IPAH. Initiation of these therapies frequently leads to increased transcapillary pressures and pulmonary edema following pulmonary arterial vasodilation and can result in rapid clinical

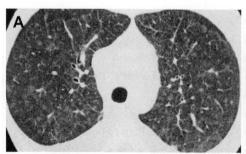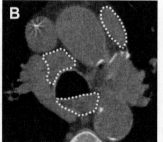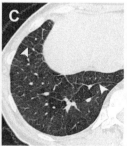

Fig. 3. Computed tomography shows (*A*) centrilobular opacities and nodules, (*B*) mediastinal lymphadenopathy, and (*C*) prominent septal lines (*arrowheads*). These findings are prominent in both PVOD and PCH. (*From* [*A, B*] Montani D, Price LC, Dorfmuller P, et al. Pulmonary veno-occlusive disease. Eur Respir J 2009;33:195, with permission; and [*C*] Frazier AA, Franks TJ, Mohammed T-LH, et al. Pulmonary veno-occlusive disease and pulmonary capillary hemangiomatosis1. Radiographics 2007;27:870, with permission.)

deterioration or death. Nonetheless, there are case reports of clinical improvement with intravenous and inhaled prostacyclins,[10,38–41] phosphodiesterase type-5 inhibitors (PDE5-I),[42–44] and endothelin receptor antagonists.[45] For this reason, experts have recommended cautious consideration of these therapies in patients with PVOD.[38] One report suggested that doses of intravenous epoprostenol greater than 6 ng/kg/min improves pulmonary venodilation, whereas lower doses principally affect precapillary vessels.[40]

Immunomodulators, including prednisone, azathioprine, and cyclophosphamide, have been used successfully in patients with sarcoidosis-associated and CTD-associated PAH under the assumption that pulmonary vascular injury in these cases has an inflammatory component.[38,46–50] Success in PVOD using these modalities is rare. Thus, these therapies are only recommended if PVOD is attributed to sarcoidosis or CTD.[38]

Platelet-derived growth factor (PDGF) pathways have been identified as an important factor in abnormal cellular proliferation and angiogenesis. Preliminary success with PDGF inhibitors in patients with both PVOD and PAH provided early enthusiasm as a new treatment option.[51–53] However, recently published data from a phase III, open-label extension study of imatinib reported significant risk of adverse events, including subdural hematoma.[54] For this reason, imatinib and other PDGF inhibitors are currently not recommended for the treatment of PAH or PVOD.

PULMONARY CAPILLARY HEMANGIOMATOSIS
History

In 1978, Wagenvoort and colleagues[55] described a 71 year old woman with features similar to PAH, including progressive dyspnea, hemoptysis, and hemorrhagic pleural effusion. However, examination of lung tissue showed atypical proliferation of capillarylike channels in the lungs, distinct from the findings seen in PAH or PVOD, leading the investigators to describe a new entity, PCH.

Pathology

The pathologic hallmark of PCH is an atypical proliferation of capillary vessels at least 2 layers thick (see **Table 1**) (**Fig. 4**).[55] The multiple layers of capillaries differentiate PCH from congested capillaries or atelectasis. Low-power microscopy shows a patchy parenchymal process often forming nodules (see **Fig. 4**A).[56] High-power microscopy may show infiltration of capillaries into bronchi, intralobular fibrous septa, and walls of small pulmonary arteries and veins (see **Fig. 4**B). Rarely capillaries proliferate into the pericardium, pleura, and mediastinal lymph nodes.[57–59] Invasion of pulmonary veins, arteries, and other tissues by capillaries also distinguishes PCH from other conditions with prominent capillaries, including PVOD.[56,60,61]

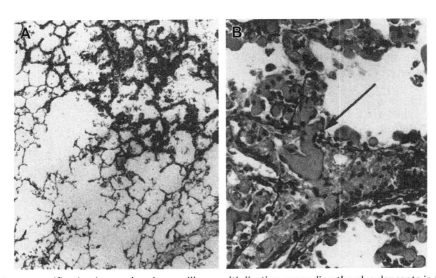

Fig. 4. (*A*) Low-magnification image showing capillary multiplication expanding the alveolar septa in PCH. To the bottom left is an area with normal capillaries and no expansion of the alveolar septa (hematoxylin and eosin, original magnification ×50). (*B*) Higher magnification image of PCH showing capillary multiplication, and invasion of capillaries into the walls of a pulmonary vein (*arrow*) (van Gieson elastic stain, original magnification ×300). (*From* Langleben D, Heneghan JM, Batten AP, et al. Familial pulmonary capillary hemangiomatosis resulting in primary pulmonary hypertension. Ann Intern Med 1988;109:106–9; with permission.)

Epidemiology

The incidence and the prevalence of PCH remain uncertain for similar reasons as in PVOD. El-Gabaly and colleagues[62] suggested a prevalence of 4 cases per million individuals. All investigators agree that PCH is a rare disorder.[56,63,64]

PCH likely occurs with equal frequency among men and women.[4] The age of onset is poorly defined. Physicians have diagnosed PCH in infancy and as late as age 71 years,[4] but most patients present for medical evaluation between the ages of 20 and 40 years, which is earlier than is typically seen with PVOD or IPAH.[56,63,64]

Risk Factors

Unlike PVOD, investigators have not identified clear risk factors for the development of PCH. Individual case reports have described the pathologic lesions of PCH in patients diagnosed with Takayasu aortoarteritis, Kartagener syndrome, scleroderma, hypertrophic cardiomyopathy, and systemic lupus erythematosus.[4,7,65] In contrast with PVOD, investigators have not reported PCH after exposure to chemotherapy, organic solvents, or stem cell transplant.

Genetic Factors

In 1988, Langleben and colleagues[56] provided the first description of familial PCH, describing a single family with 3 of 9 siblings affected, suggesting autosomal recessive inheritance. In 2013, Best and colleagues[66] identified EIF2AK4 mutations in 2 brothers affected by PCH and 2 of 10 patients with sporadic PCH. The parallel discovery by Eyries and colleagues[11] of causative EIF2AK4 mutations in patients with familial and sporadic PVOD now allows clinicians to advise patients with PVOD and PCH about guideline recommended genetic testing and counseling.[30,67]

Clinical Presentation

The symptoms and physical examination signs of PCH are similar to those seen in PVOD and PAH and largely reflect signs of hypoxemia and RV dysfunction. Investigators have suggested that hemoptysis and hemorrhagic pleural effusions are more characteristic of PCH than PVOD, occurring in about one-third of patients with PCH.[4,24,68] Cyanosis and digital clubbing are also prominent features and become more evident as arterial hypoxemia worsens.

Imaging

Chest radiographs often appear similar to those found in PVOD, with Kerley B lines and signs of interstitial edema. Often, basilar reticulonodular and micronodular opacities are seen, which are not present in PVOD.[4] However, HRCT remains an essential feature in differentiating PCH from PAH. Findings may be similar to those of PVOD, including thickened subpleural septal lines; mediastinal lymph node enlargement; and nodular, centrilobular ground-glass opacities (see **Fig. 3**).[30]

Laboratory Studies

Arterial blood gases commonly identify arterial hypoxemia with an increased alveolar-arterial oxygen tension gradient made worse with exercise. This phenomenon is typically more severe than is seen in PAH. Pulmonary function tests also show impairment and mimic patterns seen in PVOD with normal or nearly normal spirometry, but severely reduced DL_{CO}.[24,33,66] As in PVOD, cytology examination of bronchoalveolar lavage specimens may show abundant red blood cells or hemosiderin-laden macrophages.[58,69]

Hemodynamics

Pulmonary artery catheterization typically confirms severe PH with a normal pulmonary artery occlusion pressure, as in PAH and PVOD.[61]

Prognosis

The natural history of PCH remains poorly defined, but survival beyond 5 years from symptom onset is rare.[56,64] Furthermore, variability exists in onset and progression among family members with familial PCH and EIF2AK4 mutations.[66] These observations suggest that the natural history of PCH is variable, and that other factors, such as adaptation of the RV to increased pulmonary artery pressures, influence prognosis.

Therapy

Pharmacologic management of PCH remains uncertain and, like PVOD, lung transplant is the preferred option. Reports exist of catastrophic pulmonary edema following initiation of pulmonary vasodilators like calcium channel blockers or epoprostenol.[56,70,71] However, at least some patients seem to have benefitted from parenteral prostanoids.[72] Like PVOD, the rationale for the variability in prostanoid tolerance remains speculative. Individual reports also describe favorable responses to inhibitors of angiogenesis, including interferon alfa-2a,[73] imatinib,[74] and doxycycline.[75]

PULMONARY VENO-OCCLUSIVE DISEASE AND PULMONARY CAPILLARY HEMANGIOMATOSIS: SPECTRUM OF A SINGLE DISEASE OR DISTINCT ENTITIES?

As is clear from the preceding discussion, the clinical, imaging, and hemodynamic similarities between PVOD and PCH are striking (**Table 2**). In addition, there is growing evidence of marked histopathologic overlap. This overlap has prompted reclassification of PCH and PVOD into a unique subclass of group 1 PH.[76] The recent discovery of the *EIF2AK4* genetic mutation in both entities[11,66] further raises the question of whether PVOD and PCH represent different points on a spectrum of a single disease process, rather than distinct clinical entities.

Table 2
Clinical features of PAH, PVOD, and PCH

	PAH	PVOD	PCH
Demographics	• Fourth to fifth decade[24] • Female predominant	• Wide age range (most cases occur in fourth to fifth decade)[10,24] • No clear gender difference	• Wide age range, but often younger (third to fourth decade)[68] • No clear gender difference
History	• Dyspnea • Syncope • Hemoptysis rare	• Dyspnea more pronounced • Syncope • Hemoptysis rare	• Dyspnea more pronounced • Syncope • Hemoptysis in 40%[68]
Physical examination	• Findings of PH • Clubbing uncommon	• Findings of PH • Clubbing more common	• Findings of PH • Clubbing more common
Laboratory	• Decreased Pao_2 • Decreased DLco	• Lower Pao_2 • Lower DLco	• Lower Pao_2 • Lower DLco
Imaging	• Enlarged central PAs[84] • Pericardial effusions[24] • Pleural effusions in 15%[24] • No hilar and mediastinal adenopathy • No centrilobular ground-glass opacities • No septal thickening	• Enlarged central PAs[10,84] • Pericardial effusions rare[24] • Pleural effusions in 20%[24] • Hilar and mediastinal adenopathy • Centrilobular ground-glass opacities • Septal thickening	• Enlarged central PAs[84] • Pericardial effusions rare[84] • Pleural effusion in 25%[68] • Hilar and mediastinal adenopathy • Centrilobular ground-glass opacities • Septal thickening
Hemodynamics	Increased pulmonary artery pressures with normal wedge	Increased pulmonary artery pressures with normal wedge	Increased pulmonary artery pressure with normal wedge
Cytopathology	Hemosiderin-laden macrophages rare	Hemosiderin-laden macrophages more common[34,35]	Hemosiderin-laden macrophages reported[58,69]
Genetics	• Mutations in *BMPR2* found in 75% of heritable PAH cases, and 10%–20% of IPAH cases[25] • Mutations in *EIF2AK4* not reported	• Mutations in *BMPR2* reported in rare sporadic cases[21,24] • Mutations in *EIF2AK4* reported in multiple pedigrees with autosomal recessive inheritance, and 20% of sporadic cases[11]	• Mutations in *BMPR2* not reported • Mutations in *EIF2AK4* reported in 1 pedigree with autosomal recessive inheritance, and 20% of sporadic cases[66]
Clinical course	• Slower progression (mean duration from symptom onset to death of 6 y)[24] • Pulmonary edema with pulmonary vasodilator treatment not reported	• Shorter time from symptom onset to death (mean 2 y)[24] • Risk of pulmonary edema with pulmonary vasodilator treatment	• Shorter time from symptom onset to death (mean 3 y)[68] • Risk of pulmonary edema with pulmonary vasodilator treatment

Abbreviation: PA, pulmonary artery.

Histologic Overlap

Histologic changes are not always limited to the veins in PVOD, or to the capillaries in PCH. In both conditions, pulmonary arteries often show intimal thickening and medial hypertrophy, but without the plexiform lesions that characterize PAH.[8,55,77,78] Capillary engorgement and proliferation are frequently described in PVOD, and have been attributed to passive congestion related to downstream venous occlusion.[46,77,79,80] Likewise, invasion of veins by proliferating capillaries in PCH can cause secondary occlusion of veins associated with intimal fibrosis,[55,61,78] and has been hypothesized as the cause of PH in PCH.[61] In a large case series involving 35 patients diagnosed by histopathology with either PVOD (n = 30) or PCH (n = 5), 22 PVOD cases showed capillary proliferation consistent with PCH, and 4 PCH cases showed venous intimal fibrosis consistent with PVOD.[5] These findings highlight the difficulties in differentiating PVOD from PCH, and further speculation that they may represent a single disease state.

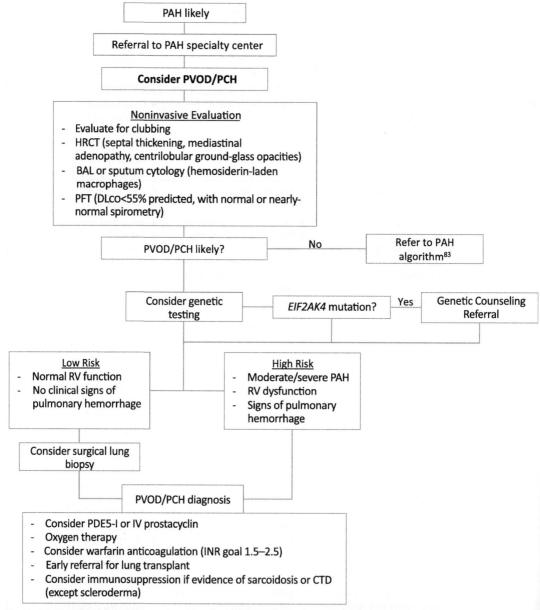

Fig. 5. Diagnostic and treatment algorithm for PVOD and PCH. BAL, bronchoalveolar lavage; IV, intravenous; INR, International Normalized Ratio.

Genetic Overlap

The identification of *EIF2AK4* mutations in both PVOD and PCH is a pivotal finding that advances the understanding of the similarities between PVOD and PCH down to the molecular level. Current understanding suggests that most *EIF2AK4* mutations that cause PVOD or PCH are either frameshift or nonsense mutations,[11,66] both of which would be expected to result in loss of protein function. Moreover, 2 of the *EIF2AK4* mutations, a single-nucleotide deletion at c1392 resulting in a frameshift, and a cytosine to thymidine substitution at c3438 resulting in a nonsense substitution, have been found in patients with PVOD and PCH.[11,66] Thus, it seems that the same molecular defect can cause both phenotypes. The reasons for this are unclear, but it suggests the presence of additional factors, such as environmental factors or additional genetic loci, that modify the effect of loss-of-function *EIF2AK4* mutations, yielding a phenotype that can range from one that predominantly shows features of PVOD to one that predominantly shows features of PCH.

PULMONARY VENO-OCCLUSIVE DISEASE AND PULMONARY CAPILLARY HEMANGIOMATOSIS: DIAGNOSTIC APPROACH

Current guidelines for the diagnosis and treatment of PH recommend a comprehensive set of investigations interpreted by physicians with expertise.[67] Clinicians must consider PVOD and PCH when the diagnosis of PAH is likely.

The definitive diagnosis of PCH or PVOD requires microscopic examination of lung tissue. However, surgical biopsy is not feasible in many cases. The authors think that diagnosis with open lung biopsy should only be considered in patients without signs of RV dysfunction, severe PH, or alveolar hemorrhage. In other patients, clinical findings, physical examination, physiologic test results (eg, DLco<55% predicted), cytology (hemosiderin-laden macrophages), HRCT imaging (eg, nodular centrilobular opacities), and genetic tests (*EIF2AK4* mutations) may be sufficient to diagnose PVOD and PCH with reasonable certainty (**Fig. 5**).

In patients with PVOD or PCH, early referral for lung transplant is essential. There is no consensus on the use of pulmonary vasodilators, but PDE5-I or intravenous prostacyclin therapy may be considered for some patients. The authors also recommend consideration of anticoagulation based on evidence of in situ thrombosis in these patients and observational data supporting the use of warfarin in PAH.[81-83] We caution providers to weigh the potential benefits against risk in patients who have evidence of prior pulmonary hemorrhage.[24,35] We recommend diuretics in patients who have signs of pulmonary edema or RV failure as well as supplemental oxygen to treat arterial hypoxemia.

SUMMARY

PVOD and PCH constitute a rare subgroup of PAH. As diagnosis and management of PAH become more common, providers must be aware of the features that distinguish PVOD and PCH from PAH. This article highlights the current understanding regarding pathology, genetics, and clinical features of PVOD and PCH and offers a guide to the diagnosis and management of such patients.

ACKNOWLEDGMENTS

The authors are grateful for the administrative assistance of Jana Johnson.

REFERENCES

1. Hora J. Zur histologie der klinischen 'primaren pulmonalsklerose'. Frankf Z Pathol 1934;47:100.
2. Heath D, Segel N, Bishop J. Pulmonary veno-occlusive disease. Circulation 1966;34:242–8.
3. Pietra GG, Capron F, Stewart S, et al. Pathologic assessment of vasculopathies in pulmonary hypertension. J Am Coll Cardiol 2004;43:25S–32S.
4. Frazier AA, Franks TJ, Mohammed T-LH, et al. Pulmonary veno-occlusive disease and pulmonary capillary hemangiomatosis1. Radiographics 2007;27:867–82.
5. Lantuejoul S, Sheppard MN, Corrin B, et al. Pulmonary veno-occlusive disease and pulmonary capillary hemangiomatosis: a clinicopathologic study of 35 cases. Am J Surg Pathol 2006;30:850–7.
6. Montani D, O'Callaghan DS, Savale L, et al. Pulmonary veno-occlusive disease: recent progress and current challenges. Respir Med 2010;104(Suppl 1):S23–32.
7. Thomas de Montpreville V, Dulmet E, Fadel E, et al. Lymph node pathology in pulmonary veno-occlusive disease and pulmonary capillary heamangiomatosis. Virchows Arch 2008;453:171–6.
8. Wagenvoort CA, Wagenvoort N. The pathology of pulmonary veno-occlusive disease. Virchows Arch A Pathol Anat Histol 1974;364:69–79.
9. Mandel J, Mark EJ, Hales CA. Pulmonary veno-occlusive disease. Am J Respir Crit Care Med 2000;162:1964–73.

10. Holcomb BW Jr, Loyd JE, Ely EW, et al. Pulmonary veno-occlusive disease: a case series and new observations. Chest 2000;118:1671–9.

11. Eyries M, Montani D, Girerd B, et al. EIF2AK4 mutations cause pulmonary veno-occlusive disease, a recessive form of pulmonary hypertension. Nat Genet 2014;46:65–9.

12. Wagenvoort CA. Pulmonary veno-occlusive disease. Entity or syndrome? Chest 1976;69:82–6.

13. Dai Z, Matsui Y. Pulmonary veno-occlusive disease: an 80-year-old mystery. Respiration 2014; 88:148–57.

14. Ranchoux B, Gunther S, Quarck R, et al. Chemotherapy-induced pulmonary hypertension: role of alkylating agents. Am J Pathol 2015;185:356–71.

15. Shahab N, Haider S, Doll DC. Vascular toxicity of antineoplastic agents. Semin Oncol 2006;33: 121–38.

16. Montani D, Lau EM, Descatha A, et al. Occupational exposure to organic solvents: a risk factor for pulmonary veno-occlusive disease. Eur Respir J 2015;46: 1721–31.

17. Voordes CG, Kuipers JR, Elema JD. Familial pulmonary veno-occlusive disease: a case report. Thorax 1977;32:763–6.

18. Davies P, Reid L. Pulmonary veno-occlusive disease in siblings: case reports and morphometric study. Hum Pathol 1982;13:911–5.

19. Rosenthal A, Vawter G, Wagenvoort CA. Intrapulmonary veno-occlusive disease. Am J Cardiol 1973;31: 78–83.

20. Loyd JE, Primm RK, Newman JH. Familial primary pulmonary hypertension: clinical patterns. Am Rev Respir Dis 1984;129:194–7.

21. Runo JR, Vnencak-Jones CL, Prince M, et al. Pulmonary veno-occlusive disease caused by an inherited mutation in bone morphogenetic protein receptor II. Am J Respir Crit Care Med 2003;167:889–94.

22. Aldred MA, Vijayakrishnan J, James V, et al. BMPR2 gene rearrangements account for a significant proportion of mutations in familial and idiopathic pulmonary arterial hypertension. Hum Mutat 2006;27:212–3.

23. Machado RD, Aldred MA, James V, et al. Mutations of the TGF-beta type II receptor BMPR2 in pulmonary arterial hypertension. Hum Mutat 2006;27: 121–32.

24. Montani D, Achouh L, Dorfmüller P, et al. Pulmonary veno-occlusive disease: clinical, functional, radiologic, and hemodynamic characteristics and outcome of 24 cases confirmed by histology. Medicine 2008;87:220–33.

25. Best DH, Austin ED, Chung WK, et al. Genetics of pulmonary hypertension. Curr Opin Cardiol 2014; 29:520–7.

26. Montani D, Kemp K, Dorfmuller P, et al. Idiopathic pulmonary arterial hypertension and pulmonary veno-occlusive disease: similarities and differences. Semin Respir Crit Care Med 2009;30:411–20.

27. Scheibel RL, Dedeker KL, Gleason DF, et al. Radiographic and angiographic characteristics of pulmonary veno-occlusive disease. Radiology 1972;103: 47–51.

28. Resten A, Maitre S, Humbert M, et al. Pulmonary hypertension: CT of the chest in pulmonary venoocclusive disease. AJR Am J Roentgenol 2004;183: 65–70.

29. Mineo G, Attina D, Mughetti M, et al. Pulmonary veno-occlusive disease: the role of CT. Radiol Med 2014;119:667–73.

30. Galie N, Humbert M, Vachiery JL, et al. 2015 ESC/ERS guidelines for the diagnosis and treatment of pulmonary hypertension: the Joint Task Force for the Diagnosis and Treatment of Pulmonary Hypertension of the European Society of Cardiology (ESC) and the European Respiratory Society (ERS): endorsed by: Association for European Paediatric and Congenital Cardiology (AEPC), International Society for Heart and Lung Transplantation (ISHLT). Eur Respir J 2015;46: 903–75.

31. Seferian A, Helal B, Jais X, et al. Ventilation/perfusion lung scan in pulmonary veno-occlusive disease. Eur Respir J 2012;40:75–83.

32. Bailey CL, Channick RN, Auger WR, et al. High probability" perfusion lung scans in pulmonary venoocclusive disease. Am J Respir Crit Care Med 2000;162:1974–8.

33. Elliott CG, Colby TV, Hill T, et al. Pulmonary veno-occlusive disease associated with severe reduction of single-breath carbon monoxide diffusing capacity. Respiration 1988; 53:262–6.

34. Lederer H, Muggli B, Speich R, et al. Haemosiderin-laden sputum macrophages for diagnosis in pulmonary veno-occlusive disease. PLoS One 2014;9: e115219.

35. Rabiller A, Jais X, Hamid A, et al. Occult alveolar haemorrhage in pulmonary veno-occlusive disease. Eur Respir J 2006;27:108–13.

36. McLaughlin VV, Archer SL, Badesch DB, et al. ACCF/AHA 2009 expert consensus document on pulmonary hypertension: a report of the American College of Cardiology Foundation Task Force on Expert Consensus Documents and the American Heart Association: developed in collaboration with the American College of Chest Physicians, American Thoracic Society, Inc., and the Pulmonary Hypertension Association. Circulation 2009;119:2250–94.

37. Wille KM, Sharma NS, Kulkarni T, et al. Characteristics of patients with pulmonary venoocclusive disease awaiting transplantation. Ann Am Thorac Soc 2014;11:1411–8.

38. Montani D, Price LC, Dorfmuller P, et al. Pulmonary veno-occlusive disease. Eur Respir J 2009; 33:189–200.

39. Okumura H, Nagaya N, Kyotani S, et al. Effects of continuous IV prostacyclin in a patient with pulmonary veno-occlusive disease. Chest 2002;122: 1096–8.

40. Davis LL, deBoisblanc BP, Glynn CE, et al. Effect of prostacyclin on microvascular pressures in a patient with pulmonary veno-occlusive disease. Chest 1995;108:1754–6.

41. Hoeper MM, Eschenbruch C, Zink-Wohlfart C, et al. Effects of inhaled nitric oxide and aerosolized iloprost in pulmonary veno-occlusive disease. Respir Med 1999;93:62–4.

42. Barreto AC, Franchi SM, Castro CR, et al. One-year follow-up of the effects of sildenafil on pulmonary arterial hypertension and veno-occlusive disease. Braz J Med Biol Res 2005;38:185–95.

43. Creagh-Brown BC, Nicholson AG, Showkathali R, et al. Pulmonary veno-occlusive disease presenting with recurrent pulmonary oedema and the use of nitric oxide to predict response to sildenafil. Thorax 2008;63:933–4.

44. Kuroda T, Hirota H, Masaki M, et al. Sildenafil as adjunct therapy to high-dose epoprostenol in a patient with pulmonary veno-occlusive disease. Heart Lung Circ 2006;15:139–42.

45. Barboza CE, Jardim CV, Hovnanian AL, et al. Pulmonary veno-occlusive disease: diagnostic and therapeutic alternatives. J Bras Pneumol 2008;34:749–52.

46. Dorfmuller P, Humbert M, Perros F, et al. Fibrous remodeling of the pulmonary venous system in pulmonary arterial hypertension associated with connective tissue diseases. Hum Pathol 2007;38: 893–902.

47. Dorfmuller P, Perros F, Balabanian K, et al. Inflammation in pulmonary arterial hypertension. Eur Respir J 2003;22:358–63.

48. Saito A, Takizawa H, Ito K, et al. A case of pulmonary veno-occlusive disease associated with systemic sclerosis. Respirology 2003;8:383–5.

49. Naniwa T, Takeda Y. Long-term remission of pulmonary veno-occlusive disease associated with primary Sjogren's syndrome following immunosuppressive therapy. Mod Rheumatol 2011;21:637–40.

50. Sanderson JE, Spiro SG, Hendry AT, et al. A case of pulmonary veno-occlusive disease responding to treatment with azathioprine. Thorax 1977;32:140–8.

51. Kataoka M, Yanagisawa R, Fukuda K, et al. Sorafenib is effective in the treatment of pulmonary veno-occlusive disease. Cardiology 2012;123: 172–4.

52. Overbeek MJ, van Nieuw Amerongen GP, Boonstra A, et al. Possible role of imatinib in clinical pulmonary veno-occlusive disease. Eur Respir J 2008;32:232–5.

53. Ghofrani HA, Morrell NW, Hoeper MM, et al. Imatinib in pulmonary arterial hypertension patients with inadequate response to established therapy. Am J Respir Crit Care Med 2010;182:1171–7.

54. Frost AE, Barst RJ, Hoeper MM, et al. Long-term safety and efficacy of imatinib in pulmonary arterial hypertension. J Heart Lung Transplant 2015;34: 1366–75.

55. Wagenvoort CA, Beetstra A, Spijker J. Capillary haemangiomatosis of the lungs. Histopathology 1978;2:401–6.

56. Langleben D, Heneghan JM, Batten AP, et al. Familial pulmonary capillary hemangiomatosis resulting in primary pulmonary hypertension. Ann Intern Med 1988;109:106–9.

57. Whittaker JS, Pickering CA, Heath D, et al. Pulmonary capillary haemangiomatosis. Diagn Histopathol 1983;6:77–84.

58. Domingo C, Encabo B, Roig J, et al. Pulmonary capillary hemangiomatosis: report of a case and review of the literature. Respiration 1992;59:178–80.

59. Vevaina JR, Mark EJ. Thoracic hemangiomatosis masquerading as interstitial lung disease. Chest 1988;93:657–9.

60. Havlik DM, Massie LW, Williams WL, et al. Pulmonary capillary hemangiomatosis-like foci. An autopsy study of 8 cases. Am J Clin Pathol 2000;113:655–62.

61. Tron V, Magee F, Wright JL, et al. Pulmonary capillary hemangiomatosis. Hum Pathol 1986;17:1144–50.

62. El-Gabaly M, Farver C, Budev M, et al. Pulmonary capillary hemangiomatosis imaging findings and literature update. J Comput Assist Tomogr 2007; 31:608–10.

63. Langleben D. Pulmonary capillary hemangiomatosis. In: Peacock AJ, Rubin LJ, editors. Pulmonary circulation: diseases and their treatment. London: Great Britain: Arnold, A member of the Hodder Headline Group; 2004. p. 366–71.

64. Langleben D. Pulmonary capillary hemangiomatosis: the puzzle takes shape. Chest 2014;145:197–9.

65. Fernandez-Alonso J, Zulueta T, Reyes-Ramirez JR, et al. Pulmonary capillary hemangiomatosis as cause of pulmonary hypertension in a young woman with systemic lupus erythematosus. J Rheumatol 1999;26:231–3.

66. Best DH, Sumner KL, Austin ED, et al. EIF2AK4 mutations in pulmonary capillary hemangiomatosis. Chest 2014;145:231–6.

67. Abman SH, Hansmann G, Archer SL, et al. Pediatric pulmonary hypertension: guidelines from the American Heart Association and American Thoracic Society. Circulation 2015;132:2037–99.

68. Almagro PMD, Julia JMD, Sanjaume MMD, et al. Pulmonary capillary hemangiomatosis associated with primary pulmonary hypertension: report of 2 new cases and review of 35 cases from the literature. Medicine 2002;81:417–24.

69. Sullivan A, Chmura K, Cool CD, et al. Pulmonary capillary hemangiomatosis: an immunohistochemical analysis of vascular remodeling. Eur J Med Res 2006;11:187–93.

70. Humbert M, Maitre S, Capron F, et al. Pulmonary edema complicating continuous intravenous prostacyclin in pulmonary capillary hemangiomatosis. Am J Respir Crit Care Med 1998;157:1681–5.

71. Gugnani MK, Pierson C, Vanderheide R, et al. Pulmonary edema complicating prostacyclin therapy in pulmonary hypertension associated with scleroderma: a case of pulmonary capillary hemangiomatosis. Arthritis Rheum 2000;43:699–703.

72. Ogawa A, Miyaji K, Yamadori I, et al. Safety and efficacy of epoprostenol therapy in pulmonary veno-occlusive disease and pulmonary capillary hemangiomatosis. Circ J 2012;76:1729–36.

73. White CW, Sondheimer HM, Crouch EC, et al. Treatment of pulmonary hemangiomatosis with recombinant interferon alfa-2a. N Engl J Med 1989;320:1197–200.

74. Nayyar D, Muthiah K, Kumarasinghe G, et al. Imatinib for the treatment of pulmonary arterial hypertension and pulmonary capillary hemangiomatosis. Pulm Circ 2014;4:342–5.

75. Ginns LC, Roberts DH, Mark EJ, et al. Pulmonary capillary hemangiomatosis with atypical endotheliomatosis: successful antiangiogenic therapy with doxycycline. Chest 2003;124:2017–22.

76. Simonneau G, Robbins IM, Beghetti M, et al. Updated clinical classification of pulmonary hypertension. J Am Coll Cardiol 2009;54:S43–54.

77. Stovin PGI, Mitchinson MJ. Pulmonary hypertension due to obstruction of the intrapulmonary veins. Thorax 1965;20:106–13.

78. Eltorky MA, Headley AS, Winer-Muram H, et al. Pulmonary capillary hemangiomatosis: a clinicopathologic review. Ann Thorac Surg 1994;57:772–6.

79. Daroca PJ Jr, Mansfield RE, Ichinose H. Pulmonary veno-occlusive disease: report of a case with pseudoangiomatous features. Am J Surg Pathol 1977;1:249–55.

80. Schraufnagel DE, Sekosan M, McGee T, et al. Human alveolar capillaries undergo angiogenesis in pulmonary veno-occlusive disease. Eur Respir J 1996;9:346–50.

81. Olsson KM, Delcroix M, Ghofrani HA, et al. Anticoagulation and survival in pulmonary arterial hypertension: results from the comparative, prospective registry of newly initiated therapies for pulmonary hypertension (COMPERA). Circulation 2014;129:57–65.

82. Johnson SR, Mehta S, Granton JT. Anticoagulation in pulmonary arterial hypertension: a qualitative systematic review. Eur Respir J 2006;28:999–1004.

83. Galie N, Corris PA, Frost A, et al. Updated treatment algorithm of pulmonary arterial hypertension. J Am Coll Cardiol 2013;62:D60–72.

84. Dufour B, Maitre S, Humbert M, et al. High-resolution CT of the chest in four patients with pulmonary capillary hemangiomatosis or pulmonary venoocclusive disease. AJR Am J Roentgenol 1998;171:1321–4.

Eosinophilic Lung Diseases

Vincent Cottin, MD, PhD[a,b,*]

KEYWORDS

- Eosinophil • Eosinophilic pneumonia • Interstitial lung disease
- Eosinophilic granulomatosis with polyangiitis • Aspergillus

KEY POINTS

- Eosinophilic lung diseases may present as eosinophilic pneumonia with chronic or acute onset, or as the more transient Löffler syndrome.
- The diagnosis of eosinophilic pneumonia is based on both characteristic clinical-imaging features and the demonstration of alveolar eosinophilia of at least 25% eosinophils at bronchoalveolar lavage.
- Peripheral blood eosinophilia is present in most eosinophilic lung disorders, but can be absent at presentation in idiopathic acute eosinophilic pneumonia and in patients receiving corticosteroid treatment.
- In Europe and North America, chronic eosinophilic pneumonia is most frequently idiopathic, whereas acute eosinophilic pneumonia is often related to drug or tobacco smoke exposure.
- All possible causes of eosinophilia (especially fungus or parasitic infection, drug or toxic exposure) must be thoroughly investigated.

DEFINITION AND CLASSIFICATION

Definition

Eosinophilic lung diseases are a group of diffuse parenchymal lung diseases[1,2] characterized by the prominent infiltration of the lung interstitium and the alveolar spaces by polymorphonuclear eosinophils, with conservation of the lung architecture. As a corollary, a common denominator of eosinophilic lung diseases is represented by a dramatic response to systemic corticosteroid therapy and healing without any sequelae in most cases, despite frequent impressive impairment of lung function at presentation.

Blood *eosinophilia* is defined by an eosinophil blood cell count greater than 0.5×10^9/L, and *hypereosinophilia* by an eosinophil blood cell count of greater than 1.5×10^9 on 2 examinations over at least a 1-month interval.[3–5] Alveolar eosinophilia is defined by differential cell count of at least 25% eosinophils at bronchoalveolar lavage (BAL), and typically greater than 40%.[4]

Classification

Eosinophilic lung disorders can present as acute or chronic pneumonia or as the transient Löffler syndrome, which is most commonly of parasitic origin (**Box 1**). The main causes include exposure to drugs or toxins and fungal infection; however, chronic eosinophilic pneumonia is most often idiopathic, and acute eosinophilic pneumonia most often is related to drugs or tobacco smoking. Eosinophilic lung disorders occurring in the

Conflicts of Interest/Financial Support: Hospices Civils de Lyon, Université Lyon I.

[a] Hospices Civils de Lyon, Louis Pradel Hospital, National Reference Center for Rare Pulmonary Diseases, Department of Respiratory Diseases, F-69677 Lyon, France; [b] Univ Lyon, Université Lyon I, INRA, UMR754, 8 avenue Rockefeller, F-69008 Lyon, France
* Hospices Civils de Lyon, Louis Pradel Hospital, National Reference Center for Rare Pulmonary Diseases, Department of Respiratory Diseases, F-69677 Lyon, France
E-mail address: vincent.cottin@chu-lyon.fr

Clin Chest Med 37 (2016) 535–556
http://dx.doi.org/10.1016/j.ccm.2016.04.015

context of systemic conditions suggest the diagnosis of eosinophilic granulomatosis with polyangiitis (EGPA) or the idiopathic hypereosinophilic syndromes.

PATHOPHYSIOLOGY
Recruitment of Eosinophils to the Lung

Blood and tissue eosinophilia have long been identified as major players in immunity against parasites and in the pathogenesis of allergic diseases.[6] Following differentiation of precursor cells in the bone marrow under the action of several cytokines, including interleukin (IL)-5, IL-3, and granulocyte macrophage colony-stimulating factor (GM-CSF),[7–9] eosinophils are recruited in the blood and tissue, including the lung in response to circulating IL-5, eotaxins, and the C-C chemokine receptor-3 (CCR3). Because recruitment of eosinophils to tissues is organ-specific, tissue and blood eosinophilia are not necessarily

associated. The prominence of IL-5 in eosinophil differentiation and recruitment has led to the development of anti–IL-5 monoclonal antibodies to selectively target the eosinophil lineage in humans with asthma.[10–14]

Eosinophils and Immunity

Eosinophils are active participants in innate immunity. They interact with basophils, endothelial cells, macrophages, platelets, fibroblasts, and mast cells through cell membrane signaling molecules and receptors including Toll-like receptors and receptors for cytokines, immunoglobulins, and complement.[7–9,15] Activated eosinophils release proinflammatory cytokines, arachidonic acid–derived mediators, enzymes, reactive oxygen species, complement proteins, chemokines, chemoattractants, metalloproteases, and cationic proteins. The latter are released by degranulation of activated eosinophils and exert a variety of effects, including direct cytotoxicity, upregulation of chemoattraction, expression of adhesion molecules, regulation of vascular permeability, and contraction of smooth muscle cells.[7–9] Activated, degranulated ("hypodense") eosinophils can be found in the bronchoalveolar lavage (BAL)[16,17] and the lung tissue[18] of patients with eosinophilic pneumonias. Tissue damage mediated by eosinophil cationic proteins is exemplified by the cardiac lesions that occur in the hypereosinophilic syndrome or in tropical eosinophilia.[15]

Eosinophils are also involved in adaptive immunity against bacteria, viruses, and tumors through interaction with T-lymphocytes.[7–9] They present antigens to T-helper-2 cells in tissues and in the draining lymph nodes in the context of major histocompatibility complex class II, thereby inducing T cell development, activation, and migration to sites of inflammation. Eosinophils secrete IL-4 and IL-13, amplifying the T-helper-2 response in the lung, and in turn are recruited and activated by T-helper-2 cell-derived cytokines (IL-4, IL-5, and IL-13).

IDIOPATHIC CHRONIC EOSINOPHILIC PNEUMONIA

First characterized by Carrington and colleagues,[19] idiopathic chronic eosinophilic pneumonia (ICEP) is characterized by the onset over a few weeks of cough, dyspnea, malaise, and weight loss, with diffuse pulmonary infiltrates.

Epidemiology and Risk Factors

Although it is a rare disease, representing fewer than 3% of cases of various interstitial lung diseases, ICEP is the most common of the eosinophilic pneumonias in nontropical areas where the prevalence of parasitic infection is low.[20] It predominates in women (2:1 female/male ratio),[21,22] and affects every age group with a mean age of 45 years at diagnosis,[21] with no genetic predisposition. Two-thirds of patients with ICEP have a prior history of asthma,[21,22] and approximately half a history of atopy, consisting in drug allergy, nasal polyposis, urticaria, and/or eczema.[21,22] In contrast with idiopathic acute eosinophilic pneumonia (IAEP), most patients with ICEP are nonsmokers.[21–23] It has been hypothesized that ICEP may occur predominantly in patients who are prone to develop a T-helper-2 response.[24]

Clinical Description

The onset of ICEP is progressive or subacute, with several weeks or months between the onset of symptoms and the diagnosis.[21,22] Shortness of breath is usually moderate and is the prominent clinical manifestation, present in 60% to 90% of patients. Cough (90%), rhinitis or sinusitis (20%), and rarely chest pain or hemoptysis (10% or less) may be present.[21,22] Wheezes or crackles are found in one-third of patients at auscultation. Respiratory failure requiring mechanical ventilation is exceptional in ICEP, in contrast to the frequent respiratory failure that occurs in IAEP.[25,26]

Approximately 75% of the patients with ICEP experience asthma at some time throughout the course of disease. Asthma frequently precedes the onset of ICEP, but occasionally occurs concomitantly with the diagnosis of ICEP (15%).[27] Asthma in ICEP is often severe and can progress to long-term persistent airflow obstruction in approximatively 10% of patients despite oral and inhaled corticosteroid therapy.[27] Follow-up of patients, including pulmonary function tests is therefore necessary.

Systemic symptoms are frequently associated, with fatigue, malaise, fever, anorexia, night sweats, and weight loss (occasionally severe).[21,22] Limited extrathoracic manifestations have been reported, including pericardial effusion, arthralgias, nonspecific skin manifestations, and altered liver function tests[19,21,28]; however, any significant extrathoracic manifestation should raise the suspicion of EGPA.

Chest Imaging

The imaging features of ICEP are often characteristic, albeit nonspecific, and are present on the chest radiograph in almost all cases before initiation of treatment.[19,21,22,29–35] They consist of bilateral alveolar infiltrates with ill-defined margins, with a typical peripheral predominance in approximately 25% of patients.[22,31,36,37] Spontaneous migration of the opacities observed in a quarter of the cases suggests the diagnosis of either ICEP or cryptogenic organizing pneumonia.[21]

On high-resolution computed tomography (HRCT), typical features consist of confluent consolidations and ground-glass opacities (**Fig. 1**),[21,30,34] almost always bilateral[21] and predominating in the upper lobes and peripheral subpleural areas.[30] Imaging abnormalities rapidly regress on corticosteroid therapy.[30] This pattern is sufficiently typical to suggest the diagnosis of ICEP in approximately 75% of cases in the appropriate setting.[33] Septal line thickening, band-like opacities parallel to the chest, mediastinal lymph node enlargement, or mild pleural effusion, may be found,[21,29] but cavitary lesions are exceedingly rare.[21,22,30]

Laboratory Findings

High-level peripheral blood eosinophilia present in most patients who have not yet received systemic corticosteroids[22] is the key to the diagnosis, with mean values of 5 to 6000/mm³ in large series, representing 20% to 30% of blood leukocytes.[21] BAL eosinophilia, defined as 25% eosinophils or

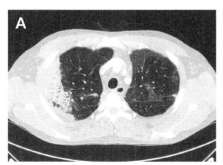
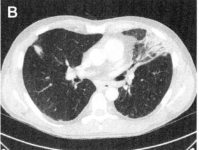

Fig. 1. Chest CT of a patient with ICEP, demonstrating peripheral airspace consolidation predominating in the upper lobes. (A) Right upper lobe; (B) lingula.

more at differential cell count, is found in all patients evaluated before any corticosteroid intake, and confirms the diagnosis of eosinophilic pneumonia, especially when eosinophils represent the predominant cell in BAL. The BAL eosinophil count is commonly greater than 40%, with a mean of 58% in large series. Sputum eosinophilia may be present but is less valuable for diagnosis. Increase in blood C-reactive protein and total immunoglobulin (Ig) E level are common but lack specificity.

Pathogenesis

The pathogenesis of ICEP is considered to be a direct consequence of lung infiltration by eosinophils, and is reversible on corticosteroid treatment. A number of studies have demonstrated the release of proinflammatory molecules and increased expression of activation markers by eosinophils from patients with ICEP.[1,9,38–40] Interestingly, recent studies have suggested a possible role for clonal blood and lung tissue T cells in ICEP,[41,42] similarly to what seen in the lymphocytic variant of the idiopathic hypereosinophilic syndrome.

Lung Function

Approximately half of patients with ICEP have airflow obstruction, and the other half have a restrictive ventilatory defect related to pulmonary infiltration. In the latter case, multiple consolidations are apparent on imaging, and reduced carbon monoxide transfer factor and coefficient are present by pulmonary function testing. In addition, many patients present with mild hypoxemia.[21,22]

Pathology

The diagnosis of ICEP does not typically require a lung biopsy. When available, pathology is characterized by prominent infiltration of the lung interstitium and the alveolar spaces by eosinophils[19,22] accompanied by a fibrinous exudate, with preservation of the lung architecture. Eosinophilic microabscesses, a non-necrotizing nongranulomatous vasculitis, and occasional multinucleated giant cells (but no granuloma) also can be found. Some histologic overlap is common with organizing pneumonia.[1] Eosinophil degranulation can be demonstrated by immunohistochemical and electron microscopic studies within the site of eosinophilic pneumonia.[17,43]

Diagnosis

Working diagnostic criteria for ICEP are found in **Box 2**.[4,5] A thorough investigation for potential causes of eosinophilia should be conducted before the condition is considered idiopathic, including drug intake, infections with parasites or

---

Box 2
Diagnostic criteria for idiopathic chronic eosinophilic pneumonia and for idiopathic acute eosinophilic pneumonia

Idiopathic chronic eosinophilic pneumonia

1. Diffuse pulmonary alveolar consolidation with air bronchogram and/or ground-glass opacities at chest imaging, especially with peripheral predominance.

2. Eosinophilia at bronchoalveolar lavage differential cell count ≥40% (or peripheral blood eosinophils ≥1000 /mm³).

3. Respiratory symptoms present for at least 2 to 4 wk.

4. Absence of other known causes of eosinophilic lung disease (especially exposure to drug susceptible to induce pulmonary eosinophilia).

Idiopathic acute eosinophilic pneumonia

1. Acute onset with febrile respiratory manifestations (≤1 mo, and especially ≤7 d duration before medical examination.

2. Bilateral diffuse infiltrates on imaging.

3. Pao_2 on room air ≤60 mm Hg (8 kPa), or Pao_2/Fio_2 ≤300 mm Hg (40 kPa), or oxygen saturation on room air <90%.

4. Lung eosinophilia, with ≥25% eosinophils at BAL differential cell count (or eosinophilic pneumonia at lung biopsy when done).

5. Absence of determined cause of acute eosinophilic pneumonia (including infection or exposure to drugs known to induce pulmonary eosinophilia). Recent onset of tobacco smoking or exposure to inhaled dusts may be present.

fungi, and exposure to toxins or illicit drugs. In the setting of a characteristic clinical and radiologic presentation, the presence of marked eosinophilia at BAL (at least 25% but usually >40% of BAL cells), or when eosinophils are more numerous than neutrophils and lymphocytes,[4] confirms the diagnosis of eosinophilic pneumonia, and obviates the need for lung biopsy.

Although performing a BAL is generally useful in patients with suspected eosinophilic pneumonia and those with diffuse alveolar opacities at imaging, the presence of markedly elevated peripheral blood eosinophilia together with typical clinical radiologic features also strongly suggest the diagnosis of ICEP. Diagnostic difficulties mainly arise in patients who are already receiving corticosteroid treatment, and therefore do not have peripheral or BAL eosinophilia at the time of clinical evaluation.

Treatment and Outcome

Although spontaneous resolution can occur, management of ICEP is based primarily on oral corticosteroids. The objective of therapy is to induce remission of disease and then to reduce the risk of relapse, while balancing the intensity of treatment with the need to minimize the side effects of corticosteroids.

There are no established dose and duration of systemic corticosteroids in ICEP.[21,23,36,44,45] A typical regimen may include treatment with an initial dose of 0.5 mg/kg per day of oral prednisone for 2 weeks, followed by 0.25 mg/kg per day for 2 weeks, then corticosteroids are progressively reduced over a total duration of approximately 6 months and stopped.[1,4] Response to corticosteroids is typically dramatic, with clinical improvement within 2 days,[22,23,46] and clearing of chest opacities within 1 week.[21,22] Most patients need corticosteroids for 6 to 12 months[21]; however, a recent study found no difference in the relapse rate between a 3-month and a 6-month treatment regimen.[47] Whether inhaled corticosteroids may be useful in nonasthmatic patients with ICEP is unknown.

Relapses occur in more than half the patients while decreasing or after stopping corticosteroids; however, they respond very well to resumed corticosteroid treatment. Relapses typically can be treated with a dose of 20 mg per day of prednisone. Patients should therefore be informed of the possibility of relapse while the corticosteroids are progressively tapered and then stopped. Such an approach reduces the overall patient's exposure to long-term corticosteroids.

There are no long-term sequelae of ICEP; however, clinical and functional follow-up is necessary to ensure that patients are asymptomatic with a normal chest radiograph and lung function.[21] Potential morbidity is related to adverse events related to oral corticosteroids, and to possible persistent airflow obstruction that may develop despite bronchodilators and inhaled corticosteroids and often oral low-dose corticosteroids.[45]

IDIOPATHIC ACUTE EOSINOPHILIC PNEUMONIA

IAEP, first described by Badesch and colleagues[48] and later individualized by Allen and colleagues,[49] is both the most dramatic and the most frequently misdiagnosed of eosinophilic pneumonias, because it mimics infectious pneumonia or acute respiratory distress syndrome in previously healthy individuals. It differs from ICEP by its acute onset, the severity of hypoxemia, the usual lack of increased blood eosinophils at the onset of disease, and the absence of relapse.

Epidemiology and Risk Factors

IAEP occurs acutely in previously healthy young adults, with a mean age of approximately 30 years, and with male predominance.[48–53] Two-thirds of patients are smokers, but there is usually no history of asthma. The disease can be triggered by various respiratory exposures, especially a recent initiation of tobacco smoking (as in military or new college student settings[52]). A change in smoking habits,[53,54] smoking large quantities of cigarettes (or cigars), reintroduction to smoking ("rechallenge"),[50,53–62] or even short-term passive smoking[54,63] also can trigger IAEP. A variety of nonspecific environmental inhaled contaminants also have been demonstrated to induce IAEP.[1] Whether this condition should be termed "idiopathic" acute eosinophilic pneumonia in cases clearly related to tobacco smoking or other exposures is debatable.[4]

Clinical Description

IAEP is characterized by acute onset of dyspnea (100% of patients), fever that is usually moderate (100%), cough (80%–100%), and pleuritic thoracic pain (50%–70%), myalgias (30%–50%), or abdominal complaints (25%).[46,50–52,54,64–72] Acute onset is an important criterion for the diagnosis of IAEP (see **Box 2**), with a delay between the first symptoms and hospital admission of less than 1 month and usually less than 7 days.[50,51] Acute respiratory failure is frequent,[53] often meeting criteria for acute respiratory distress syndrome,[73] and admission to the intensive care unit and mechanical ventilation are often required.[50,52] Crackles are present in most patients at lung auscultation.

Chest Imaging

The chest radiograph shows bilateral infiltrates, with mixed alveolar and interstitial opacities, especially Kerley lines.[51,66,71] Chest HRCT demonstrates the typical combination of poorly defined nodules of ground-glass attenuation (100%), interlobular septal thickening (90%), bilateral pleural effusion (76%), and airspace consolidation (55%),[74] which suggests the diagnosis in the appropriate setting. Thickening of bronchovascular bundles, lymph node enlargement, and centrilobular nodules also may be found.

Laboratory Findings

In contrast to other eosinophilic pneumonias, blood eosinophil count is *normal* at presentation in most cases of IAEP,[51,52] a feature that contributes to misdiagnosis of IAEP as infectious pneumonia. Within days after presentation, the eosinophil count rises to high values[46,50–52]; a finding that should suggest the diagnosis of IAEP. Given the usual lack of initial blood eosinophilia, BAL eosinophilia is often the key to the diagnosis of IAEP, with 37% to 54% eosinophils on average.[50–52] BAL bacterial cultures are sterile. BAL eosinophilia usually resolves with corticosteroid therapy, but may persist for several weeks.[75]

Biomarkers, especially serum levels of CCL17/TARC and KL6 (Krebs von den Lungen-6), have been proposed to discriminate IAEP from noneosinophilic causes of acute lung injury,[76] but have not been validated. Thoracentesis when performed may show nonspecific pleural eosinophilia.

Lung Function

Pulmonary function tests are practical only in less severe cases, but typically reveal a mild restrictive ventilatory defect, with reduced carbon monoxide transfer capacity, and increased alveolar-arterial oxygen gradient of Po_2. Arterial blood gas demonstrates hypoxemia, which can be severe due to right-to-left shunting in areas of alveolar consolidation. Patients often meet diagnostic criteria for acute lung injury (including a Pao_2/Fio_2 $\leq$300 mm Hg) or for acute respiratory distress syndrome (Pao_2/Fio_2 $\leq$200 mm Hg).

Pathology

A lung biopsy is performed only in rare cases when the diagnosis of eosinophilic pneumonia has not been suspected. When performed, it shows acute and organizing diffuse alveolar damage together with interstitial-alveolar and bronchiolar infiltration by eosinophils, intra-alveolar eosinophils, and interstitial edema.[51,72,77]

Diagnosis

BAL can both establish the presence of alveolar eosinophilia and exclude infection. Current working diagnostic criteria for IAEP and characteristics that differ between IAEP and ICEP are listed in **Box 2** and **Table 1**, respectively. Some patients with moderate disease severity may not fit established criteria.[78]

A variety of causes must be investigated, especially in the setting of acute-onset disease, including parasites, fungi,[79–83] viruses,[84] red spiders,[85] drugs, over-the-counter drugs, and illicit drugs.[86,87] The etiologic enquiry shall be repeated

---

Table 1
Distinctive features of idiopathic chronic eosinophilic pneumonia (ICEP) and idiopathic acute eosinophilic pneumonia (IAEP)

Characteristic	ICEP	IAEP
Onset	>2–4 wk	<1 mo
History of asthma	Yes	No
Smoking history	10% of smokers	2/3 smokers, often recent initiation
Respiratory failure	Rare	Usual
Initial blood eosinophilia	Yes	Often No (typically delayed)
Bronchoalveolar lavage eosinophilia	>25%	>25%
Chest imaging	Homogeneous peripheral airspace consolidation	Bilateral patchy areas of ground-glass attenuation, airspace consolidation, interlobular septal thickening, bilateral pleural effusion
Relapse	Yes	No

in case of poor response to therapy. AEP also may occur after allogeneic hematopoietic stem cell transplantation[88] or in the context of acquired immunodeficiency virus infection.[89]

Treatment and Outcome

Most patients receive systemic corticosteroids. A treatment duration of 2 weeks may be sufficient, with a starting dose of oral prednisone of 30 mg per day, or 1 to 2 mg/kg per day of intravenous methylprednisolone in patients with respiratory failure.[53] Clinical recovery occurs within 3 days on corticosteroid treatment.[53,90] Imaging[50,51,53,71] and pulmonary function abnormalities[50,51] resolve within less than a month. In contrast with ICEP, IAEP does not relapse. Patients should be informed about the etiologic role of tobacco in the disease process and should be strongly encouraged to quit.

Extrapulmonary organ failure or shock is exceptional, and only a couple of lethal cases have been reported.[52,91] Extracorporeal membrane oxygenation has been used occasionally.[86]

EOSINOPHILIC GRANULOMATOSIS WITH POLYANGIITIS
Definition

EGPA (formerly, Churg-Strauss syndrome), described in 1951,[92] mainly from autopsied cases, is a systemic disease associated with asthma, eosinophilia, and eosinophil-rich and granulomatous inflammation involving the respiratory tract and a small-vessel, necrotizing small to medium-sized vessel necrotizing vasculitis.[93] EGPA is associated in approximately 40% of cases with antineutrophil cytoplasmic antibodies (ANCA) and therefore belongs to the pulmonary ANCA-associated vasculitides.

Epidemiology and Risk Factors

EGPA predominates in the fourth or fifth decade, with no gender predominance.[94–97] It is a rare condition, with an incidence of 0.5 to 6.8 cases per million inhabitants per year, and a prevalence of 10.7 to 13.0 cases per million inhabitants.[98] A genetic predisposition has been linked to the major histopathology complex DRB4 allele.[99] Familial EGPA has been reported.[100]

Association with a history of allergy is weak, as allergy can be evidenced by specific serum IgE with corresponding clinical history in fewer than one-third of patients.[101] When present, allergy in EGPA mainly consists of perennial allergies, especially to *Dermatophagoides*, whereas seasonal allergies are less frequent than in control individuals with asthma.[101]

Although the pathogenesis of EGPA is largely unknown,[98] several triggering or adjuvant factors have been identified or suspected,[1,98,102] including infectious agents (*Aspergillus*, *Candida*, *Ascaris*, *Actinomyces*), bird exposure, cocaine, and drugs (sulfonamides used together with antiserum, diflunisal, macrolides, diphenylhydantoin, and omalizumab),[103–108] as well as allergic hyposensitization and vaccinations.[109] Clonal T cells may play a role.[110]

The possible link between leukotriene-receptor antagonists (montelukast, zafirlukast, pranlukast) and the development of EGPA is controversial.[111–115] EGPA may instead arise in patients taking these drugs due to the flare of smouldering preexisting disease as oral or inhaled corticosteroids are tapered rather than to a direct effect on the pathogenesis of vasculitis.[98,114] However, a direct effect of montelukast cannot be excluded in individual cases,[111,113,115] and it is reasonable to avoid leukotriene-receptor antagonists in asthmatic patients with eosinophilia and/or extrapulmonary manifestations compatible with smouldering EGPA.

Clinical Description

The natural course of EGPA has been described to follow 3 phases,[95] with rhinosinusitis and asthma, blood and tissue eosinophilia, and eventually systemic vasculitis, but these often overlap in time. Asthma is always present in EGPA, occurring at a mean age of approximately 35 years, generally severe and becoming rapidly corticosteroid dependent,[95,97,116–119] and often preceding the onset of the vasculitis by 3 to 9 years.[94–97,119,120] Asthma may become attenuated after the onset of the vasculitis,[95,120] likely reflecting the effect of systemic corticosteroids prescribed for EGPA.[121,122]

Eosinophilic pneumonia is the main pulmonary manifestation of EGPA other than asthma. It is often similar to ICEP in presentation, but may be acute in onset.[1] The frequency of eosinophilic pneumonia may be underestimated in some series of EGPA, as it rapidly resolves on corticosteroid treatment, and because extrathoracic manifestations may be prominent clinically.

Chronic rhinitis or rhinosinusitis is present in approximately 75% of cases but lacks specificity. It may consist of chronic paraseptal sinusitis, crusty rhinitis, nasal obstruction, and nasal polyposis, often with eosinophilic infiltration at histopathology.[95,97,123–126] Septal nasal perforation does not occur in EGPA as opposed to granulomatosis with polyangiitis.

General symptoms are present in two-thirds of patients (asthenia, weight loss, fever, arthralgias, myalgias). Any organ system can be affected by the systemic disease through eosinophilic infiltration and/or granulomatous vasculitis.[98,127] Heart and kidney involvement are frequently insidious and must be systematically investigated due to potential morbidity and mortality.

Cardiac involvement is often asymptomatic but can lead to sudden death or acute or chronic cardiac failure[95–97,119,120,128,129] due to eosinophilic myocarditis and less commonly from coronary arteritis.[130,131] Heart transplantation may be required.[132] Therefore, any patient with suspected EGPA should undergo a systematic cardiac evaluation with electrocardiogram, echocardiography, N-terminal pro–brain natriuretic peptide, and serum level of troponin I. MRI of the heart is currently the preferred investigation when cardiac involvement is suspected.[129,133–135] However, the clinical significance of subclinical abnormalities detected by MRI[129,134,136] or echocardiography[134,137] is unknown. Patients with EGPA are also at greater risk of venous thromboembolic events.[92]

Chest Imaging

Chest imaging abnormalities in patients with EGPA are twofold:

- Pulmonary infiltrates (50%–70%) corresponding to eosinophilic pneumonia and consisting of ill-defined opacities, sometimes migratory, with peripheral predominance or random distribution, and density varying from ground-glass opacities to airspace consolidation[95,97,120,138–142] (**Fig. 2**). These abnormalities rapidly disappear on corticosteroid therapy.

- Airways abnormalities, including centrilobular nodules, bronchial wall thickening, and bronchiectasis.[1,33,35,140]

Interlobular septal thickening, hilar or mediastinal lymphadenopathy, pleural effusion, or pericardial effusion also may be seen.[35,139,140,142,143] Pleural effusion may correspond to eosinophilic pleural effusion or to a transudate caused by cardiomyopathy (see **Fig. 2B**).

Laboratory Findings

Peripheral blood eosinophilia is a major feature of EGPA, with mean values generally between 5 and 20,000/mm^3 at diagnosis.[95,97,120] It is accompanied by BAL eosinophilia greater than 25% and usually greater than 40%.[144] Increase in serum IgE and C-reactive protein levels is nonspecific. Biomarkers to reflect eosinophil degranulation and disease activity in vivo await prospective validation.[145–147]

Although EGPA is one of the ANCA-associated pulmonary vasculitides, ANCAs are found in only 40% of patients, and their absence does not exclude the diagnosis of EGPA. They are mainly perinuclear-ANCA with myeloperoxidase specificity.[96,97,148–150] When present, ANCAs support the diagnosis of EGPA; however, their titer does not correlate with the activity of disease. Different clinical phenotypes of disease have been reported in ANCA-positive and ANCA-negative patients[148–152] (**Box 3**), possibly with a genetic correlate.[99,153]

Lung Function

Airflow obstruction is present in 70% of patients at diagnosis despite inhaled bronchodilator and high-dose inhaled corticosteroid therapy for asthma.[121] Lung function improves with oral corticosteroid therapy given for the systemic disease; however,

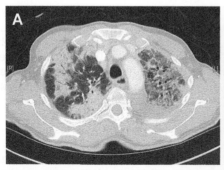
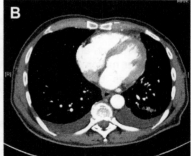

Fig. 2. Chest CT of a patient with EGPA. (*A*) Lung window demonstrating alveolar opacities and ground-glass attenuation; (*B*) mediastinal window showing bilateral pleural effusion due to eosinophilic myocarditis with heart failure.

Box 3
Working diagnostic for eosinophilic granulomatosis with polyangiitis

1. Asthma

2. Peripheral blood eosinophilia greater than 1500/mm^3 and/or alveolar eosinophilia greater than 25%

3. Extrapulmonary clinical manifestations of disease (other than rhinosinusitis), with at least 1 of the following:

   a. Systemic manifestation typical of the disease: mononeuritis multiplex; or cardiomyopathy confidently attributed to the eosinophilic disorder; or palpable purpura;

   b. Any extrapulmonary manifestation with histopathological evidence of vasculitis as demonstrated especially by skin, muscle, or nerve biopsy;

   c. Any extrapulmonary manifestation with evidence of antineutrophil cytoplasmic antibodies with antimyeloperoxidase or antiproteinase 3 specificity.

Note: When a single extrarespiratory manifestation attributable to the systemic disease is present, disease may be called "forme fruste of EGPA."

---

mild airflow obstruction may persist.[121,122] Low-dose long-term oral corticosteroids are required for asthma in most patients in addition to inhaled therapy,[95,97,121] causing significant morbidity and susceptibility to infections. Persistent airflow obstruction may be present in 30% to 40% of patients with long-term follow-up.[121]

Pathology

The diagnosis of EGPA is frequently based on the clinical presentation and marked eosinophilia, and lung biopsy is seldom necessary. Biopsy of more accessible tissues, such as skin, nerve, or muscle, has a better safety profile and can be useful.[97] A single tissue specimen[154,155] rarely contains all 3 defining characteristics; vasculitis (necrotizing or not, involving mainly the medium-sized pulmonary arteries), granulomata, and eosinophilic tissue infiltration (with palisading histiocytes and giant cells).

Diagnosis

Although the diagnosis is typically straightforward in patients with acute or chronic eosinophilic pneumonia and true vasculitis with positive ANCA, it may be more difficult in those with asthma, blood eosinophilia, negative ANCA, and mild extrathoracic manifestations; those with the so-called "forme fruste" of EGPA; or in subjects receiving corticosteroid treatment.[118,156,157] Diagnostic difficulties thus largely depend on the stage of disease, yet it is crucial that this diagnosis be established before severe organ involvement develops, especially cardiac disease.

The diagnostic criteria proposed by Lanham and colleagues[95] include (1) asthma, (2) eosinophilia exceeding 1.5 × 10^9/L, and (3) systemic vasculitis of 2 or more extrapulmonary organs; however,

they are not applicable to patients with limited disease or those without a biopsy. Classification criteria have been established by the American College of Rheumatology[158]; however, they can be applied only in cases with established systemic vasculitis. Working diagnostic criteria are proposed (**Table 2**), which include the diagnostic contribution of ANCA when present.

Treatment and Outcome

Corticosteroids remain the mainstay of treatment of EGPA, with oral prednisone typically initiated at a dose of 1 mg/kg per day for 3 to 4 weeks, then tapered to reach 5 to 10 mg per day by 12 months of therapy.[98] An initial methylprednisolone bolus (15 mg/kg per day for 1–3 days) may be indicated in the most severe cases. Cyclophosphamide therapy (0.6–0.7 g/m^2 intravenously at days 1, 15, and 30, then every 3 weeks) should be added to corticosteroids to induce remission in patients with manifestations that could result in mortality or severe morbidity,[159] especially heart failure,[160,161] with 1 or more of the following "poor prognostic" criteria: age older than 65 years; cardiac symptoms; gastrointestinal involvement; renal insufficiency with serum creatinine greater than 150 μg/L; and absence of ear, nose, and throat manifestations.[159,162] Subcutaneous interferon-α, high-dose intravenous immunoglobulins, plasma exchange, cyclosporine,[2] and rituximab[163–171] have been used successfully in a few cases refractory to corticosteroids. However, experience with rituximab is limited, and bronchospasm has been reported[172]; rituximab should therefore not be used routinely in EGPA.[98]

Once remission has been achieved, prolonged maintenance therapy is necessary to prevent

Table 2
Distinct subtypes of eosinophilic granulomatosis with polyangiitis

Characteristic	Vasculitic Phenotype	Eosinophilic Tissue Disease Phenotype
Respective frequency	~40%	~60%
ANCA	Present (mostly p-ANCA with anti-MPO specificity)	Absent
Predominant manifestations	Glomerular renal disease Peripheral neuropathy Purpura Biopsy-proven vasculitis	Cardiac involvement (eosinophilic myocarditis) Eosinophilic pneumonia Fever

Abbreviations: ANCA, antineutrophil cytoplasmic antibodies; MPO, myeloperoxidase.

relapses. Patients without poor prognosis criteria are generally treated by corticosteroids alone; the possible benefit of azathioprine to maintain remission in this setting (especially in patients who relapse despite 20 mg per day of prednisone or more) is currently being evaluated. In patients with poor prognostic criteria, maintenance therapy for 18 to 24 months (after remission has been obtained using cyclophosphamide) is generally based on azathioprine, which has a favorable risk/benefit ratio.[98]

Promising preliminary results have been obtained using the anti–IL-5 antibody mepolizumab.[13,173,174] Drugs that target the eosinophil cell line may become part of the treatment strategy in the near future.[175] In a retrospective multicenter study of 17 patients who received omalizumab for severe steroid-dependent asthma, alone or in association with other immunosuppressive agents, omalizumab treatment resulted in some efficacy and corticosteroid sparing effect, but severe flares occurred in a quarter of patients.[176]

Approximately 25% of patients experience at least 1 relapse, generally with peripheral eosinophilia, with or without new-onset systemic manifestations. The 5-year overall survival in EGPA is currently greater than 95%,[159,177,178] with most deaths occurring during the first year of treatment due to cardiac involvement.[179] Treatment-related side effects especially related to corticosteroids are the main cause of long-term morbidity. Difficult asthma and persistent airflow obstruction also cause significant morbidity.[121,178]

ALLERGIC BRONCHOPULMONARY ASPERGILLOSIS
Epidemiology and Pathogenesis

Allergic bronchopulmonary aspergillosis (ABPA) occurs almost exclusively in subjects with a prior history of chronic bronchial disease. It may occur in up to 1% to 2% of asthmatic adults and in up to 7% to 10% of patients with cystic fibrosis.[180,181] Isolated cases have been reported in patients with chronic obstructive pulmonary disease, and in workers in bagasse-containing sites in sugarcane mills.[182]

Chronic bronchial disease is associated with viscid mucus, which with exposure to fungal spores predisposes to this condition. In response to the presence of *Aspergillus* growing in mucous plugs in the airways of patients with asthma, complex chronic immune and inflammatory reactions develop in the bronchi and the surrounding lung parenchyma, causing local damage and impairment of the mucociliary clearance.[183] Both type I hypersensitivity mediated by IgE antibodies, and type III hypersensitivity responses (with the participation of IgG and IgA antibodies and of exaggerated Th2 CD4+ T-cell–mediated immune response) are involved in the immunologic process. Excessive B-cell response, immunoglobulin production, and high levels of circulating IL-4 play a key role.[183]

As ABPA does not develop in all patients with asthma, genetic predisposition may have a role in conjunction with environmental exposure.[183] An increased prevalence of heterozygotic cystic fibrosis transmembrane conductance regulator (CFTR) gene mutations has been demonstrated in patients with ABPA without cystic fibrosis,[184] as well as a polymorphism within the IL-4 receptor alpha-chain gene, the IL-10 promoter, and the surfactant protein A genes,[185–187] and an association with HLA DR2/5 subtypes.[188–190] Familial cases have been reported.[191]

ABPA may be associated with allergic *Aspergillus* sinusitis,[192] resulting in a syndrome called sinobronchial allergic aspergillosis.[193]

Clinical Description

Patients with ABPA experience chronic cough, dyspnea, expectoration of brown or tan sputum plugs, low-grade fever, and chronic rhinitis. The course of disease is chronic with repeated exacerbations,[183,194] and does not necessarily follow the 5 classic stages of ABPA (acute, remission, recurrent exacerbations, corticosteroid-dependent asthma, and fibrotic end stage). Pulmonary infiltrates or peripheral blood eosinophilia may be only present during the acute phase or recurrent exacerbations of the disease. ABPA rarely progresses to chronic respiratory failure requiring oxygen supplementation.

Sputum production may be abundant in patients with bronchiectasis, with sputum cultures often positive for *Pseudomonas aeruginosa*, *Staphylococcus aureus*, *Aspergillus fumigatus*, and/or nontuberculous mycobacteria.[195]

Chest Imaging

Imaging abnormalities often suggest the diagnosis.[33] Bronchial abnormalities are prominent at HRCT and include central cylindrical bronchiectasis (including in the upper lobes), bronchial wall thickening, mucous plugging (mucoid impaction) with "finger-in-glove" pattern,[196,197] ground-glass attenuation, and airspace consolidation.[33,198–200] The "finger-in-glove" sign present in approximately 25% of patients corresponds to bronchial mucous impaction radiating from the hilum to the periphery.[199] Features of bronchiolitis are common, with centrilobular nodules and tree-in-bud pattern[198,200] (**Figs. 3** and **4**). Eosinophilic pneumonia can occur during the early course of the disease, but airspace consolidation should be differentiated from segmental or lobar atelectasis caused by mucus plugging[194] (see **Fig. 4**).

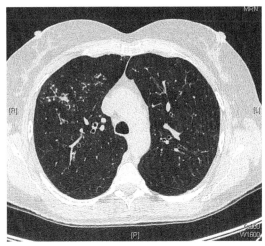

Fig. 4. Chest CT of a patient with ABPA, showing tree-in-bud pattern.

Laboratory Findings

Blood eosinophils are usually greater than 1000/mm³ in the absence corticosteroid treatment. Serum levels of total IgE may be particularly high and lead to suspicion of ABPA in patients with asthma.[183] Skin-prick testing, and serum IgE and IgG (precipitin) reactions to *A fumigatus*, including antibodies specific for recombinant *Aspergillus* allergens (especially *Asp f4* and *Asp f6*), corroborate the diagnosis. Specific IgE against *A fumigatus* may be used to screen for ABPA in patients with asthma.[201,202] Total and *Aspergillus*-specific IgE levels generally increase during exacerbations of ABPA.[203] Fungal mycelia can be found by direct examination of sputum plugs.

Pathology

A lung biopsy is seldom necessary in patients with ABPA. Analysis of specimens from limited resection performed because of chronic pulmonary consolidation or atelectasis demonstrates bronchiectasis with mucous or mucopurulent plugs containing fungal hyphae, granulomatous inflammation of the bronchiolar wall, peribronchiolar chronic eosinophilic infiltrates with areas of eosinophilic pneumonia, exudative bronchiolitis, and mucous impaction of bronchi.[204]

Diagnosis

The current primary diagnostic criteria are listed (**Box 4**).[205] Cases without typical proximal bronchiectasis are designated ABPA-seropositive[206] and may correspond to a distinct variant.[207]

Allergic bronchopulmonary syndromes similar to ABPA can be associated with yeasts or other

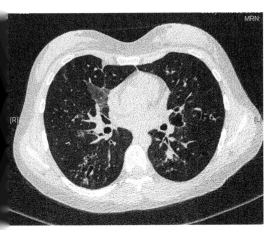

Fig. 3. Chest CT of a patient with ABPA, showing proximal bronchiectasis, bronchial wall thickening, ground-glass attenuation, centrilobular nodules.

Box 4
Minimal essential diagnostic criteria of allergic bronchopulmonary aspergillosis

Patients with asthma and central bronchiectasis

1. Asthma

2. Central bronchiectasis (inner 2/3 of chest CT field)

3. Immediate cutaneous reactivity to *Aspergillus*

4. Total serum IgE concentration greater than 417 kU/L (1000 mg/mL)

5. Elevated serum IgE-*Aspergillus fumigatus* and/or IgG-*A fumigatus* (infiltrates on chest radiograph and serum precipitating antibodies to *A fumigatus* may be present but are not minimal essential diagnostic criteria)

Patients with asthma (ABPA seropositive)

Patients with the preceding criteria 1, 3, 4, and 5 (infiltrates on chest radiograph may be present but are not a minimal essential diagnostic criteria)

Patients with cystic fibrosis

1. Clinical deterioration (increased cough, wheezing, exercise intolerance, increase sputum, decrease in pulmonary function)

2. Immediate cutaneous reactivity to *Aspergillus* or presence of IgE-*A fumigatus*

3. Total serum IgE concentration $\geq$1000 kU/L

4. Precipitating antibodies to *A fumigatus* or serum IgG-*A fumigatus*

5. Abnormal chest radiograph (infiltrates, mucus plugging, or a change from earlier films)

Abbreviations: ABPA, allergic bronchopulmonary aspergillosis; CT, computed tomography; Ig, immunoglobulin.

---

fungi[1,208]; the diagnosis is particularly challenging and based on repeated culture of the offending microorganism and serology if available.

Treatment and Outcome

Goals of treatment for ABPA includes the management of asthma exacerbations and prevention of progression to bronchiectasis and severe fibrotic lung disease while minimizing corticosteroid side effects.

The mainstay of treatment for ABPA is the use of corticosteroids during ABPA exacerbations. Oral prednisone is preferred to intravenous methylprednisolone for typical episodes.[209] Medium-dose oral glucocorticoids (oral prednisolone 0.5 mg kg^{-1} day^{-1} for 2 weeks followed by 0.5 mg kg^{-1} on alternate days for 8 weeks, then taper by 5 mg every 2 weeks and discontinue after 3–5 months) are as effective and safer than higher doses in acute-onset ABPA.[210] Intravenous pulses of high-dose methylprednisolone may be used in refractory ABPA exacerbations.[211] Long-term oral corticosteroids are maintained only in patients with frequent symptomatic attacks or evidence of progressive lung damage. Treatment of episodes of pulmonary consolidation may prevent the progression of ABPA to fibrotic end-stage disease.[212]

Inhaled corticosteroids may reduce the need for long-term oral corticosteroids; however, persistent airflow obstruction may develop over years.

Oral itraconazole prescribed for 16 to 32 weeks to reduce the burden of fungal colonization in the lung is a useful adjunct to corticosteroids,[213,214] allowing steroid dose reductions, and decreasing the frequency of exacerbations.[213,214] Total serum IgE level is often used to monitor therapy.[183] Experience with voriconazole in ABPA is limited. The anti-IgE recombinant antibody omalizumab may be useful especially in subjects with difficult asthma in ABPA.[215–219]

OTHER EOSINOPHILIC LUNG DISEASES
Idiopathic Hypereosinophilic Syndromes

The idiopathic hypereosinophilic syndromes, historically defined as a persistent eosinophilia greater than 1500/mm^3 for longer than 6 months, without a known cause of eosinophilia, and with presumptive signs and symptoms of organ involvement,[220] now encompass 2 variants[221,222]: (1) the "lymphocytic variant" (approximately 30% of cases), resulting from clonal Th2 lymphocytes bearing an aberrant antigenic surface phenotype[223]; and (2) chronic eosinophilic leukemia or the "myeloproliferative variant" (approximately

20% of cases) due to an interstitial chromosomal deletion in 4q12 encoding a constitutively activated tyrosine kinase fusion protein (*Fip1L1-PDGFRα*).[224] At least half of the cases remain idiopathic and unclassified. Imatinib is used as first-line therapy in chronic eosinophilic leukemia,[222,224,225] and can be stopped without relapse in some but not all patients.[226] Corticosteroids are the mainstay of treatment of the lymphocytic variant. Mepolizumab is increasingly used.[10,227,228]

Clinical manifestations mainly comprise fatigue, weight loss, and nonrespiratory involvement, especially targeting the skin, mucosa, heart, and nervous system.[222] In older series, respiratory manifestations present in up to 40% of patients were nonspecific and included cough, dyspnea, and patchy ground-glass attenuation, consolidation, and small nodules at chest imaging.[220] In more recent studies using current diagnostic standards, respiratory manifestations are generally of mild severity, with rare eosinophilic pneumonia if any.[229] Chronic dry cough can be remarkable and may be a presenting feature.[230]

Idiopathic Hypereosinophilic Obliterative Bronchiolitis

Hypereosinophilic obliterative bronchiolitis is a recently individualized entity,[231] currently defined by demonstration of bronchiolitis, peripheral blood and/or alveolar eosinophilia, and persistent airflow obstruction despite high-dose inhaled bronchodilators and corticosteroids. Demonstration of a bronchiolitis may be obtained by lung biopsy[231–235] and/or HRCT showing direct signs of bronchiolitis (eg, centrilobular nodules and branching opacities).[231] Hypereosinophilic obliterative bronchiolitis can be idiopathic, but may also occur in the setting of EGPA, ABPA, drug-induced eosinophilic lung disease (such as minocycline), and possibly in severe asthma.[231]

Patients report cough and exercise dyspnea but generally do not present with intermittent asthma symptoms or wheezes. The blood eosinophil cell count (with a mean value of 2.7×10^9/L), and the eosinophil differential percentage at BAL (with a mean value of 63%) are elevated.[231] Airflow obstruction is often severe but reversible in all cases with oral corticosteroid therapy[231,236]; however, clinical and functional manifestations often recur when the daily dose of oral prednisone is tapered to less than 10 to 15 mg. Unrecognized untreated hypereosinophilic obliterative bronchiolitis might be a cause of irreversible airflow obstruction in chronic eosinophilic respiratory diseases. Notably, whitish tracheal and bronchial granulations or bronchial ulcerative lesions can be present with prominent tissue eosinophils on bronchial biopsy.[231]

Eosinophilic Pneumonias in Parasitic Diseases

Parasitic infection it is the main cause of eosinophilic pneumonia in the world. However, it is less common in Europe and North America, and the diagnosis may be missed, especially because clinical and radiologic manifestations are nonspecific. Presentation is rarely as typical as that of ICEP or IAEP.[1,237]

A detailed description can be found elsewhere.[1] Briefly, infection with the nematode *Ascaris lumbricoides* mainly causes Löffler syndrome; for example, mild eosinophilic pneumonia with transient cough, wheezing, fever, high blood eosinophilia, and pulmonary infiltrates. Visceral larva migrans syndrome caused by *Toxocara canis* that occurs throughout the world causes fever, seizures, fatigue, blood eosinophilia, and transient pulmonary manifestations (cough, dyspnea, wheezes or crackles at pulmonary auscultation, and pulmonary infiltrates at chest radiograph). Hyperinfection syndrome caused by *Strongyloides stercoralis* is a severe disease in immunocompromised patients, which can affect all organs. Tropical pulmonary eosinophilia is caused by the filarial parasites *Wuchereria bancrofti* and *Brugia malayi*.

Eosinophilic Pneumonias Induced by Drugs and Toxics

A diligent search for the etiology of eosinophilic lung diseases is of paramount importance, as the identification of a potential cause may have practical consequences, especially when the disease is caused by drugs.[1] When present, pleural effusion and extrapulmonary manifestations, including cutaneous rash, further suggest the possibility of drug-induced eosinophilic pneumonia.[1] Therefore, a thorough investigation must be conducted for drugs taken in the weeks or days before an eosinophilic lung disease.

Although many drugs have been incriminated (www.pneumotox.com), causality has been established for approximately 20 agents.[102] Those are mostly antibiotics (ethambutol, fenbufen, minocycline, nitrofurantoin, penicillins, pyrimethamine, sulfamides, sulfonamides, trimethoprim-sulfamethoxazole) and nonsteroidal anti-inflammatory drugs and related drugs (acetylsalicylic acid, diclofenac, ibuprofen, naproxen, phenylbutazone, piroxicam, sulindac, tolfenamic acid).[102] Other drugs can be involved, such as captopril, carbamazepine, or granulocyte-monocyte colony-stimulating factor.

An acute onset similar to the presentation to IAEP is common, especially with minocycline[238] or nitrofurantoin,[239] but the differential often includes chronic eosinophilic pneumonia. Presentation may be similar to that of ICEP, or have an acute onset similar to IAEP. Acute eosinophilic pneumonia may occur in the context of drug rash with eosinophilia and systemic symptoms.[240]

Eosinophilic lung disease of varying presentation may be due to illicit drugs, especially cocaine or heroin, but also cannabis.[86,87] The eosinophilia-myalgia syndrome that developed in 1989 in the United States was linked to impurities in L-tryptophan preparations in genetically susceptible hosts.[241–243] One new case has been recently reported in a patient who had been taking L-tryptophan for 3 weeks, as well as other dietary supplements.[244] The toxic-oil syndrome that affected approximately 20,000 people in Spain in 1981[245] is a sclerodermalike disorder characterized in the acute phase by diffuse parenchymal lung disease and possibly respiratory failure with interstitial-alveolar pattern on chest imaging and blood eosinophilia.

Radiation Therapy

A condition similar to ICEP has been reported after radiation therapy for breast cancer in women (similar to the syndrome of radiation-induced organizing pneumonia), with a median delay of 3.5 months after completion of radiotherapy.[24,246,247] Relapse can occur after withdrawal of corticosteroid therapy.[24]

Miscellaneous

ICEP may overlap with or mimic cryptogenic organizing pneumonia. Eosinophilia may be found in other bronchopulmonary disorders in which eosinophilic pneumonia is not prominent,[1] including the eosinophilic phenotype of asthma,[248] asthma with marked blood eosinophilia (ie, >1500/mm^3) or "hypereosinophilic asthma,"[249] eosinophilic bronchitis (without asthma), bronchocentric granulomatosis, isolated cases of idiopathic interstitial pneumonias (idiopathic pulmonary fibrosis/usual interstitial pneumonia, nonspecific interstitial pneumonia, and desquamative interstitial pneumonia), pulmonary Langerhans cell histiocytosis, sarcoidosis, and in lung transplant recipients.[250]

PRACTICAL APPROACH TO DIAGNOSIS AND TREATMENT

The diagnosis of eosinophilic lung diseases usually relies primarily on characteristic clinical-imaging features and the demonstration of alveolar eosinophilia, and lung biopsy is generally not necessary.

Peripheral blood eosinophilia is an excellent diagnostic biomarker but may be absent at presentation, especially in IAEP and in patients who have already received corticosteroid treatment.

Defining the etiology of eosinophilic lung diseases has practical implications for therapeutic intervention, including interruption of a medicinal or illicit drugs, exposure to toxins, or treatment of infections with parasites or fungi.[5] Laboratory investigations for parasites must take into account the epidemiology of parasites. Biological investigations for ABPA should be prompted by the presence of proximal bronchiectasis in patients with asthma or cystic fibrosis. When no cause is found, the eosinophilic lung disease is considered idiopathic. Extrathoracic manifestations are key to the diagnosis of EGPA. The diagnosis of ICEP or IAEP is considered only once all known causes of eosinophilia have been excluded.

Treatment of eosinophilic lung diseases involves oral corticosteroids in most cases, and withdrawal of the offending agent when appropriate. Cyclophosphamide treatment may be required in severe cases of EGPA. The development of therapies that more specifically target the differentiation, activation, or recruitment of eosinophils to the lungs is a promising new research direction for the eosinophilic lung diseases.

REFERENCES

1. Cordier JF, Cottin V. Eosinophilic pneumonias. In: Schwarz MI, King TE Jr, editors. Interstitial lung disease. 5th edition. Shelton (CT): People's Medical Publishing House-USA; 2011. p. 833–93.
2. Cottin V, Cordier JF. Eosinophilic pneumonias. Allergy 2005;60:841–57.
3. Valent P, Klion AD, Horny HP, et al. Contemporary consensus proposal on criteria and classification of eosinophilic disorders and related syndromes. J Allergy Clin Immunol 2012;130:607–12.
4. Cottin V, Cordier JF. Eosinophilic pneumonia. In: Cottin V, Cordier JF, Richeldi L, editors. Orphan lung diseases: a clinical guide to rare lung disease. London: Springer-Verlag; 2015. p. 227–51.
5. Cottin V, Cordier JF. Eosinophilic pneumonia. In: Mason RJ, Ernst JD, King TE Jr, et al, editors. Murray and Nadel's textbook of respiratory medicine. 6th edition. Philadelphia: Elsevier Saunders; 2016. p. 1221–42.
6. Walsh ER, August A. Eosinophils and allergic airway disease: there is more to the story. Trends Immunol 2010;31:39–44.
7. Hogan SP, Rosenberg HF, Moqbel R, et al. Eosinophils: biological properties and role in health and disease. Clin Exp Allergy 2008;38:709–50.

8. Rothenberg ME, Hogan SP. The eosinophil. Annu Rev Immunol 2006;24:147–74.

9. Blanchard C, Rothenberg ME. Biology of the eosinophil. Adv Immunol 2009;101:81–121.

10. Rothenberg ME, Klion AD, Roufosse FE, et al. Treatment of patients with the hypereosinophilic syndrome with mepolizumab. N Engl J Med 2008; 358:1215–28.

11. Nair P, Pizzichini MM, Kjarsgaard M, et al. Mepolizumab for prednisone-dependent asthma with sputum eosinophilia. N Engl J Med 2009;360: 985–93.

12. Haldar P, Brightling CE, Hargadon B, et al. Mepolizumab and exacerbations of refractory eosinophilic asthma. N Engl J Med 2009;360:973–84.

13. Kim S, Marigowda G, Oren E, et al. Mepolizumab as a steroid-sparing treatment option in patients with Churg-Strauss syndrome. J Allergy Clin Immunol 2010;125:1336–43.

14. Wechsler ME, Fulkerson PC, Bochner BS, et al. Novel targeted therapies for eosinophilic disorders. J Allergy Clin Immunol 2012;130:563–71.

15. Akuthota P, Weller PF. Eosinophils and disease pathogenesis. Semin Hematol 2012;49:113–9.

16. Prin L, Capron M, Gosset P, et al. Eosinophil lung disease: immunological studies of blood and alveolar eosinophils. Clin Exp Immunol 1986;63: 249–57.

17. Janin A, Torpier G, Courtin P, et al. Segregation of eosinophil proteins in alveolar macrophage compartments in chronic eosinophilic pneumonia. Thorax 1993;48:57–62.

18. Fox B, Seed WA. Chronic eosinophilic pneumonia. Thorax 1980;35:570–80.

19. Carrington CB, Addington WW, Goff AM, et al. Chronic eosinophilic pneumonia. N Engl J Med 1969;280:787–98.

20. Thomeer MJ, Costabe U, Rizzato G, et al. Comparison of registries of interstitial lung diseases in three European countries. Eur Respir J Suppl 2001;32: 114s–8s.

21. Marchand E, Reynaud-Gaubert M, Lauque D, et al. Idiopathic chronic eosinophilic pneumonia. A clinical and follow-up study of 62 cases. The Groupe d'Etudes et de Recherche sur les Maladies "Orphelines" Pulmonaires (GERM"O"P). Medicine (Baltimore) 1998;77:299–312.

22. Jederlinic PJ, Sicilian L, Gaensler EA. Chronic eosinophilic pneumonia. A report of 19 cases and a review of the literature. Medicine (Baltimore) 1988;67:154–62.

23. Naughton M, Fahy J, FitzGerald MX. Chronic eosinophilic pneumonia. A long-term follow-up of 12 patients. Chest 1993;103:162–5.

24. Cottin V, Frognier R, Monnot H, et al. Chronic eosinophilic pneumonia after radiation therapy for breast cancer. Eur Respir J 2004;23:9–13.

25. Libby DM, Murphy TF, Edwards A, et al. Chronic eosinophilic pneumonia: an unusual cause of acute respiratory failure. Am Rev Respir Dis 1980;122: 497–500.

26. Ivanick MJ, Donohue JF. Chronic eosinophilic pneumonia: a cause of adult respiratory distress syndrome. South Med J 1986;79:686–90.

27. Marchand E, Etienne-Mastroianni B, Chanez P, et al. Idiopathic chronic eosinophilic pneumonia and asthma: how do they influence each other? The Groupe d'Etudes et de Recherche sur les Maladies "Orphelines" Pulmonaires (GERM"O"P). Eur Respir J 2003;22:8–13.

28. Weynants P, Riou R, Vergnon JM, et al. Pneumopathies chroniques à éosinophiles. Etude de 16 cas. Rev Mal Respir 1985;2:63–8.

29. Mayo JR, Muller NL, Road J, et al. Chronic eosinophilic pneumonia: CT findings in six cases. AJR Am J Roentgenol 1989;153:727–30.

30. Ebara H, Ikezoe J, Johkoh T, et al. Chronic eosinophilic pneumonia: evolution of chest radiograms and CT features. J Comput Assist Tomogr 1994; 18:737–44.

31. Gaensler E, Carrington C. Peripheral opacities in chronic eosinophilic pneumonia: the photographic negative of pulmonary edema. AJR Am J Roentgenol 1977;128:1–13.

32. Robertson CL, Shackelford GD, Armstrong JD. Chronic eosinophilic pneumonia. Radiology 1971; 101:57–61.

33. Johkoh T, Muller NL, Akira M, et al. Eosinophilic lung diseases: diagnostic accuracy of thin-section CT in 111 patients. Radiology 2000;216:773–80.

34. Arakawa H, Kurihara Y, Niimi H, et al. Bronchiolitis obliterans with organizing pneumonia versus chronic eosinophilic pneumonia: high-resolution CT findings in 81 patients. AJR Am J Roentgenol 2001;176:1053–8.

35. Furuiye M, Yoshimura N, Kobayashi A, et al. Churg-Strauss syndrome versus chronic eosinophilic pneumonia on high-resolution computed tomographic findings. J Comput Assist Tomogr 2010; 34:19–22.

36. Bancal C, Sadoun D, Valeyre D, et al. Chronic idiopathic eosinophilic pneumopathy. Carrington's disease. Presse Med 1989;18:1695–8 [in French].

37. Zimhony O. Photographic negative shadow of pulmonary oedema. Lancet 2002;360:33.

38. Cottin V, Cordier JF. Idiopathic eosinophilic pneumonias. Eur Respir Mon 2012;134:118–39.

39. Cottin V, Deviller P, Tardy F, et al. Urinary eosinophil-derived neurotoxin/protein X: a simple method for assessing eosinophil degranulation in vivo. J Allergy Clin Immunol 1998;101:116–23.

40. Ono E, Taniguchi M, Mita H, et al. Increased urinary leukotriene E4 concentration in patients with eosinophilic pneumonia. Eur Respir J 2008;32:437–42.

41. Shimizudani N, Murata H, Kojo S, et al. Analysis of T cell receptor V(beta) gene expression and clonality in bronchoalveolar fluid lymphocytes from a patient with chronic eosinophilic pneumonitis. Lung 2001;179:31–41.

42. Freymond N, Kahn JE, Legrand F, et al. Clonal expansion of T cells in patients with eosinophilic lung disease. Allergy 2011;66:1506–8.

43. Grantham JG, Meadows JA 3rd, Gleich GJ. Chronic eosinophilic pneumonia. Evidence for eosinophil degranulation and release of major basic protein. Am J Med 1986;80:89–94.

44. Pearson DL, Rosenow EC 3rd. Chronic eosinophilic pneumonia (Carrington's): a follow-up study. Mayo Clin Proc 1978;53:73–8.

45. Durieu J, Wallaert B, Tonnel AB. Long term follow-up of pulmonary function in chronic eosinophilic pneumonia. Eur Respir J 1997;10:286–91.

46. Hayakawa H, Sato A, Toyoshima M, et al. A clinical study of idiopathic eosinophilic pneumonia. Chest 1994;105:1462–6.

47. Oyama Y, Fujisawa T, Hashimoto D, et al. Efficacy of short-term prednisolone treatment in patients with chronic eosinophilic pneumonia. Eur Respir J 2015;45:1624–31.

48. Badesch DB, King TE, Schwartz MI. Acute eosinophilic pneumonia: a hypersensitivity phenomenon? Am Rev Respir Dis 1989;139:249–52.

49. Allen JN, Pacht ER, Gadek JE, et al. Acute eosinophilic pneumonia as a reversible cause of noninfectious respiratory failure. N Engl J Med 1989; 321:569–74.

50. Philit F, Etienne-Mastroianni B, Parrot A, et al. Idiopathic acute eosinophilic pneumonia: a study of 22 patients. The Groupe d'Etudes et de Recherche sur les Maladies "Orphelines" Pulmonaires (GERM"O"P). Am J Respir Crit Care Med 2002;166:1235–9.

51. Pope-Harman AL, Davis WB, Allen ED, et al. Acute eosinophilic pneumonia. A summary of 15 cases and review of the literature. Medicine (Baltimore) 1996;75:334–42.

52. Shorr AF, Scoville SL, Cersovsky SB, et al. Acute eosinophilic pneumonia among US military personnel deployed in or near Iraq. JAMA 2004; 292:2997–3005.

53. Rhee CK, Min KH, Yim NY, et al. Clinical characteristics and corticosteroid treatment of acute eosinophilic pneumonia. Eur Respir J 2013;41:402–9.

54. Uchiyama H, Suda T, Nakamura Y, et al. Alterations in smoking habits are associated with acute eosinophilic pneumonia. Chest 2008;133:1174–80.

55. Nakajima M, Manabe T, Niki Y, et al. A case of cigarette smoking-induced acute eosinophilic pneumonia showing tolerance. Chest 2000;118:1517–8.

56. Nakajima M, Manabe T, Niki Y, et al. Cigarette smoke-induced acute eosinophilic pneumonia. Radiology 1998;207:829–31.

57. Shintani H, Fujimura M, Ishiura Y, et al. A case of cigarette smoking-induced acute eosinophilic pneumonia showing tolerance. Chest 2000;117: 277–9.

58. Shintani H, Fujimura M, Yasui M, et al. Acute eosinophilic pneumonia caused by cigarette smoking. Intern Med 2000;39:66–8.

59. Vahid B, Marik PE. An 18-year-old woman with fever, diffuse pulmonary opacities, and rapid onset of respiratory failure: idiopathic acute eosinophilic pneumonia. Chest 2006;130:1938–41.

60. Bok GH, Kim YK, Lee YM, et al. Cigarette smoking-induced acute eosinophilic pneumonia: a case report including a provocation test. J Korean Med Sci 2008;23:134–7.

61. Dujon C, Guillaud C, Azarian R, et al. Pneumopathie aiguë à éosinophiles: rôle d'un tabagisme récemment débuté. Rev Mal Resp 2004;21:825–7.

62. Al-Saieg N, Moammar O, Kartan R. Flavored cigar smoking induces acute eosinophilic pneumonia. Chest 2007;131:1234–7.

63. Komiya K, Teramoto S, Kawashima M, et al. A case of acute eosinophilic pneumonia following short-term passive smoking: an evidence of very high level of urinary cotinine. Allergol Int 2010;59:421–3.

64. Buchheit J, Eid N, Rodgers G Jr, et al. Acute eosinophilic pneumonia with respiratory failure: a new syndrome? Am Rev Respir Dis 1992;145:716–8.

65. Davis WB, Wilson HE, Wall RL. Eosinophilic alveolitis in acute respiratory failure. A clinical marker for a non-infectious etiology. Chest 1986;90:7–10.

66. Cheon JE, Lee KS, Jung GS, et al. Acute eosinophilic pneumonia: radiographic and CT findings in six patients. AJR Am J Roentgenol 1996;167:1195–9.

67. Chiappini J, Arbib F, Heyraud JD, et al. Subacute idiopathic eosinophilic pneumopathy with favorable outcome without corticotherapy. Rev Mal Respir 1995;12:25–8 [in French].

68. Elcadi T, Morcos E, Lancrenon C, et al. Abdominal pain syndrome disclosing acute eosinophilic pneumonia. Presse Med 1997;26:416 [in French].

69. Balbi B, Fabiano F. A young man with fever, dyspnoea and nonproductive cough. Eur Respir J 1996; 9:619–21.

70. Ogawa H, Fujimura M, Matsuda T, et al. Transient wheeze. Eosinophilic bronchobronchiolitis in acute eosinophilic pneumonia. Chest 1993;104:493–6.

71. King MA, Pope-Harman AL, Allen JN, et al. Acute eosinophilic pneumonia: radiologic and clinical features. Radiology 1997;203:715–9.

72. Tazelaar HD, Linz LJ, Colby TV, et al. Acute eosinophilic pneumonia: histopathologic findings in nine patients. Am J Respir Crit Care Med 1997;155: 296–302.

73. Thompson BT, Moss M. A new definition for the acute respiratory distress syndrome. Semin Respir Crit Care Med 2013;34:441–7.

74. Daimon T, Johkoh T, Sumikawa H, et al. Acute eosinophilic pneumonia: thin-section CT findings in 29 patients. Eur J Radiol 2008;65:462–7.

75. Taniguchi H, Kadota J, Fujii T, et al. Activation of lymphocytes and increased interleukin-5 levels in bronchoalveolar lavage fluid in acute eosinophilic pneumonia. Eur Respir J 1999;13:217–20.

76. Miyazaki E, Nureki S, Ono E, et al. Circulating thymus- and activation-regulated chemokine/CCL17 is a useful biomarker for discriminating acute eosinophilic pneumonia from other causes of acute lung injury. Chest 2007;131:1726–34.

77. Mochimaru H, Kawamoto M, Fukuda Y, et al. Clinicopathological differences between acute and chronic eosinophilic pneumonia. Respirology 2005;10:76–85.

78. Perng DW, Su HT, Tseng CW, et al. Pulmonary infiltrates with eosinophilia induced by nimesulide in an asthmatic patient. Respiration 2005;72:651–3.

79. Matsuno O, Ueno T, Takenaka R, et al. Acute eosinophilic pneumonia caused by Candida albicans. Respir Med 2007;101:1609–12.

80. Miyazaki E, Sugisaki K, Shigenaga T, et al. A case of acute eosinophilic pneumonia caused by inhalation of Trichosporon terrestre. Am J Respir Crit Care Med 1995;151:541–3.

81. Swartz J, Stoller JK. Acute eosinophilic pneumonia complicating Coccidioides immitis pneumonia: a case report and literature review. Respiration 2009;77:102–6.

82. Ricker DH, Taylor SR, Gartner JC Jr, et al. Fatal pulmonary aspergillosis presenting as acute eosinophilic pneumonia in a previously healthy child. Chest 1991;100:875–7.

83. Trawick D, Kotch A, Matthay R, et al. Eosinophilic pneumonia as a presentation of occult chronic granulomatous disease. Eur Respir J 1997;10:2166–70.

84. Jeon EJ, Kim KH, Min KH. Acute eosinophilic pneumonia associated with 2009 influenza A (H1N1). Thorax 2010;65:268–70.

85. Godeau B, Brochard L, Theodorou I, et al. A case of acute eosinophilic pneumonia with hypersensitivity to "red spider" allergens. J Allergy Clin Immunol 1995;95:1056–8.

86. Sauvaget E, Dellamonica J, Arlaud K, et al. Idiopathic acute eosinophilic pneumonia requiring ECMO in a teenager smoking tobacco and cannabis. Pediatr Pulmonol 2010;45:1246–9.

87. Brander PE, Tukiainen P. Acute eosinophilic pneumonia in a heroin smoker. Eur Respir J 1993;6:750–2.

88. Wagner T, Dhedin N, Philippe B, et al. Acute eosinophilic pneumonia after allogeneic hematopoietic stem cell transplantation. Ann Hematol 2006;85:202–3.

89. Glazer CS, Cohen LB, Schwarz MI. Acute eosinophilic pneumonia in AIDS. Chest 2001;120:1732–5.

90. Jhun BW, Kim SJ, Kim K, et al. Outcomes of rapid corticosteroid tapering in acute eosinophilic pneumonia patients with initial eosinophilia. Respirology 2015;20:1241–7.

91. Kawayama T, Fujiki R, Morimitsu Y, et al. Fatal idiopathic acute eosinophilic pneumonia with acute lung injury. Respirology 2002;7:373–5.

92. Churg J, Strauss L. Allergic granulomatosis, allergic angiitis, and periarteritis nodosa. Am J Pathol 1951;27:277–301.

93. Jennette JC, Falk RJ, Bacon PA, et al. 2012 revised international Chapel Hill consensus conference nomenclature of vasculitides. Arthritis Rheum 2013;65:1–11.

94. Mouthon L, le Toumelin P, Andre MH, et al. Polyarteritis nodosa and Churg-Strauss angiitis: characteristics and outcome in 38 patients over 65 years. Medicine (Baltimore) 2002;81:27–40.

95. Lanham JG, Elkon KB, Pusey CD, et al. Systemic vasculitis with asthma and eosinophilia: a clinical approach to the Churg-Strauss syndrome. Medicine (Baltimore) 1984;63:65–81.

96. Keogh KA, Specks U. Churg-Strauss syndrome: clinical presentation, antineutrophil cytoplasmic antibodies, and leukotriene receptor antagonists. Am J Med 2003;115:284–90.

97. Guillevin L, Cohen P, Gayraud M, et al. Churg-Strauss syndrome. Clinical study and long-term follow-up of 96 patients. Medicine (Baltimore) 1999;78:26–37.

98. Dunogué B, Pagnoux C, Guillevin L. Churg-Strauss syndrome: clinical symptoms, complementary investigations, prognosis and outcome, and treatment. Semin Respir Crit Care Med 2011;32:298–309.

99. Vaglio A, Martorana D, Maggiore U, et al. HLA-DRB4 as a genetic risk factor for Churg-Strauss syndrome. Arthritis Rheum 2007;56:3159–66.

100. Tsurikisawa N, Morita S, Tsuburai T, et al. Familial Churg-Strauss syndrome in two sisters. Chest 2007;131:592–4.

101. Bottero P, Bonini M, Vecchio F, et al. The common allergens in the Churg-Strauss syndrome. Allergy 2007;62:1288–94.

102. Cottin V, Bonniaud P. Drug-induced infiltrative lung disease. Eur Respir Mon 2009;46:287–318.

103. Ruppert AM, Averous G, Stanciu D, et al. Development of Churg-Strauss syndrome with controlled asthma during omalizumab treatment. J Allergy Clin Immunol 2008;121:253–4.

104. Winchester DE, Jacob A, Murphy T. Omalizumab for asthma. N Engl J Med 2006;355:1281–2.

105. Puechal X, Rivereau P, Vinchon F. Churg-Strauss syndrome associated with omalizumab. Eur J Internmed 2008;19:364–6.

106. Bargagli E, Madioni C, Olivieri C, et al. Churg-Strauss vasculitis in a patient treated with omalizumab. J Asthma 2008;45:115–6.

107. Wechsler ME, Wong DA, Miller MK, et al. Churg-Strauss syndrome in patients treated with omalizumab. Chest 2009;136:507–18.

108. Hamilos DL, Christensen J. Treatment of Churg-Strauss syndrome with high-dose intravenous immunoglobulin. J Allergy Clin Immunol 1991;88: 823–4.

109. Guillevin L, Guittard T, Bletry O, et al. Systemic necrotizing angiitis with asthma: causes and precipitating factors in 43 cases. Lung 1987;165: 165–72.

110. Boita M, Guida G, Circosta P, et al. The molecular and functional characterization of clonally expanded CD8+ TCR BV T cells in eosinophilic granulomatosis with polyangiitis (EGPA). Clin Immunol 2014;152: 152–63.

111. Nathani N, Little MA, Kunst H, et al. Churg-Strauss syndrome and leukotriene antagonist use: a respiratory perspective. Thorax 2008;63:883–8.

112. Harrold LR, Patterson MK, Andrade SE, et al. Asthma drug use and the development of Churg-Strauss syndrome (CSS). Pharmacoepidemiol Drug Saf 2007;16:620–6.

113. Beasley R, Bibby S, Weatherall M. Leukotriene receptor antagonist therapy and Churg-Strauss syndrome: culprit or innocent bystander? Thorax 2008; 63:847–9.

114. Hauser T, Mahr A, Metzler C, et al. The leukotriene-receptor antagonist montelukast and the risk of Churg-Strauss syndrome: a case-crossover study. Thorax 2008;63(8):677–82.

115. Bibby S, Healy B, Steele R, et al. Association between leukotriene receptor antagonist therapy and Churg-Strauss syndrome: an analysis of the FDA AERS database. Thorax 2010;65:132–8.

116. Della Rossa A, Baldini C, Tavoni A, et al. Churg-Strauss syndrome: clinical and serological features of 19 patients from a single Italian centre. Rheumatology (Oxford) 2002;41:1286–94.

117. Solans R, Bosch JA, Perez-Bocanegra C, et al. Churg-Strauss syndrome: outcome and long-term follow-up of 32 patients. Rheumatology (Oxford) 2001;40:763–71.

118. Churg A, Brallas M, Cronin SR, et al. Formes frustes of Churg-Strauss syndrome. Chest 1995; 108:320–3.

119. Reid AJ, Harrison BD, Watts RA, et al. Churg-Strauss syndrome in a district hospital. QJM 1998;91:219–29.

120. Chumbley LC, Harrison EG Jr, DeRemee RA. Allergic granulomatosis and angiitis (Churg-Strauss syndrome). Report and analysis of 30 cases. Mayo Clin Proc 1977;52:477–84.

121. Cottin V, Khouatra C, Dubost R, et al. Persistent airflow obstruction in asthma of patients with Churg-Strauss syndrome and long-term follow-up. Allergy 2009;64:589–95.

122. Szczeklik W, Sokolowska BM, Zuk J, et al. The course of asthma in Churg-Strauss syndrome. J Asthma 2011;48:183–7.

123. Bacciu A, Bacciu S, Mercante G, et al. Ear, nose and throat manifestations of Churg-Strauss syndrome. Acta Otolaryngol 2006;126:503–9.

124. Bacciu A, Buzio C, Giordano D, et al. Nasal polyposis in Churg-Strauss syndrome. Laryngoscope 2008;118:325–9.

125. Olsen KD, Neel HB, De Remee RA, et al. Nasal manifestations of allergic granulomatosis and angiitis (Churg-Strauss syndrome). Otolaryngol Head Neck Surg 1995;88:85–9.

126. Srouji I, Lund V, Andrews P, et al. Rhinologic symptoms and quality-of-life in patients with Churg-Strauss syndrome vasculitis. Am J Rhinol 2008; 22:406–9.

127. Cottin V, Cordier JF. Churg-Strauss syndrome. Allergy 1999;54:535–51.

128. Vinit J, Bielefeld P, Muller G, et al. Heart involvement in Churg-Strauss syndrome: retrospective study in French Burgundy population in past 10 years. Eur J Intern Med 2010;21:341–6.

129. Neumann T, Manger B, Schmid M, et al. Cardiac involvement in Churg-Strauss syndrome: impact of endomyocarditis. Medicine (Baltimore) 2009; 88:236–43.

130. Ginsberg F, Parrillo JE. Eosinophilic myocarditis. Heart Fail Clin 2005;1:419–29.

131. Kajihara H, Tachiyama Y, Hirose T, et al. Eosinophilic coronary periarteritis (vasospastic angina and sudden death), a new type of coronary arteritis: report of seven autopsy cases and a review of the literature. Virchows Arch 2013;462:239–48.

132. Groh M, Masciocco G, Kirchner E, et al. Heart transplantation in patients with eosinophilic granulomatosis with polyangiitis (Churg-Strauss syndrome). J Heart Lung Transplant 2014;33:842–50.

133. Courand PY, Croisille P, Khouatra C, et al. Churg-Strauss syndrome presenting with acute myocarditis and cardiogenic shock. Heart Lung Circ 2012;21:178–81.

134. Dennert RM, van Paassen P, Schalla S, et al. Cardiac involvement in Churg-Strauss syndrome. Arthritis Rheum 2010;62:627–34.

135. Yune S, Choi DC, Lee BJ, et al. Detecting cardiac involvement with magnetic resonance in patients with active eosinophilic granulomatosis with polyangiitis. Int J Cardiovasc Imaging 2016. [Epub ahead of print].

136. Marmursztejn J, Vignaux O, Cohen P, et al. Impact of cardiac magnetic resonance imaging for

assessment of Churg-Strauss syndrome: a cross-sectional study in 20 patients. Clin Exp Rheumatol 2009;27:S70–6.

137. Pela G, Tirabassi G, Pattoneri P, et al. Cardiac involvement in the Churg-Strauss syndrome. Am J Cardiol 2006;97:1519–24.

138. Degesys GE, Mintzer RA, Vrla RF. Allergic granulomatosis: Churg-Strauss syndrome. AJR Am J Roentgenol 1980;135:1281–2.

139. Choi YH, Im JG, Han BK, et al. Thoracic manifestation of Churg-Strauss syndrome: radiologic and clinical findings. Chest 2000;117:117–24.

140. Kim YK, Lee KS, Chung MP, et al. Pulmonary involvement in Churg-Strauss syndrome: an analysis of CT, clinical, and pathologic findings. Eur Radiol 2007;17:3157–65.

141. Chung MP, Yi CA, Lee HY, et al. Imaging of pulmonary vasculitis. Radiology 2010;255:322–41.

142. Johkoh T. Imaging of idiopathic interstitial pneumonias. Clin Chest Med 2008;29:133–47, vi.

143. Worthy SA, Muller NL, Hansell DM, et al. Churg-Strauss syndrome: the spectrum of pulmonary CT findings in 17 patients. AJR Am J Roentgenol 1998;170:297–300.

144. Wallaert B, Gosset P, Prin L, et al. Bronchoalveolar lavage in allergic granulomatosis and angiitis. Eur Respir J 1993;6:413–7.

145. Cottin V, Tardy F, Gindre D, et al. Urinary eosinophil-derived neurotoxin in Churg-Strauss syndrome. J Allergy Clin Immunol 1995;96:261–4.

146. Vaglio A, Strehl JD, Manger B, et al. IgG4 immune response in Churg-Strauss syndrome. Ann Rheum Dis 2012;71:390–3.

147. Dallos T, Heiland GR, Strehl J, et al. CCL17/thymus and activation-related chemokine in Churg-Strauss syndrome. Arthritis Rheum 2010;62:3496–503.

148. Sablé-Fourtassou R, Cohen P, Mahr A, et al. Antineutrophil cytoplasmic antibodies and the Churg-Strauss syndrome. Ann Intern Med 2005;143:632–8.

149. Sinico RA, Di Toma L, Maggiore U, et al. Prevalence and clinical significance of antineutrophil cytoplasmic antibodies in Churg-Strauss syndrome. Arthritis Rheum 2005;52:2926–35.

150. Healy B, Bibby S, Steele R, et al. Antineutrophil cytoplasmic autoantibodies and myeloperoxidase autoantibodies in clinical expression of Churg-Strauss syndrome. J Allergy Clin Immunol 2013; 131:571–6.e1–6.

151. Comarmond C, Pagnoux C, Khellaf M, et al. Eosinophilic granulomatosis with polyangiitis (Churg-Strauss): clinical characteristics and long-term followup of the 383 patients enrolled in the French Vasculitis Study Group cohort. Arthritis Rheum 2013;65:270–81.

152. Sokolowska BM, Szczeklik WK, Wludarczyk AA, et al. ANCA-positive and ANCA-negative phenotypes of eosinophilic granulomatosis with polyangiitis (EGPA): outcome and long-term follow-up of 50 patients from a single Polish center. Clin Exp Rheumatol 2014;32:S41–7.

153. Wieczorek S, Hellmich B, Arning L, et al. Functionally relevant variations of the interleukin-10 gene associated with antineutrophil cytoplasmic antibody-negative Churg-Strauss syndrome, but not with Wegener's granulomatosis. Arthritis Rheum 2008;58:1839–48.

154. Katzenstein AL. Diagnostic features and differential diagnosis of Churg-Strauss syndrome in the lung. A review. Am J Clin Pathol 2000;114:767–72.

155. Churg A. Recent advances in the diagnosis of Churg-Strauss syndrome. Mod Pathol 2001;14: 1284–93.

156. Lie JT. Limited forms of Churg-Strauss syndrome. Pathol Annu 1993;28:199–220.

157. Wechsler ME, Garpestad E, Flier SR, et al. Pulmonary infiltrates, eosinophilia, and cardiomyopathy following corticosteroid withdrawal in patients with asthma receiving zarfirlukast. JAMA 1998;279:455–7.

158. Masi AT, Hunder GG, Lie JT, et al. The American College of Rheumatology 1990 criteria for the classification of Churg-Strauss syndrome (allergic granulomatosis and angiitis). Arthritis Rheum 1990;33:1094–100.

159. Guillevin L, Pagnoux C, Seror R, et al. The Five-Factor Score revisited: assessment of prognoses of systemic necrotizing vasculitides based on the French Vasculitis Study Group (FVSG) cohort. Medicine (Baltimore) 2011;90:19–27.

160. Moosig F, Richardt G, Gross WL. A fatal attraction: eosinophils and the heart. Rheumatology (Oxford) 2013;52:587–9.

161. Samson M, Puechal X, Devilliers H, et al. Long-term outcomes of 118 patients with eosinophilic granulomatosis with polyangiitis (Churg-Strauss syndrome) enrolled in two prospective trials. J Autoimmun 2013;43:60–9.

162. Groh M, Pagnoux C, Baldini C, et al. Eosinophilic granulomatosis with polyangiitis (Churg-Strauss) (EGPA) Consensus Task Force recommendations for evaluation and management. Eur J Intern Med 2015;26(7):545–53.

163. Cartin-Ceba R, Keogh KA, Specks U, et al. Rituximab for the treatment of Churg-Strauss syndrome with renal involvement. Nephrol Dial Transplant 2011;26:2865–71.

164. Donvik KK, Omdal R. Churg-Strauss syndrome successfully treated with rituximab. Rheumatol Int 2011;31:89–91.

165. Kaushik VV, Reddy HV, Bucknall RC. Successful use of rituximab in a patient with recalcitrant Churg-Strauss syndrome. Ann Rheum Dis 2006; 65:1116–7.

166. Koukoulaki M, Smith KG, Jayne DR. Rituximab in Churg-Strauss syndrome. Ann Rheum Dis 2006; 65:557–9.

167. Najem CE, Yadav R, Carlson E. Successful use of rituximab in a patient with recalcitrant multisystemic eosinophilic granulomatosis with polyangiitis. BMJ Case Rep 2015;2015. http://dx.doi.org/10.1136/bcr-2014-206421.

168. Pepper RJ, Fabre MA, Pavesio C, et al. Rituximab is effective in the treatment of refractory Churg-Strauss syndrome and is associated with diminished T-cell interleukin-5 production. Rheumatology (Oxford) 2008;47:1104–5.

169. Saech J, Owczarczyk K, Rosgen S, et al. Successful use of rituximab in a patient with Churg-Strauss syndrome and refractory central nervous system involvement. Ann Rheum Dis 2010;69:1254–5.

170. Thiel J, Hassler F, Salzer U, et al. Rituximab in the treatment of refractory or relapsing eosinophilic granulomatosis with polyangiitis (Churg-Strauss syndrome). Arthritis Res Ther 2013;15:R133.

171. Umezawa N, Kohsaka H, Nanki T, et al. Successful treatment of eosinophilic granulomatosis with polyangiitis (EGPA; formerly Churg-Strauss syndrome) with rituximab in a case refractory to glucocorticoids, cyclophosphamide, and IVIG. Mod Rheumatol 2014;24:685–7.

172. Bouldouyre MA, Cohen P, Guillevin L. Severe bronchospasm associated with rituximab for refractory Churg-Strauss syndrome. Ann Rheum Dis 2009; 68:606.

173. Kahn JE, Grandpeix-Guyodo C, Marroun I, et al. Sustained response to mepolizumab in refractory Churg-Strauss syndrome. J Allergy Clin Immunol 2010;125:267–70.

174. Moosig F, Gross WL, Herrmann K, et al. Targeting interleukin-5 in refractory and relapsing Churg-Strauss syndrome. Ann Intern Med 2011;155:341–3.

175. Rosenwasser LJ, Rothenberg ME. IL-5 pathway inhibition in the treatment of asthma and Churg-Strauss syndrome. J Allergy Clin Immunol 2010;125:1245–6.

176. Jachiet M, Samson M, Cottin V, et al, French Vasculitis Study Group (FVSG). Anti-IgE monoclonal antibody in refractory and relapsing eosinophilic granulomatosis with polyangiitis (Churg-Strauss): data from 17 patients. Arthritis Rheum 2016. [Epub ahead of print].

177. Cohen P, Pagnoux C, Mahr A, et al. Treatment of Churg-Strauss syndrome (CSS) without poor prognosis factor at baseline with corticosteroids (CS) alone. Preliminary results of a prospective multicenter trial. Arthritis Rheum 2003;48:S209.

178. Ribi C, Cohen P, Pagnoux C, et al. Treatment of Churg-Strauss syndrome without poor-prognosis factors: a multicenter, prospective, randomized, open-label study of seventy-two patients. Arthritis Rheum 2008;58:586–94.

179. Bourgarit A, Le Toumelin P, Pagnoux C, et al. Deaths occurring during the first year after treatment onset for polyarteritis nodosa, microscopic polyangiitis, and Churg-Strauss syndrome: a retrospective analysis of causes and factors predictive of mortality based on 595 patients. Medicine (Baltimore) 2005;84:323–30.

180. Geller DE, Kaplowitz H, Light MJ, et al. Allergic bronchopulmonary aspergillosis in cystic fibrosis: reported prevalence, regional distribution, and patient characteristics. Chest 1999; 116:639–46.

181. Mastella G, Rainisio M, Harms HK, et al. Allergic bronchopulmonary aspergillosis in cystic fibrosis. A European epidemiological study. Epidemiologic Registry of Cystic Fibrosis. Eur Respir J 2000;16: 464–71.

182. Mehta SK, Sandhu RS. Immunological significance of Aspergillus fumigatus in cane-sugar mills. Arch Environ Health 1983;38:41–6.

183. Bains SN, Judson MA. Allergic bronchopulmonary aspergillosis. Clin Chest Med 2012;33:265–81.

184. Marchand E, Verellen-Dumoulin C, Mairesse M, et al. Frequency of cystic fibrosis transmembrane conductance regulator gene mutations and 5T allele in patients with allergic bronchopulmonary aspergillosis. Chest 2001;119:762–7.

185. Knutsen AP, Kariuki B, Consolino JD, et al. IL-4 alpha chain receptor (IL-4Ralpha) polymorphisms in allergic bronchopulmonary aspergillosis. Clin Mol Allergy 2006;4:3.

186. Brouard J, Knauer N, Boelle PY, et al. Influence of interleukin-10 on Aspergillus fumigatus infection in patients with cystic fibrosis. J Infect Dis 2005; 191:1988–91.

187. Saxena S, Madan T, Shah A, et al. Association of polymorphisms in the collagen region of SP-A2 with increased levels of total IgE antibodies and eosinophilia in patients with allergic bronchopulmonary aspergillosis. J Allergy Clin Immunol 2003; 111:1001–7.

188. Chauhan B, Santiago L, Kirschmann DA, et al. The association of HLA-DR alleles and T cell activation with allergic bronchopulmonary aspergillosis. J Immunol 1997;159:4072–6.

189. Chauhan B, Santiago L, Hutcheson PS, et al. Evidence for the involvement of two different MHC class II regions in susceptibility or protection in allergic bronchopulmonary aspergillosis. J Allergy Clin Immunol 2000;106:723–9.

190. Chauhan B, Knutsen A, Hutcheson PS, et al. T cell subsets, epitope mapping, and HLA-restriction in patients with allergic bronchopulmonary aspergillosis. J Clin Invest 1996;97:2324–31.

191. Shah A, Khan ZU, Chaturvedi S, et al. Concomitant allergic Aspergillus sinusitis and allergic bronchopulmonary aspergillosis associated with familial

occurrence of allergic bronchopulmonary aspergillosis. Ann Allergy 1990;64:507–12.

192. Leonard CT, Berry GJ, Ruoss SJ. Nasal-pulmonary relations in allergic fungal sinusitis and allergic bronchopulmonary aspergillosis. Clin Rev Allergy Immunol 2001;21:5–15.

193. Venarske DL, deShazo RD. Sinobronchial allergic mycosis: the SAM syndrome. Chest 2002;121:1670–6.

194. Agarwal R. Allergic bronchopulmonary aspergillosis. Chest 2009;135:805–26.

195. Mussaffi H, Rivlin J, Shalit I, et al. Nontuberculous mycobacteria in cystic fibrosis associated with allergic bronchopulmonary aspergillosis and steroid therapy. Eur Respir J 2005;25:324–8.

196. Agarwal R, Gupta D, Aggarwal AN, et al. Clinical significance of hyperattenuating mucoid impaction in allergic bronchopulmonary aspergillosis: an analysis of 155 patients. Chest 2007;132:1183–90.

197. Logan PM, Muller NL. High-attenuation mucous plugging in allergic bronchopulmonary aspergillosis. Can Assoc Radiol J 1996;47:374–7.

198. Agarwal R, Gupta D, Aggarwal AN, et al. Allergic bronchopulmonary aspergillosis: lessons from 126 patients attending a chest clinic in north India. Chest 2006;130:442–8.

199. Martinez S, Heyneman LE, McAdams HP, et al. Mucoid impactions: finger-in-glove sign and other CT and radiographic features. Radiographics 2008;28:1369–82.

200. Ward S, Heyneman L, Lee MJ, et al. Accuracy of CT in the diagnosis of allergic bronchopulmonary aspergillosis in asthmatic patients. AJR Am J Roentgenol 1999;173:937–42.

201. Agarwal R, Maskey D, Aggarwal AN, et al. Diagnostic performance of various tests and criteria employed in allergic bronchopulmonary aspergillosis: a latent class analysis. PLoS One 2013;8:e61105.

202. Sehgal IS, Agarwal R. Specific IgE is better than skin testing for detecting Aspergillus sensitization and allergic bronchopulmonary aspergillosis in asthma. Chest 2015;147:e194.

203. Rosenberg M, Patterson R, Roberts M, et al. The assessment of immunologic and clinical changes occurring during corticosteroid therapy for allergic bronchopulmonary aspergillosis. Am J Med 1978;64:599–606.

204. Bosken C, Myers J, Greenberger P, et al. Pathologic features of allergic bronchopulmonary aspergillosis. Am J Surg Pathol 1988;12:216–22.

205. Agarwal R, Chakrabarti A, Shah A, et al. Allergic bronchopulmonary aspergillosis: review of literature and proposal of new diagnostic and classification criteria. Clin Exp Allergy 2013;43:850–73.

206. Greenberger PA. Allergic bronchopulmonary aspergillosis. J Allergy Clin Immunol 2002;110:685–92.

207. Agarwal R, Garg M, Aggarwal AN, et al. Serologic allergic bronchopulmonary aspergillosis (ABPA-S): long-term outcomes. Respir Med 2012;106:942–7.

208. Chowdhary A, Agarwal K, Kathuria S, et al. Allergic bronchopulmonary mycosis due to fungi other than Aspergillus: a global overview. Crit Rev Microbiol 2014;40:30–48.

209. Moss RB. Treatment options in severe fungal asthma and allergic bronchopulmonary aspergillosis. Eur Respir J 2014;43:1487–500.

210. Agarwal R, Aggarwal AN, Dhooria S, et al. A randomised trial of glucocorticoids in acute-stage allergic bronchopulmonary aspergillosis complicating asthma. Eur Respir J 2016;47:385–7.

211. Singh Sehgal I, Agarwal R. Pulse methylprednisolone in allergic bronchopulmonary aspergillosis exacerbations. Eur Respir Rev 2014;23:149–52.

212. Patterson R, Greenberger PA, Lee TM, et al. Prolonged evaluation of patients with corticosteroid-dependent asthma stage of allergic bronchopulmonary aspergillosis. J Allergy Clin Immunol 1987;80:663–8.

213. Salez F, Brichet A, Desurmont S, et al. Effects of itraconazole therapy in allergic bronchopulmonary aspergillosis. Chest 1999;116:1665–8.

214. Wark P. Pathogenesis of allergic bronchopulmonary aspergillosis and an evidence-based review of azoles in treatment. Respir Med 2004;98:915–23.

215. van der Ent CK, Hoekstra H, Rijkers GT. Successful treatment of allergic bronchopulmonary aspergillosis with recombinant anti-IgE antibody. Thorax 2007;62:276–7.

216. Zirbes JM, Milla CE. Steroid-sparing effect of omalizumab for allergic bronchopulmonary aspergillosis and cystic fibrosis. Pediatr Pulmonol 2008;43:607–10.

217. Kanu A, Patel K. Treatment of allergic bronchopulmonary aspergillosis (ABPA) in CF with anti-IgE antibody (omalizumab). Pediatr Pulmonol 2008;43:1249–51.

218. Tillie-Leblond I, Germaud P, Leroyer C, et al. Allergic bronchopulmonary aspergillosis and omalizumab. Allergy 2011;66:1254–6.

219. Perez-de-Llano LA, Vennera MC, Parra A, et al. Effects of omalizumab in Aspergillus-associated airway disease. Thorax 2011;66:539–40.

220. Chusid MJ, Dale DC, West BC, et al. The hypereosinophilic syndrome: analysis of fourteen cases with review of the literature. Medicine (Baltimore) 1975;54:1–27.

221. Klion A. Hypereosinophilic syndrome: current approach to diagnosis and treatment. Annu Rev Med 2009;60:293–306.

222. Ogbogu PU, Bochner BS, Butterfield JH, et al. Hypereosinophilic syndrome: a multicenter, retrospective analysis of clinical characteristics and

response to therapy. J Allergy Clin Immunol 2009; 124:1319–25.e3.

223. Simon HU, Plotz SG, Dummer R, et al. Abnormal clones of T cells producing interleukin-5 in idiopathic eosinophilia. N Engl J Med 1999;341: 1112–20.

224. Cools J, DeAngelo DJ, Gotlib J, et al. A tyrosine kinase created by fusion of the PDGFRA and FIP1L1 genes as a therapeutic target of imatinib in idiopathic hypereosinophilic syndrome. N Engl J Med 2003;348:1201–14.

225. Griffin JH, Leung J, Bruner RJ, et al. Discovery of a fusion kinase in EOL-1 cells and idiopathic hypereosinophilic syndrome. Proc Natl Acad Sci U S A 2003;100:7830–5.

226. Legrand F, Renneville A, Macintyre E, et al. The spectrum of FIP1L1-PDGFRA-associated chronic eosinophilic leukemia: new insights based on a survey of 44 cases. Medicine (Baltimore) 2013. [Epub ahead of print].

227. Roufosse F, de Lavareille A, Schandene L, et al. Mepolizumab as a corticosteroid-sparing agent in lymphocytic variant hypereosinophilic syndrome. J Allergy Clin Immunol 2010;126:828–35.e3.

228. Roufosse FE, Kahn JE, Gleich GJ, et al. Long-term safety of mepolizumab for the treatment of hypereosinophilic syndromes. J Allergy Clin Immunol 2013;131:461–7.e1–5.

229. Dulohery MM, Patel RR, Schneider F, et al. Lung involvement in hypereosinophilic syndromes. Respir Med 2011;105:114–21.

230. Chung KF, Hew M, Score J, et al. Cough and hypereosinophilia due to FIP1L1-PDGFRA fusion gene with tyrosine kinase activity. Eur Respir J 2006;27: 230–2.

231. Cordier JF, Cottin V, Khouatra C, et al. Hypereosinophilic obliterative bronchiolitis: a distinct, unrecognised syndrome. Eur Respir J 2013;41:1126–34.

232. Takayanagi N, Kanazawa M, Kawabata Y, et al. Chronic bronchiolitis with associated eosinophilic lung disease (eosinophilic bronchiolitis). Respiration 2001;68:319–22.

233. Fukushima Y, Kamiya K, Tatewaki M, et al. A patient with bronchial asthma in whom eosinophilic bronchitis and bronchiolitis developed during treatment. Allergol Int 2010;59:87–91.

234. Kobayashi T, Inoue H, Mio T. Hypereosinophilic obliterative bronchiolitis clinically mimicking diffuse panbronchiolitis: four-year follow-up. Intern Med 2015;54:1091–4.

235. Tang TT, Cheng HH, Zhang H, et al. Hypereosinophilic obliterative bronchiolitis with an elevated level of serum CEA: a case report and a review of the literature. Eur Rev Med Pharmacol Sci 2015; 19:2634–40.

236. Wang LH, Tsai YS, Yan JJ, et al. Reversing rapidly deteriorating lung function in eosinophilic bronchiolitis by pulse steroid and anti-IgE therapy. J Formos Med Assoc 2014;113:326–7.

237. Kunst H, Mack D, Kon OM, et al. Parasitic infections of the lung: a guide for the respiratory physician. Thorax 2011;66:528–36.

238. Sitbon O, Bidel N, Dussopt C, et al. Minocycline pneumonitis and eosinophilia. A report on eight patients. Arch Intern Med 1994;154:1633–40.

239. Sovijarvi AR, Lemola M, Stenius B, et al. Nitrofurantoin-induced acute, subacute and chronic pulmonary reactions. Scand J Respir Dis 1977;58:41–50.

240. Favrolt N, Bonniaud P, Collet E, et al. [Severe drug rash with eosinophilia and systemic symptoms after treatment with minocycline]. Rev Mal Respir 2007;24:892–5 [in French].

241. Belongia EA, Hedberg CW, Gleich GJ, et al. An investigation of the cause of the eosinophilia-myalgia syndrome associated with tryptophan use. N Engl J Med 1990;323:357–65.

242. Hertzman PA, Blevins WL, Mayer J, et al. Association of the eosinophilia-myalgia syndrome with the ingestion of tryptophan. N Engl J Med 1990;322: 869–73.

243. Silver RM, Heyes MP, Maize JC, et al. Scleroderma, fasciitis, and eosinophilia associated with the ingestion of tryptophan. N Engl J Med 1990;322: 874–81.

244. Allen JA, Peterson A, Sufit R, et al. Post-epidemic eosinophilia myalgia syndrome associated with L-Tryptophan. Blood 2011;63(11):3633–9.

245. Alonso-Ruiz A, Calabozo M, Perez-Ruiz F, et al. Toxic oil syndrome. A long-term follow-up of a cohort of 332 patients. Medicine (Baltimore) 1993; 72:285–95.

246. Miranowski AC, Ditto AM. A 59-year-old woman with fever, cough, and eosinophilia. Ann Allergy Asthma Immunol 2006;96:483–8.

247. Cottin V, Cordier JF. Eosinophilic pneumonia in a patient with breast cancer: idiopathic or not? Ann Allergy Asthma Immunol 2006;97:557–8.

248. Pavord ID. Eosinophilic phenotypes of airway disease. Ann Am Thorac Soc 2013;10(Suppl):S143–9.

249. Cordier JF. Asthmes hyperéosinophiliques. Rev Fr Allergol Immunol Clin 2004;44:92–5.

250. Verleden SE, Ruttens D, Vandermeulen E, et al. Elevated bronchoalveolar lavage eosinophilia correlates with poor outcome after lung transplantation. Transplantation 2014;97:83–9.

Hyper-IgE Syndromes and the Lung

Alexandra F. Freeman, MD*, Kenneth N. Olivier, MD, MPH

KEYWORDS

- Hyper-IgE syndromes • Pulmonary manifestations • Job syndrome • DOCK8 deficiency
- PGM3 deficiency • STAT3

KEY POINTS

- The hyper-IgE syndromes (HIES) comprise distinct primary immunodeficiencies characterized by eczema, recurrent skin and lung infections, and high serum IgE.
- STAT3-deficient patients with HIES frequently develop pneumatoceles that become secondarily infected.
- DOCK8 deficiency is associated with increased viral infections, typically of the skin, and recurrent lung infections that often lead to bronchiectasis.
- PGM3 deficiency is a glycosylation disorder characterized by neurologic abnormalities, cytopenias, and significant bronchiectasis.

INTRODUCTION

IgE is a type of antibody linked with host defense against parasitic infection. However, in most countries with a low incidence of parasitic infection, high IgE is more commonly associated with disorders of immune dysregulation, such as atopy. There are various pulmonary conditions associated with high serum IgE. IgE is one of the drivers of asthma associated with atopy, which led to the development of omalizumab, an anti-IgE monoclonal antibody, as an asthma therapy.[1] High serum IgE is associated with allergic bronchopulmonary aspergillosis, which complicates cystic fibrosis and asthma; monitoring the fall of IgE is helpful to assess therapeutic response.[2] Peripheral and pulmonary eosinophilia along with high serum IgE is associated with parasitic infections, such as *Strongyloides* and *Ascaris* leading to Löffler syndrome. Pulmonary eosinophilia and high serum IgE can also be associated with inflammatory conditions, such as eosinophilic granulomatosis with polyangiitis (Churg-Strauss syndrome), which frequently manifests with pulmonary infiltrates, asthma, and chronic rhinosinusitis.[3] Finally, recurrent pneumonias and bronchiectasis with high serum IgE may result from several primary immunodeficiencies.

The hyper-IgE syndromes (HIES) are grouped together because of symptoms of eczema, recurrent lung and skin infections, and high serum IgE. Mutations in STAT3 (Signal Transducer and Activator 3), DOCK8 (Dedicator of Cytokinesis 8), and PGM3 (Phosphogucomutase 3) lead to three distinct disease entities that have been classified as HIES.[4–9] This article discusses the clinical features of these primary immunodeficiencies with a particular focus on the pulmonary manifestations and discussion of the genetics, pathogenesis, and approaches to therapy.

This work was supported in part by the Intramural Research Programs of the NIAID and NHLBI, NIH.
Laboratory of Clinical Infectious Diseases, NIAID, NHLBI, National Institutes of Health, Bethesda, MD, USA
* Corresponding author. National Institutes of Health, Building 10, Room 12C103, 9000 Rockville Pike, Bethesda, MD 20892.
E-mail address: freemaal@mail.nih.gov

AUTOSOMAL-DOMINANT HYPER-IGE SYNDROMES (JOB SYNDROME)

Job syndrome was initially described in two patients with recurrent skin abscesses that were reminiscent of the boils described in the Bible as affecting the prophet Job.[10] Several years later, IgE was identified and high serum levels were associated with this syndrome of eczema and recurrent infections.[11] Over the next few decades, the clinical spectrum of this syndrome broadened to include many diverse features, the genetics were described, and the understanding of the pathogenesis increased dramatically.[12]

Pulmonary Features

Recurrent pyogenic pneumonias caused by *Staphylococcus aureus, Streptococcus pneumoniae* and *Haemophilus influenzae* typically begin in the first several years of life.[12] The systemic signs of infection are often diminished leading to delayed diagnosis of pneumonia. For instance, *S aureus* lobar pneumonia may present with minimal fever, normal peripheral white blood cell count, and fairly normal inflammatory markers. Despite the lack of systemic signs of inflammation, airway inflammation is prominent and mucus production may be especially tenacious (**Fig. 1**). Bronchoscopy may be helpful not only to identify the cause of infection but to assist in airway clearance. The pyogenic pneumonias typically respond well to appropriate antibiotics, but because of the frequent delay in diagnosis, there may be complications, such as empyema, pneumatocele formation, and bronchiectasis. AD-HIES seems to be associated with impaired epithelial repair, which likely explains the high frequency of pneumatoceles and parenchymal abnormalities, encountered in approximately 70% of patients.[12]

Once the parenchyma of the lungs in AD-HIES has been altered by pyogenic pneumonias, the list of infecting microbes expands to include nontuberculous mycobacteria; molds, such as *Aspergillus fumigatus*; and persistent gram-negative bacilli, such as *Pseudomonas* (**Fig. 2**). In our series, 16% of our relatively large AD-HIES cohort met the American Thoracic Society/Infectious Disease Society of America criteria for nontuberculous mycobacteria infection, prevalence similar to that seen in cystic fibrosis.[13] Molds and gram-negative bacilli cause chronic infection even more commonly. These chronic infections are the cause of significant morbidity and mortality for these individuals because they may cause significant hemoptysis and/or become increasingly resistant to antimicrobial agents with time.[14,15]

Most pulmonary mold infections occur in areas of pre-existing pneumatoceles and bronchiectasis, leading to chronic airway infection.[16] Occasionally, however, features of allergic bronchopulmonary mycosis are seen. This is difficult to diagnose because the serum IgE is high and antigen-specific serologies may be falsely positive to many allergens. The typical imaging findings can lead to this diagnosis and corticosteroid, antifungal, or omalizumab treatment initiated (**Fig. 3**). Generally, however, long-term steroid administration is not recommended because of the high incidence of bone fractures (discussed later).

Other Clinical Features

The first manifestation of disease is typically a rash, which is present at birth or develops within the first few weeks.[17–19] The rash is typically diagnosed as neonatal acne or erythema toxicum neonatorum, and predominates on the head and upper body. If scraped, eosinophils are typically present. The rash evolves into an eczematous dermatitis that is usually driven by *S aureus* colonization and chronic infection, and therefore

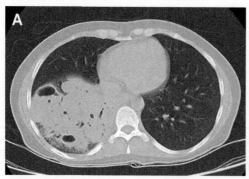 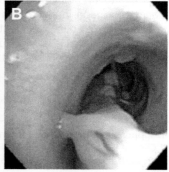

Fig. 1. Chest computed tomography (CT) demonstrating a lobar infiltrate caused by methicillin-resistant *Staphylococcus aureus* in a 37 year old with AD-HIES (*A*). Bronchoscopy of right bronchus intermedius showed tenacious mucus extending from the right lower lobe (*B*).

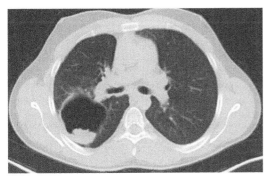

Fig. 2. Large pneumatocele with an aspergilloma seen on chest CT of a 23 year old with AD-HIES. The patient had recurrent episodes of hemoptysis that improved with systemic antifungal therapy.

frequently clears if antistaphylococcal antibiotics are given. Skin abscesses, or boils, frequently appear in the first few years of life, and, similar to the pyogenic pneumonias, often are associated with minimal systemic symptoms, such as fever and pain. If drained, however, the abscesses are purulent, and *S aureus* predominates. Sinus and ear infections are also common.

Mucocutaneous candidiasis is another common feature, often manifesting as thrush or nail infections. Endemic fungal infections occur, but may have atypical presentations.[20] For instance, histoplasmosis may manifest as a gastrointestinal (GI) tract infection, with minimal pulmonary findings, mimicking inflammatory bowel disease.[21–23] *Cryptococcus* has been reported to cause meningitis, but also isolated GI infection, and *Coccidiodes* has been associated with meningitis.[24–26] *Pneumocystis jirovecii* pneumonia is a rare cause of initial pneumonia in infants.[27] Although molds can cause significant pulmonary disease, these are usually airway-based and dissemination is rare.

What makes AD-HIES unique among many primary immunodeficiencies is the multisystem involvement with vascular, GI, and musculoskeletal manifestations. There is a typical facial appearance that usually manifests during adolescence and includes a prominent forehead, deep-set eyes, a broad nose, and porous skin.[12] The skull often has some degree of craniosynostosis. A high arched palate is usually present. Primary teeth are generally not shed and, if not surgically removed before emergence of secondary teeth, dental crowding may be noted.[28] Scoliosis is present in most patients and may be severe enough to require surgical correction. Skeletal fractures can occur following minimal trauma, with or without concurrent osteoporosis. The joints are typically very flexible, and in adulthood, significant arthritis and degenerative spinal disease frequently develop. Middle-sized arterial abnormalities have most frequently been recognized as coronary artery aneurysm and tortuousity, with an increasing prevalence with age.[29,30] Other vascular manifestations include cerebral aneurysm, which can present as subarachnoid hemorrhage[31]; and pulmonary hemorrhage, which may be caused in part by tortuous and dilated bronchial arteries adjacent to areas of chronic airway inflammation. GI manifestations include eosinophilic esophagitis and dysmotility, diverticulosis, and infrequently GI perforations without clearly associated pathology. The incidence of lymphoma is increased, and there have been several cases of extranodal B cell disease.[32]

Although higher than the general population, rates of allergy and anaphylaxis are considerably less common than in other conditions with similarly elevated IgE levels.[33] Asthma, although present in some, is generally not that severe or difficult to manage (**Box 1**).

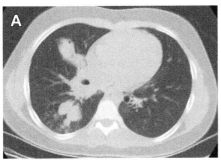
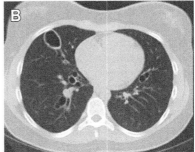

Fig. 3. Chest CT of a 15 year old with AD-HIES who presented with increased cough and wheezing (*A*). CT revealed proximal airway dilation with mucus plugging characteristic of allergic bronchopulmonary aspergillosis and sputum cultures grew *Aspergillus fumigatus*. Patient responded to systemic antifungals and corticosteroids, although had persistent airway dilation (*B*).

Laboratory Findings

As is evident from the name of the syndrome, the most consistent laboratory finding is a high serum IgE. The peak is typically greater than 2000 IU/mL, but in adulthood, the level can decrease and even normalize. The IgE level does not necessarily correlate with disease activity. Eosinophilia also is common. The complete blood count is frequently normal, but the white blood cell count may be low with a relative neutropenia. The white blood cell count often fails to increase as expected during bacterial infection. Serum immunoglobulins are usually normal, but specific antibody protection is variable. Lymphocyte phenotyping typically reveals low memory T and B lymphocytes, and interleukin (IL)-17 producing T cells (Th17 cells) are very diminished.[34–36]

Genetics and Pathogenesis

Dominant negative mutations in STAT3 were identified as the cause of AD-HIES in 2007.[4,5] Sporadic mutations are fairly common, which then are passed down in an autosomal-dominant pattern. The mutations are missense or small in-frame deletions that allow for normal protein expression but diminished function. STAT3 is a key signal transduction molecule for many cytokines including, among others, IL-6, IL-10, IL-21, and IL-17. On binding to their receptors, the JAK-STAT pathway is activated and STAT3 dimerizes and enters the nucleus to initiate transcription of many genes involved in immunity, wound healing, oncogenesis, embryogenesis, and cell survival. Absence of STAT3 is embryonically lethal in mice.

STAT3 signaling is required for the differentiation of naive T lymphocytes into Th17 lymphocytes. Shortly after STAT3 mutations were identified as causing AD-HIES, these patients were found to have a lack of differentiation of T cells into CD4+Th17 cells. Th17 lymphocytes secrete IL-17 and IL-22, cytokines that were shown initially in mice and later in humans to be associated with *Candida* mucosal susceptibility.[35,37] After this discovery in AD-HIES, several other primary immunodeficiencies with *Candida* susceptibility were noted to have disruption of this pathway. Increased IL-17 and IL-22 activity leads to upregulation of antimicrobial peptides at mucosal borders, which are involved in the killing of *Candida*. The saliva of STAT3-deficient patients has been shown to be deficient in some of these antimicrobial peptides including β-defensin 2 and histatins.[38] However, although the diminished antimicrobial peptides likely explain the *Candida* susceptibility in AD-HIES, the susceptibility to *S aureus* infections remains unclear. The *S aureus* infections are also at epithelial borders in AD-HIES, but the lack of recurrent *S aureus* infections in other diseases with disruption of this pathway remains puzzling.

Other aspects of the immunodeficiency of AD-HIES are explained by low numbers of memory T and B lymphocytes, with preservation of the naive lymphocyte subsets. Individuals with AD-HIES typically handle viral infections without complications; however, there is a higher incidence of viral reactivation manifesting as uncomplicated zoster or asymptomatic Epstein-Barr virus (EBV) infection.[36] This is thought to be caused by the poor maturation of T lymphocytes leading to decreased numbers of memory T lymphocytes. Memory B lymphocyte numbers also are low, and combined with impaired T follicular helper cell function and IL-21 signaling, likely explain the variable production of specific antibodies by patients with AD-HIES.[34,39]

Several clinical manifestations seem consistent with defective tissue remodeling. Most apparent is the frequent occurrence of pneumatoceles, and prolonged bronchopleural fistulae after lung surgery or spontaneous pneumothoraces.[40] Although normal STAT3 signaling in mouse models is not essential for lung development, it is required for normal repair of bronchiolar and alveolar epithelium after damage.[41] With epithelial injury, basal cells are thought to multiply to cover the denuded epithelium and produce IL-6 locally. The subsequent IL-6/STAT3 signaling promotes basal cell differentiation into ciliated cells and inhibits secretory cell differentiation by inhibiting Notch 1 expression and up-regulating cilia biogenesis genes, such as *Mcidas* and *Foxj1*.[41] These ciliated and secretory cells are key components of the mucociliary clearance apparatus. Following epithelial damage during infection-driven airway inflammation in AD-HIES, altered regulation of these normal repair mechanisms might partially explain the marked buildup of tenacious secretions, which can firmly adhere to the airway walls (see **Fig. 1**). Abnormal tissue remodeling likely also explains the middle-sized arterial aneurysms. STAT3 is involved in the regulation of matrix metalloproteinases, and plasma levels of matrix metalloproteinases have been found to be abnormal in STAT3-deficient patients compared with control subjects.[42]

Management

Prophylactic antimicrobials to prevent pyogenic pneumonias and early recognition and treatment of infection are essential to try and prevent development of pneumatoceles and bronchiectasis. Trimethoprim/sulfamethoxasole (given once or twice daily) is frequently used because of its long-term tolerability and activity against *S aureus*, including most community-acquired methicillin-resistant strains. Dilute bleach baths or other antiseptics can improve the skin disease remarkably. Prophylactic antifungals, such as fluconazole, are used if chronic or frequent recurrences of *Candida* infections occur. In areas with a high incidence of endemic mycoses, antifungal prophylaxis, such as fluconazole for *Coccidioides* or itraconazole for *Histoplasma*, should be considered. It is not clear if antimold prophylaxis, such as with itraconazole, prevents colonization and infection of molds inside pneumatoceles, but this can be considered. Immunoglobulin replacement is frequently given because of the variable specific antibody production, and in one series, reduced the rate of pneumonias by about two-thirds.[43]

Management of lung disease in the setting of chronic infection with bronchiectasis and pneumatoceles is more difficult, and proving efficacy of therapeutic interventions is limited by the rare nature of the disease. Airway clearance techniques, such as nebulized hypertonic saline and secretion clearance devices (eg, percussive vest, cough assist, or hand-held oscillatory PEP [positive expiratory pressure]), should generally be considered as in other patients with bronchiectasis. However, it should be noted that in some patients with AD-HIES, especially those with extensive bronchiectasis, chronically infected pneumatoceles, or mycetomas, hemoptysis is a significant cause of morbidity and mortality, likely from abnormal vasculature associated with the chronic infection.[14] In addition to optimizing antimicrobial treatment and withholding inhaled airway irritants during acute episodes of hemoptysis, bronchial arterial embolization or surgical resection may be required. Patients should be counseled about bleeding thresholds for seeking emergent

evaluation. Minimal trauma fractures are fairly frequent, and include rib fractures with coughing, thus limiting such techniques as percussive vests for some. In our experience, azithromycin seems to be helpful in decreasing the frequency of exacerbations for many with AD-HIES and bronchiectasis. This has the advantage of offering some antibacterial prophylaxis as well, and may be given daily for this purpose. Evaluating the QTc interval on electrocardiogram is prudent when combining an azole antifungal and azithromycin, especially because these patients also may receive intermittent fluoroquinolones. When chronic fungal infection of pneumatoceles or bronchiectatic airways is present, long-term administration of a mold-active antifungal, such as posaconazole, seems to minimize spread of infection and associated bleeding. If voriconazole is used, consideration of long-term toxicities, such as phototoxicity, skin cancers, and hyperfluorosis, is important.[44]

Antifungals are not always effective in treating aspergillomas that form inside pneumatoceles. Resection is the generally accepted therapy; however, it has unique challenges in patients with AD-HIES. In a published series of lung surgeries performed in STAT3-deficient patients in the United States and Germany, there was a complication rate of approximately 50%, with frequent prolonged bronchopleural fistulae, often persisting for months and causing complicated empyema and at times the need for further lung surgery.[40] Prolonged bronchopleural fistulae also can complicate pneumonias; in one case, prompt resolution occurred after bronchoscopic placement of one-way endobronchial valves.[45] Although bone and joint surgeries seem to heal well, complications have been reported after open GI surgeries, suggesting that surgery involving epithelial borders may have more healing complications.[46]

Several successful hematopoietic stem cell transplants (HSCT) in patients with AD-HIES have been published, prompting increased consideration of this option.[47,48] The immune defect corrects, but it is unclear how many of the somatic features will improve. There is a suggestion that the bone phenotype may improve. Lung transplantation has only been reported in one patient whose lungs were chronically infected with *Mycobacterium abscessus*, *A fumigatus*, and *Stenotrophomonas maltophilia* entering transplant (**Fig. 4**). Unfortunately, the surgery was complicated and posttransplantation, there were multiple *Asperillus* infections including supradiaphragmatic abscesses and endobronchial infection of the right-sided anastomosis that likely extended into the adjacent hilar and mediastinal space and

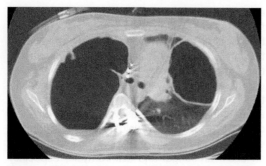

Fig. 4. A 27 year old with AD-HIES and large pneumatoceles chronically infected with *Mycobacterium abscessus*, *Aspergillus fumigatus*, and *Stenotrophomonas maltophilia*.

obstructed the right pulmonary artery.[49] The patient died approximately 3 years after lung transplantation with signs of transplant vasculopathy. Posttransplantation, she was maintained on prophylactic antibiotics and immunoglobulin replacement and did not experience the typical AD-HIES-associated recurrent bacterial pneumonias. She did have asymptomatic airway infection caused by WU polyomavirus.[50]

DOCK8 DEFICIENCY

In 2009, homozygous and compound heterozygous mutations in the DOCK8 gene were identified in patients previously described as having autosomal-recessive HIES.[6] Besides the recessive inheritance pattern, several clinical features set DOCK8 deficiency apart from those with AD-HIES, including a lack of the nonimmunologic features and a higher incidence of viral skin infections and malignancy.

Clinical Features

DOCK8 deficiency typically presents in infancy or early childhood with rash and recurrent sinopulmonary infections.[19,51–53] The eczema ranges from mild to much more severe than is seen in AD-HIES. Atopy is more common in DOCK8 deficiency and significant food allergies and asthma may be present. Viral skin infections are common including recurrent or chronic mucocutaneous herpes simplex virus, recurrent zoster, and severe and often disfiguring human papilloma virus and molluscum contagiosum infection. Although cutaneous viral infections predominate, there are rare severe systemic viral infections including JC virus–associated progressive multifocal leukoencephalopathy. The long-term prognosis with DOCK8 deficiency is worse than with AD-HIES with only about 50% of affected individuals living

beyond 20 years.[52] In part, this is caused by infection, but this also reflects the tendency to develop malignancy at young ages. Malignancy is frequently driven by chronic viral infections, including human papilloma virus–associated squamous cell carcinomas and EBV-associated lymphoma. Non-EBV lymphomas also occur.

Bronchiectasis is the most common lung finding caused by recurrent bacterial and viral pneumonias (**Fig. 5**). Pneumocystis pneumonia also occurs. Eosinophilic pneumonia has been described[54]; however, it is prudent to search thoroughly for an etiologic agent causing the eosinophilic infiltration, and to minimize corticosteroid use because corticosteroid therapy can worsen the cutaneous viral infections and potentially increase the malignancy risk. Asthma is common.

Vasculitis and vasculopathy of the cerebral arteries and aorta have been described, the latter rarely resulting in aortic aneurysm and calcification.[55] The cause of most of the vascular defects remains unknown, although one case of zoster vasculitis was described.[56] Hepatic disease is also seen in some patients, which particularly affects the biliary system.[57] In some but not all cases, this is caused by chronic cryptosporidia infection (**Box 2**).

Laboratory Findings

Serum IgE is usually elevated in DOCK8 deficiency and there typically is eosinophilia, which can be elevated in the range of hypereosinophilic syndromes. Serum IgG is usually normal, but specific antibody production is often poor; serum IgM is frequently low and serum IgA is variable.[6] There is usually some degree of lymphopenia, particularly of the T lymphocytes, but this is often progressive and so in young children may not be as

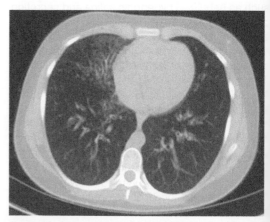

Fig. 5. A 15 year old with DOCK8 deficiency and bronchiectasis after recurrent pneumonias.

Box 2
Distinctive features of DOCK8 deficiency

- Viral cutaneous infections
- Malignancies including lymphoma and squamous cell carcinoma
- Vasculopathy of aorta with early calcification (infrequent)
- Decreased serum IgM
- Progressive lymphopenia over time

---

pronounced. If there has been past EBV infection, chronic EBV viremia is common.

Genetics and Pathogenesis

Homozygous or compound heterozygous mutations typically lead to lack of DOCK8 expression.[6] Diagnosis is by gene sequencing, with comparative genomic hybridization frequently being used to detect large deletions. Flow assays to detect DOCK8 protein are being developed to allow for easier screening because the DOCK8 gene is large and sequencing is not widely available.

DOCK8 is involved in actin cytoskeleton organization for cell migration and synapse formation.[58–61] Lymphocytes deficient in DOCK8 have trouble migrating through collagen gel matrices, which is thought to be one of the factors in the high incidence of severe cutaneous viral infections.[61] DOCK8 is also involved in the survival of T, B, and natural killer cells.

Management

HSCT is the accepted treatment of DOCK8 deficiency because of the high rates of morbidity and mortality at a young age.[62–66] DOCK8 is more of a pure immune deficiency than AD-HIES, and therefore HSCT is thought to be curative. Unfortunately, the diagnosis is often not made until

end-organ damage has occurred, such as bronchiectasis. It is important to optimize airway clearance and minimize chronic infection in preparation for HSCT. Frequently with engraftment there is worsening of mucus production and airway clearance measures may need to be intensified.

Prophylactic antimicrobials and immunoglobulin supplementation is the mainstay of therapies until HSCT is performed. Trimethoprim/sulfamethoxazole offers bacterial and *Pneumocystis* prophylaxis. If there is a history of herpes simplex virus or varicella zoster virus infection, acyclovir prophylaxis should be considered. Interferon-α therapy has been used at times to treat recalcitrant viral infections,[67,68] but there are significant side effects, such as depression and cytopenias, which need to be monitored.

PGM3 DEFICIENCY

Homozygous and compound heterozygous mutations in PGM3 were identified in 2014 as causing a HIES phenotype.[7–9] PGM3 is a proximal enzyme in the glycosylation pathway to decorate proteins with sugars.

Clinical Features

Because PGM3 deficiency is a congenital disorder of glycosylation, many proteins throughout the body with diverse functions are affected leading to multisystem abnormalities. Similar to STAT3 and DOCK8 deficiencies, PGM3 deficiency is associated with eczema, recurrent sinopulmonary infections, and high IgE. Asthma and food allergy may be present. In contrast to the other syndromes discussed here, neurologic abnormalities, such as cognitive and motor delays, are usually present. Autoimmunity also may be seen, such as vasculitis, psoriasis, and glomerulonephritis. Hodgkin lymphoma has been seen and musculoskeletal abnormalities, such as scoliosis and hypotonia, have been described.[7–9]

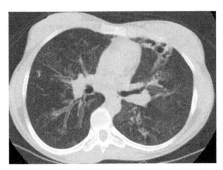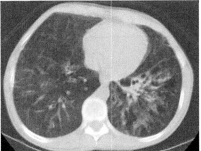

Fig. 6. A 25 year old with PGM3 deficiency with severe bronchiectasis before successful bilateral lung transplantation.

Lung disease can be severe with recurrent pneumonias leading to severe bronchiectasis. In one family, one member died in early adulthood because of progressive lung disease, and another had a successful bilateral lung transplant (**Fig. 6**).[7] Allergic bronchopulmonary aspergillosis also has been seen (**Box 3**, **Fig. 7**).

Laboratory Findings

In addition to high serum IgE and frequent eosinophilia, cytopenias are common in PGM3 deficiency. Neutropenia has been fairly common, although not usually associated with sepsis. Lymphopenia is frequent and is predominantly a result of a decrease in CD8 T lymphocytes. Early onset with a severe combined immunodeficiency–like phenotype also has been described.[9] In contrast to AD-HIES, Th17 lymphocytes are increased, which is consistent with the increased finding of autoimmunity. Serum IgA, IgM, and IgG are increased, but specific antibody production is variable.[7] Diagnosis of PGM3 deficiency is suggested by glycan profiling of urine and serum, with both O- and N-linked glycans being abnormal.

Genetics and Pathogenesis

Hypomorphic homozygous and compound heterozygous mutations have been reported to cause PGM3 deficiency.[7–9] Protein is made but is hypofunctional, because protein-negative mutations would be embryonic lethal. PGM3 is an early step in many glycosylation pathways, responsible for converting GlcNAc-6-phosphate to GlcNAc-1-phosophate, which then converts to UDP-GlcNAc. Glycosylation is required for adequate function of most proteins. The pathogenesis of the multiple features of this disease is still being investigated.

Management

The management of patients with PGM3 deficiency is still being defined. The described treatments have generally been supportive, including antibiotic prophylaxis, eczema management, and treatment of infections and autoinflammatory

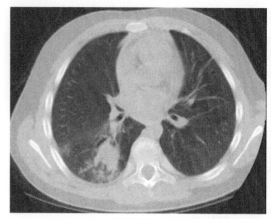

Fig. 7. Chest CT of a 13 year old with PGM3 deficiency showing proximal airway dilation with mucus plugging characteristic of allergic bronchopulmonary aspergillosis. Sputum cultures grew *Aspergillus flavus*.

conditions as they arise. However, several children have been described with severe combined immunodeficiency–like presentations and pancytopenia who received early and successful HSCT.[9] It remains unclear if HSCT will correct the neurologic and other somatic features. Other congenital disorders of glycosylation have been treated with dietary supplementation to bypass the pathway abnormalities.[69] Potential supplementation is being explored in PGM3 deficiency.

SUMMARY

Elevated serum IgE has many causes including parasitic infection, allergy and asthma, malignancy, and immune dysregulation. The HIES caused by mutations in STAT3, DOCK8, and PGM3 are monogenic primary immunodeficiencies that are associated with high IgE, eczema, and recurrent infections. All of these primary immunodeficiencies are associated with recurrent pneumonias leading to bronchiectasis; however, each has unique features and genetic diagnosis is essential in guiding therapy, discussing family planning, and defining prognosis. STAT3-mutated HIES is unique with respect to its multiorgan features and frequent pneumatocele formation. DOCK8 deficiency is characterized by severe cutaneous viral infections and early mortality. PGM3 deficiency is newly defined and is distinct in having neurologic abnormalities and cytopenias.

REFERENCES

1. Schulman ES. Development of a monoclonal anti-immunoglobulin E antibody (omalizumab) for the

---

> **Box 3**
> **Distinctive features of PGM3 deficiency**
>
> - Neurologic abnormalities including cognitive delay
> - Frequent neutropenia
> - Autoimmunity, such as vasculitis, glomerulonephritis
> - CD8 lymphopenia

treatment of allergic respiratory disorders. Am J Respir Crit Care Med 2001;164(8 Pt 2):S6–11.

2. Hogan C, Denning DW. Allergic bronchopulmonary aspergillosis and related allergic syndromes. Semin Respir Crit Care Med 2011;32(6):682–92.

3. Lally L, Spiera RF. Pulmonary vasculitis. Rheum Dis Clin North Am 2015;41(2):315–31.

4. Minegishi Y, Saito M, Tsuchiya S, et al. Dominant-negative mutations in the DNA-binding domain of STAT3 cause hyper-IgE syndrome. Nature 2007; 448(7157):1058–62.

5. Holland SM, DeLeo FR, Elloumi HZ, et al. STAT3 mutations in the hyper-IgE syndrome. N Engl J Med 2007;357(16):1608–19.

6. Zhang Q, Davis JC, Lamborn IT, et al. Combined immunodeficiency associated with DOCK8 mutations. N Engl J Med 2009;361(21):2046–55.

7. Zhang Y, Yu X, Ichikawa M, et al. Autosomal recessive phosphoglucomutase 3 (PGM3) mutations link glycosylation defects to atopy, immune deficiency, autoimmunity, and neurocognitive impairment. J Allergy Clin Immunol 2014;133(5):1400–9, 1409.e1–5.

8. Sassi A, Lazaroski S, Wu G, et al. Hypomorphic homozygous mutations in phosphoglucomutase 3 (PGM3) impair immunity and increase serum IgE levels. J Allergy Clin Immunol 2014;133(5):1410–9, 1419.e1–e13.

9. Stray-Pedersen A, Backe PH, Sorte HS, et al. PGM3 mutations cause a congenital disorder of glycosylation with severe immunodeficiency and skeletal dysplasia. Am J Hum Genet 2014;95(1):96–107.

10. Davis SD, Schaller J, Wedgwood RJ. Job's syndrome. Recurrent, "cold", staphylococcal abscesses. Lancet 1966;1(7445):1013–5.

11. Buckley RH, Wray BB, Belmaker EZ. Extreme hyperimmunoglobulinemia E and undue susceptibility to infection. Pediatrics 1972;49(1):59–70.

12. Grimbacher B, Holland SM, Gallin JI, et al. Hyper-IgE syndrome with recurrent infections: an autosomal dominant multisystem disorder. N Engl J Med 1999;340(9):692–702.

13. Melia E, Freeman AF, Shea YR, et al. Pulmonary nontuberculous mycobacterial infections in hyper-IgE syndrome. J Allergy Clin Immunol 2009;124(3): 617–8.

14. Freeman AF, Kleiner DE, Nadiminti H, et al. Causes of death in hyper-IgE syndrome. J Allergy Clin Immunol 2007;119(5):1234–40.

15. Sowerwine KJ, Holland SM, Freeman AF. Hyper-IgE syndrome update. Ann N Y Acad Sci 2012; 1250:25–32.

16. Vinh DC, Sugui JA, Hsu AP, et al. Invasive fungal disease in autosomal-dominant hyper-IgE syndrome. J Allergy Clin Immunol 2010;125(6):1389–90.

17. Chamlin SL, McCalmont TH, Cunningham BB, et al. Cutaneous manifestations of hyper-IgE syndrome in infants and children. J Pediatr 2002;141(4):572–5.

18. Eberting CL, Davis J, Puck JM, et al. Dermatitis and the newborn rash of hyper-IgE syndrome. Arch Dermatol 2004;140(9):1119–25.

19. Chu EY, Freeman AF, Jing H, et al. Cutaneous manifestations of DOCK8 deficiency syndrome. Arch Dermatol 2012;148(1):79–84.

20. Odio CD, Milligan KL, McGowan K, et al. Endemic mycoses in patients with STAT3-mutated hyper-IgE (Job) syndrome. J Allergy Clin Immunol 2015; 136(5):1411–3.e1–2.

21. Steiner SJ, Kleiman MB, Corkins MR, et al. Ileocecal histoplasmosis simulating Crohn disease in a patient with hyperimmunoglobulin E syndrome. Pediatr Infect Dis J 2009;28(8):744–6.

22. Cappell MS, Manzione NC. Recurrent colonic histoplasmosis after standard therapy with amphotericin B in a patient with Job's syndrome. Am J Gastroenterol 1991;86(1):119–20.

23. Alberti-Flor JJ, Granda A. Ileocecal histoplasmosis mimicking Crohn's disease in a patient with Job's syndrome. Digestion 1986;33(3):176–80.

24. Hutto JO, Bryan CS, Greene FL, et al. Cryptococcosis of the colon resembling Crohn's disease in a patient with the hyperimmunoglobulinemia E-recurrent infection (Job's) syndrome. Gastroenterology 1988;94(3):808–12.

25. Jacobs DH, Macher AM, Handler R, et al. Esophageal cryptococcosis in a patient with the hyperimmunoglobulin E-recurrent infection (Job's) syndrome. Gastroenterology 1984;87(1):201–3.

26. Powers AE, Bender JM, Kumánovics A, et al. Coccidioides immitis meningitis in a patient with hyperimmunoglobulin E syndrome due to a novel mutation in signal transducer and activator of transcription. Pediatr Infect Dis J 2009;28(7):664–6.

27. Freeman AF, Davis J, Anderson VL, et al. *Pneumocystis jiroveci* infection in patients with hyperimmunoglobulin E syndrome. Pediatrics 2006; 118(4):e1271–1275.

28. Freeman AF, Domingo DL, Holland SM. Hyper IgE (Job's) syndrome: a primary immune deficiency with oral manifestations. Oral Dis 2009;15(1):2–7.

29. Chandesris MO, Azarine A, Ong KT, et al. Frequent and widespread vascular abnormalities in human signal transducer and activator of transcription 3 deficiency. Circ Cardiovasc Genet 2012;5(1):25–34.

30. Freeman AF, Avila EM, Shaw PA, et al. Coronary artery abnormalities in hyper-IgE syndrome. J Clin Immunol 2011;31(3):338–45.

31. Fathi AR, Vortmeyer A, Holland SM, et al. Intracranial aneurysms associated with hyperimmunoglobulinaemia E (Job) syndrome: report of two cases. J Neurol Neurosurg Psychiatry 2011;82(6):704–6.

32. Leonard GD, Posadas E, Herrmann PC, et al. Non-Hodgkin's lymphoma in Job's syndrome: a case report and literature review. Leuk Lymphoma 2004; 45(12):2521–5.

33. Siegel AM, Stone KD, Cruse G, et al. Diminished allergic disease in patients with STAT3 mutations reveals a role for STAT3 signaling in mast cell degranulation. J Allergy Clin Immunol 2013;132(6):1388–96.

34. Speckmann C, Enders A, Woellner C, et al. Reduced memory B cells in patients with hyper IgE syndrome. Clin Immunol 2008;129(3):448–54.

35. Renner ED, Rylaarsdam S, Anover-Sombke S, et al. Novel signal transducer and activator of transcription 3 (STAT3) mutations, reduced T(H)17 cell numbers, and variably defective STAT3 phosphorylation in hyper-IgE syndrome. J Allergy Clin Immunol 2008;122(1):181–7.

36. Siegel AM, Heimall J, Freeman AF, et al. A critical role for STAT3 transcription factor signaling in the development and maintenance of human T cell memory. Immunity 2011;35(5):806–18.

37. Milner JD, Brenchley JM, Laurence A, et al. Impaired T(H)17 cell differentiation in subjects with autosomal dominant hyper-IgE syndrome. Nature 2008; 452(7188):773–6.

38. Conti HR, Baker O, Freeman AF, et al. New mechanism of oral immunity to mucosal candidiasis in hyper-IgE syndrome. Mucosal Immunol 2011;4(4): 448–55.

39. Ma CS, Avery DT, Chan A, et al. Functional STAT3 deficiency compromises the generation of human T follicular helper cells. Blood 2012;119(17): 3997–4008.

40. Freeman AF, Renner ED, Henderson C, et al. Lung parenchyma surgery in autosomal dominant hyper-IgE syndrome. J Clin Immunol 2013;33(5):896–902.

41. Tadokoro T, Wang Y, Barak LS, et al. IL-6/STAT3 promotes regeneration of airway ciliated cells from basal stem cells. Proc Natl Acad Sci U S A 2014; 111(35):E3641–9.

42. Sekhsaria V, Dodd LE, Hsu AP, et al. Plasma metalloproteinase levels are dysregulated in signal transducer and activator of transcription 3 mutated hyper-IgE syndrome. J Allergy Clin Immunol 2011; 128(5):1124–7.

43. Chandesris MO, Melki I, Natividad A, et al. Autosomal dominant STAT3 deficiency and hyper-IgE syndrome: molecular, cellular, and clinical features from a French national survey. Medicine 2012; 91(4):e1–19.

44. Goyal RK. Voriconazole-associated phototoxic dermatoses and skin cancer. Expert Rev Anti Infect Ther 2015;13(12):1537–46.

45. Olivier KN, Barnhart L, Brown DT, et al. Management of persistent bronchopleural fistula in Job's syndrome. Am J Respir Crit Care Med 2013;187:A5870.

46. Langan RC, Sherry RM, Avital I, et al. Safety of major abdominal surgical procedures in patients with hyperimmunoglobulinemia E (Job's syndrome): a changing paradigm? J Gastrointest Surg 2013; 17(5):1009–14.

47. Goussetis E, Constantoulakis P, Kitra V, et al. Successful bone marrow transplantation in a pediatric patient with chronic myeloid leukemia from a HLA-identical sibling selected by preimplantation HLA testing. Pediatr Blood Cancer 2011;57(2):345–7.

48. Patel NC, Gallagher JL, Torgerson TR, et al. Successful haploidentical donor hematopoietic stem cell transplant and restoration of STAT3 function in an adolescent with autosomal dominant hyper-IgE syndrome. J Clin Immunol 2015;35(5):479–85.

49. Kim T, Jancel T, Kumar P, et al. Drug-drug interaction between isavuconazole and tacrolimus: a case report indicating the need for tacrolimus drug-level monitoring. J Clin Pharm Ther 2015. [Epub ahead of print].

50. Siebrasse EA, Pastrana DV, Nguyen NL, et al. WU polyomavirus in respiratory epithelial cells from lung transplant patient with Job syndrome. Emerg Infect Dis 2015;21(1):103–6.

51. Zhang Q, Davis JC, Dove CG, et al. Genetic, clinical, and laboratory markers for DOCK8 immunodeficiency syndrome. Dis Markers 2010;29(3–4):131–9.

52. Aydin SE, Kilic SS, Aytekin C, et al. DOCK8 deficiency: clinical and immunological phenotype and treatment options: a review of 136 patients. J Clin Immunol 2015;35(2):189–98.

53. Engelhardt KR, Gertz ME, Keles S, et al. The extended clinical phenotype of 64 patients with dedicator of cytokinesis 8 deficiency. J Allergy Clin Immunol 2015;136(2):402–12.

54. Tsuge I, Ito K, Ohye T, et al. Acute eosinophilic pneumonia occurring in a dedicator of cytokinesis 8 (DOCK8) deficient patient. Pediatr Pulmonol 2014; 49(3):E52–5.

55. Al Mutairi M, Al-Mousa H, AlSaud B, et al. Grave aortic aneurysmal dilatation in DOCK8 deficiency. Mod Rheumatol 2014;24(4):690–3.

56. Sabry A, Hauk PJ, Jing H, et al. Vaccine strain varicella-zoster virus-induced central nervous system vasculopathy as the presenting feature of DOCK8 deficiency. J Allergy Clin Immunol 2014; 133(4):1225–7.

57. Alsum Z, Hawwari A, Alsmadi O, et al. Clinical, immunological and molecular characterization of DOCK8 and DOCK8-like deficient patients: single center experience of twenty-five patients. J Clin Immunol 2013;33(1):55–67.

58. McGhee SA, Chatila TA. DOCK8 immune deficiency as a model for primary cytoskeletal dysfunction. Dis Markers 2010;29(3–4):151–6.

59. Mizesko MC, Banerjee PP, Monaco-Shawver L, et al. Defective actin accumulation impairs human natural killer cell function in patients with dedicator of cytokinesis 8 deficiency. J Allergy Clin Immunol 2013; 131(3):840–8.

60. Randall KL, Lambe T, Johnson AL, et al. Dock8 mutations cripple B cell immunological synapses,

germinal centers and long-lived antibody production. Nat Immunol 2009;10(12):1283–91.

61. Zhang Q, Dove CG, Hor JL, et al. DOCK8 regulates lymphocyte shape integrity for skin antiviral immunity. J Exp Med 2014;211(13):2549–66.

62. Barlogis V, Galambrun C, Chambost H, et al. Successful allogeneic hematopoietic stem cell transplantation for DOCK8 deficiency. J Allergy Clin Immunol 2011;128(2):420 2.o2.

63. Bittner TC, Pannicke U, Renner ED, et al. Successful long-term correction of autosomal recessive hyper-IgE syndrome due to DOCK8 deficiency by hematopoietic stem cell transplantation. Klin Padiatr 2010; 222(6):351–5.

64. Boztug H, Karitnig-Weiß C, Ausserer B, et al. Clinical and immunological correction of DOCK8 deficiency by allogeneic hematopoietic stem cell transplantation following a reduced toxicity conditioning regimen. Pediatr Hematol Oncol 2012;29(7):585–94.

65. Cuellar-Rodriguez J, Freeman AF, Grossman J, et al. Matched related and unrelated donor hematopoietic stem cell transplantation for DOCK8 deficiency. Biol Blood Marrow Transplant 2015;21(6):1037–45.

66. Metin A, Tavil B, Azık F, et al. Successful bone marrow transplantation for DOCK8 deficient hyper IgE syndrome. Pediatr Transplant 2012;16(4):398–9.

67. Al-Zahrani D, Raddadi A, Massaad M, et al. Successful interferon-alpha 2b therapy for unremitting warts in a patient with DOCK8 deficiency. Clin Immunol 2014;153(1):104–8.

68. Keles S, Jabara HH, Reisli I, et al. Plasmacytoid dendritic cell depletion in DOCK8 deficiency: rescue of severe herpetic infections with IFN-alpha 2b therapy. J Allergy Clin Immunol 2014;133(6):1753–5.e3.

69. Tegtmeyer LC, Rust S, van Scherpenzeel M, et al. Multiple phenotypes in phosphoglucomutase 1 deficiency. N Engl J Med 2014;370(6):533–42.

Immunoglobulin G4-Related Disease and the Lung

Jay H. Ryu, MD[a],*, Eunhee S. Yi, MD[b]

KEYWORDS

- Immunoglobulin G4 • Fibroinflammatory • Pseudotumor • Interstitial lung disease • Pleuritis
- Lymphadenopathy

KEY POINTS

- Immunoglobulin (Ig)G4-related disease (RD) is an immune-mediated fibroinflammatory disorder that can affect virtually any organ or tissue in the body.
- Any compartment in the thorax can be involved in IgG4-RD, with or without associated extrathoracic manifestations.
- In patients presenting with fibroinflammatory disease of obscure cause, the possibility of IgG4-RD should be considered.
- Although the etiology of IgG4-RD remains unclear, early diagnosis and treatment can effectively manage most patients with this corticosteroid-responsive disorder.

INTRODUCTION

Immunoglobulin G4-related disease (IgG4-RD) is a recently recognized systemic fibroinflammatory disease with protean manifestations involving virtually any organ in the body. IgG4-RD has been previously referred to as "IgG4-related sclerosing disease" or "hyper-IgG4 disease."[1,2] At initial clinical presentation, 1 or multiple organs may be involved with the disease process. It has become apparent in recent years that many disorders previously considered idiopathic (eg, inflammatory pseudotumors, Mikulicz's syndrome, Küttner's tumor, Riedel's thyroiditis) belong, at least in part, under the spectrum of IgG4-RD.[3,4]

Initial descriptions of IgG4-RD focused on pancreatic disease. For example, Hamano and colleagues[5] described in 2001 the association of high serum IgG4 levels with a form of sclerosing pancreatitis characterized by lymphoplasmacytic infiltrates containing IgG4+ plasma cells (currently named type 1 autoimmune pancreatitis). It has since become clear that IgG4-RD can cause an immune-mediated fibroinflammatory process, commonly manifesting as mass-like lesions, in various regions of the body including intrathoracic structures.[2,4,6,7] This pathologic process is characterized by infiltration of IgG4+ plasma cells and a propensity to fibrosis leading to organ dysfunction.

EPIDEMIOLOGY

Although the majority of earlier reports described IgG4-RD in the Japanese population, it is clear that those in the Western hemisphere are affected as well.[3,4,8–10] It is a rare disease with an annual incidence in Japan estimated to be approximately 1 per 100,000.[11] An increasing number of cases are being recognized in recent years with true

Funding: None.
Disclosure: None for all authors.
[a] Division of Pulmonary and Critical Care Medicine, Mayo Clinic, Gonda 18 South, 200 First Street Southwest, Rochester, MN 55905, USA; [b] Division of Anatomic Pathology, Mayo Clinic, Hilton Building 11, 200 First Street Southwest, Rochester, MN 55905, USA
* Corresponding author.
E-mail address: ryu.jay@mayo.edu

Clin Chest Med 37 (2016) 569–578
http://dx.doi.org/10.1016/j.ccm.2016.04.017
0272-5231/16/$ – see front matter © 2016 Elsevier Inc. All rights reserved.

incidence and prevalence figures remaining to be defined. It affects mainly adults who are more commonly men (60%–80%) than women.[4,7] The median age at diagnosis is 60 to 65 years.[7,12]

PATHOGENESIS
Immunologic Mechanisms

The etiology of IgG4-RD remains obscure. Immunologic mechanisms are likely involved in the pathogenesis of this disorder, but the target antigens and the exact role of IgG4 (the smallest subclass of IgG) remain to be defined. The immunologic profile of IgG4-RD manifests characteristics of a predominantly type 2 helper cell immune response and infiltration by regulatory T cells, which produce interleukin-10.[13–15] This cytokine imbalance is thought to potentiate IgG4 production and promote IgG4-RD. There is also evidence of expanded plasmablast (stage of B lymphocyte development between activated B cell and plasma cell) population that is oligoclonal in nature.[16]

Immunoglobulin G4

High serum levels of IgG4 are found commonly in patients with IgG4-RD. However, IgG4 is generally thought to function as an antiinflammatory antibody. Thus, the elevated serum IgG4 level may reflect a response to the inflammatory process rather than a pathogenic role. Similarly, various forms of circulating autoantibodies that are found in some patients with IgG4-RD are considered nonspecific, with no direct role in the pathogenesis of IgG4-RD.[13,15]

Genetic Predisposition

In genetic association studies, some susceptibility genes for IgG4-RD have been identified. For example, studies in Japanese and Korean patients with type 1 autoimmune pancreatitis have implicated several HLA haplotypes and non-HLA genes, for example, CTLA4.[13,17] These findings implicate genes related to immune response in susceptibility to IgG4-RD.

Microorganisms

Microorganisms, such as Helicobacter pylori, have been investigated as potential triggers for immune processes in IgG4-RD.[4,13] However, the potential role of microorganisms in inciting IgG4-RD remains speculative.

PATHOLOGY

IgG4-RD is associated with tumefactive (swelling) lesions in various organs, such as renal mass in IgG4-related kidney disease. Similarly, there are histopathologic features that are characteristic of IgG4-RD. These are dense lymphoplasmacytic infiltrate, fibrosis (often in storiform pattern), and obliterative phlebitis (**Fig. 1**). Immunohistochemical staining identifies elevated numbers of IgG4+ plasma cells within the fibroinflammatory infiltrate (**Fig. 2**). Increased numbers of eosinophils and obliterative arteritis may also be seen (see **Fig. 1**D). However, as discussed elsewhere in this paper, none of these findings is specific for IgG4-RD diagnosis.

Although there are general similarities in histopathologic findings, site-specific features have also been noted for some organs including the lung, which often does not show distinct storiform fibrosis when involved with IgG4-RD.[18,19] Similarly, the density of IgG4+ plasma cells in involved organs varies and influences the quantitative cutoff values used for number of IgG4+ plasma cell per high-power field and IgG4+/IgG+ cell ratio in the histopathologic diagnosis of IgG4-RD.[20,21]

Clinical Manifestations

Although the initial description of IgG4-RD focused on its presentation as a pancreatic disease, it is now apparent that affected patients can present with a wide array of extrapancreatic manifestations. Aside from the pancreas, other sites commonly involved include the hepatobiliary tract, salivary and lacrimal glands, lymph nodes, orbital tissues, retroperitoneum, kidney, and lung.[1,7,11,12]

Clinical manifestations attributable to this disorder continue to expand. Patients with IgG4-RD commonly present with multiorgan manifestations, although single-organ involvement is noted in approximately 40% of patients.[3,4,7,8,12,21,22] During the clinical course of active IgG4-RD, various organs may become involved metachronously.

Symptoms

Symptoms associated with IgG4-related lung disease are nonspecific and include cough (most common), chest pain, and dyspnea. Systemic symptoms such as low-grade fever and weight loss may be present, but are uncommon. In patients presenting with symptomatic extrapulmonary IgG4-RD, asymptomatic lung involvement may be detected on imaging studies. Overall, approximately one-half of patients with IgG4-related lung disease will manifest respiratory symptoms.[2,22–25]

Immunoglobulin G4-Related Lung Disease

Pulmonary involvement (excluding intrathoracic lymphadenopathy) in IgG4-RD is reported to

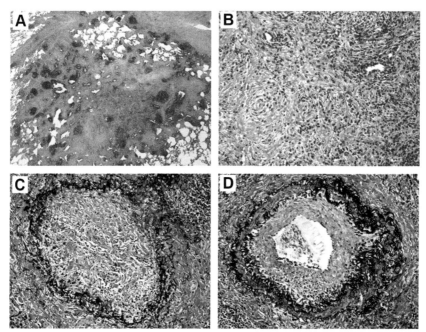

Fig. 1. Histopathology of immunoglobulin (Ig)G4-related lung disease. (*A*) Low-power view of IgG4-related lung disease characterized by mass-like fibroinflammatory lesion with heavy lymphoplasmacytic infiltrates and thickening in the interlobular septa shown in the upper left and right corners. (*B*) Cellular fibrosis with vague storiform pattern accompanied by numerous plasma cells (hematoxylin and eosin staining; original magnification ×20 and ×200 for *A* and *B*, respectively). (*C*) Obliterative pulmonary phlebitis and (*D*) pulmonary arteritis with marked luminal narrowing owing to intimal fibroinflammatory changes (Verhoeff van Gieson staining; original magnification ×200 for *C* and *D*).

occur in 5% to 18% of affected patients.[7–9,26] For example, Wallace and colleagues[8] recently reported 125 patients with IgG4-RD, among whom 17.6% had evidence of lung involvement and 8% had lung "damage." Pulmonary

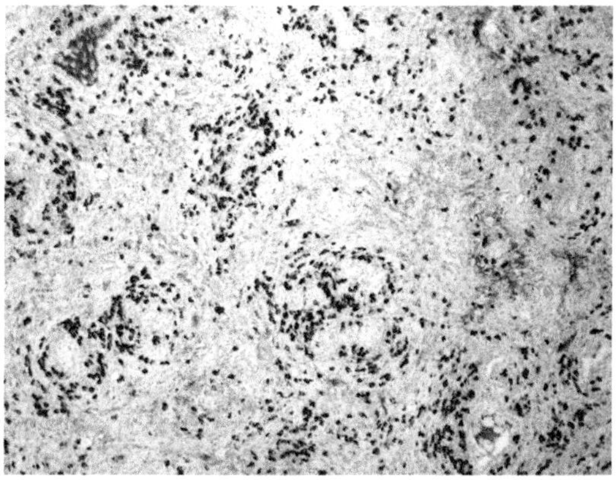

Fig. 2. Immunoglobulin (Ig)G4 immunostain of IgG4-related lung disease. Diffusely increased IgG4-positive plasma cells greater than 100 per high-power field (IgG4 immunostaining; original magnification ×100) with a high IgG4⁺/IgG⁺ cell ratio greater than 50% on IgG immunostaining (not shown).

manifestations in IgG4-RD are diverse but can be categorized according to anatomic compartments (**Box 1**).[2,7,19,24,27,28]

Parenchymal Lung Manifestations

Pulmonary parenchymal involvement is most commonly manifest radiographically as a focal opacity (**Fig. 3**) and often appears mass-like mimicking a neoplasm.[23,24,27] Lesions of IgG4-RD commonly demonstrate uptake on ^{18}F-fluorodeoxyglucose PET, which may further heighten concern for a malignancy.[29] It now seems that IgG4-RD accounts for some cases previously diagnosed as inflammatory pseudotumor (plasma cell granuloma) in the lung.[30]

Interstitial lung disease, often diffuse, is another parenchymal manifestation of IgG4-RD.[18,19,23–25,27,31–34] Histopathologically, parenchymal lung disease in IgG4-RD may resemble nonspecific interstitial pneumonia, organizing pneumonia, or lymphoid interstitial pneumonia.[18,19,35,36] Rarely, usual interstitial pneumonia may be encountered.[27] Given that these patterns are not specific, it is only when an excess numbers of plasma cells are noted, and IgG4 staining is performed, that the diagnosis of

<table>
<tr><td>

Box 1
Pulmonary manifestations of immunoglobulin G4-related disease

Parenchyma
- Focal opacities (nodules, masses)
- Interstitial lung disease

Airway
- Stenosis/endobronchial mass
- Bronchospastic disease

Vasculature
- Vasculitis
- Pulmonary hypertension

Mediastinum
- Lymphadenopathy
- Fibrosing mediastinitis

Pleural
- Thickening or mass
- Effusion

</td></tr>
</table>

IgG4-RD is established. On computed tomography imaging, widely varying radiologic patterns of interstitial lung infiltrates may be seen, including reticular opacities, patchy ground-glass opacities, alveolar consolidation, and thickening of the bronchovascular bundles and interlobular septa.[2,23,24,32,35,37–39] Interstitial lung disease occurring with IgG4-RD is associated with a restrictive pattern accompanied by a

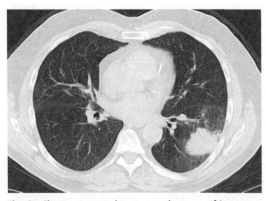

Fig. 3. Chest computed tomography scan of immunoglobulin (Ig)G4-related lung disease. Mass-like consolidative opacity is present in the left lower lobe posterolaterally in this 68-year-old man with type 1 autoimmune pancreatitis. The lung lesion was resected for suspected malignancy and revealed IgG4-related lung disease.

reduced diffusing capacity on pulmonary function testing.[2]

Airway Manifestations

Airway disease in IgG4-RD has included an asthma-like syndrome, airway stenosis, and endobronchial tumor.[40–43] For example, Ito and colleagues[44] described a middle-aged woman with autoimmune pancreatitis who presented with cough and exhibited tracheobronchial stenosis associated with mediastinal and hilar lymphadenopathy. Bronchial biopsy demonstrated diffuse inflammatory infiltrates consisting mainly of IgG4+ plasma cells, lymphocytes, and scattered eosinophils with fibrosis. Prednisone treatment led to a dramatic improvement of the airway disease and associated airflow obstruction.

Pulmonary Vascular Manifestations

Several cases of pulmonary vascular involvement with dense lymphoplasmacytic infiltrates around muscular pulmonary arteries resulting in pulmonary hypertension have been reported.[45,46] As noted, obliterative phlebitis and/or obliterative arteritis are relatively common histopathologic findings seen on surgical lung biopsy specimens.[18,19,27]

Mediastinal Manifestations

In the mediastinum, IgG4-RD can manifest as lymphadenopathy or fibrosing mediastinitis **(Fig. 4)**.[23,27,47–50] Intrathoracic lymphadenopathy is observed commonly on computed tomography scanning in patients with intrathoracic or extrathoracic IgG4-RD.[7,37,51] Occasionally, lymphadenopathy may be the primary presenting manifestation.[52]

Pleural Manifestations

IgG4-related pleural disease can occur alone or with accompanying parenchymal lung lesions or extrapulmonary manifestations of IgG4-RD. Pleural features have included pleural mass, pleuritis with fibrosis (nodular or diffuse pleural thickening), and pleural effusion.[23,27,53–55] Occasionally, pleural effusion may be bilateral and massive.[56] Pleural fluid is exudative with cellular constituents composed mainly of lymphocytes and plasma cells.[57,58] Pleural biopsy reveals fibrinous pleuritis with lymphoplasmacytic inflammation including many IgG4+ plasma cells and fibrosis.

DIAGNOSTIC EVALUATION

In general, the diagnosis of IgG4-RD requires judicious correlation of clinicoradiologic findings with

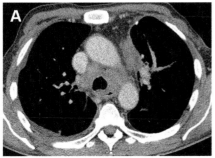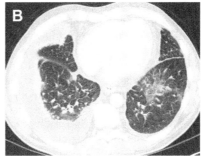

Fig. 4. Chest computed tomography scan of immunoglobulin G4-related lung disease in a 59-year-old man demonstrates (*A*) mediastinal adenopathy and confluent soft tissue thickening surrounding the trachea, extending into the hilar regions. (*B*) Interlobular septal thickening, patchy ground-glass opacities, and bilateral pleural effusions (greater on the right) are seen.

histopathologic features, which should include dense lymphoplasmacytic infiltrates, a storiform pattern of fibrosis, and obliterative phlebitis combined with an increased number of IgG4+ plasma cells (**Box 2**).[2,3,6,20,21] None of the histopathologic features or laboratory findings, including a high serum IgG4 level, is specific for the diagnosis of IgG4-RD. Similarly, increased numbers of IgG4+ plasma cells can be seen in other disorders including granulomatosis with polyangiitis (Wegener's) and rheumatoid synovitis (**Box 3**).[18,59,60] In addition, storiform pattern of fibrosis may not be a prominent feature in the IgG4-related lung disease.

Immunoglobulin G4 Immunostain

Suggested cutoff values for quantitating IgG4+ plasma cells in the diagnosis of IgG4-RD vary depending on the organ, according to the current consensus statement on pathologic analysis.[20] For the lung, greater than 20 or greater than 50 IgG4+ plasma cells per high-power field in nonsurgical biopsy and surgical biopsy specimens,

---

Box 2
Diagnostic criteria for IgG4-related disease

Clinicoradiologic features compatible with IgG4-related disease

Characteristic histopathologic features

- Dense lymphoplasmacytic infiltrates
- Storiform pattern of fibrosis
- Obliterative phlebitis
- Increased number of IgG4+ plasma cells (>10/hpf and IgG4+/IgG+ cell ratio >40%)[a]

Other supportive findings

- Serum IgG4 level greater than 135 mg/dL

Exclude other identifiable diseases with overlapping clinicoradiologic and/or histopathologic features.

Abbreviations: hpf, high-power field; Ig, immunoglobulin.
[a] See text for additional details in the text regarding diagnostic cutoff values for IgG4+ plasma cells on lung and pleural biopsy specimens.

Box 3
Differential diagnosis for IgG4-related lung disease

Diseases with similar pulmonary presentations

- Neoplastic disorders, including lymphoma (nodular opacities)
- Infections, including lung abscess (nodular opacities ± cavitation)
- Interstitial pneumonias (interstitial infiltrates)
- Asthma (airway disease)

Diseases with multisystem involvement

- Connective tissue diseases with lung involvement
- Vasculitis, especially granulomatosis with polyangiitis (Wegener)
- Sarcoidosis

Diseases with pulmonary inflammation and increased IgG4+ plasma cells

- Granulomatosis with polyangiitis (Wegener)
- Eosinophilic granulomatous with polyangiitis (Churg-Strauss)
- Multicentric Castleman's disease
- Rosai-Dorfman disease

Abbreviation: Ig, immunoglobulin.

respectively, with an $IgG4^+/IgG^+$ plasma cell ratio of greater than 40% for both types of specimens have been proposed. The respective cutoff values for the pleura are greater than 50 $IgG4^+$ plasma cells per high-power field and greater than 40% $IgG4^+/IgG^+$ plasma cell ratio.[20]

To identify the characteristic histopathologic features of IgG4-RD within the thorax, a surgical biopsy specimen is generally needed. However, bronchoscopic or transthoracic needle biopsy may sometimes yield features suggestive of IgG4-RD while allowing exclusion of competing diagnoses.[2,20,21]

Although histopathologic data are important in confirming the diagnosis of IgG4-related lung disease, lung or pleural biopsy may not be necessary in achieving this diagnosis if an extrapulmonary organ has already been biopsied to confirm the presence of IgG4-RD. In the absence of another more likely explanation for the intrathoracic lesion, the diagnosis of IgG4-RD can be assumed in most such cases. A subsequent clinical course that is atypical, such as progressive lung disease despite treatment, may warrant additional diagnostic evaluation including lung biopsy.

Serum Immunoglobulin G4 Level

Earlier studies describing patients with IgG4-RD emphasized the association with elevated serum IgG4 levels. Although serum IgG4 level is often elevated (>135 mg/dL) in patients with IgG4-RD, this laboratory finding is not an adequately sensitive or specific for diagnostic purposes.[3,21,61–63] Serum IgG4 level has been reported to be elevated in 50% to 95% of patients with active IgG4-RD.[8,61,63,64] Conversely, only 10% to 20% of patients with an elevated serum IgG4 level in clinical practice have IgG4-RD.[62,65,66] Thus, an elevated serum IgG4 level is supportive of the diagnosis of IgG4-RD but not necessary nor sufficient.

Other Laboratory Tests

Other laboratory abnormalities that may be observed in patients with IgG4-RD include mild-to-moderate peripheral eosinophilia, elevated C-reactive protein level and erythrocyte sedimentation rate, polyclonal hypergammaglobulinemia, antinuclear autoantibodies, rheumatoid factor, and hypocomplementemia.[3,8,20,21,32] Recent studies have suggested that circulating plasmablast levels are elevated in patients with IgG4-RD and may correlate with disease activity.[16,67] Circulating plasmablast level may become an important biomarker in IgG4-RD.

BRONCHOALVEOLAR LAVAGE

Bronchoalveolar lavage (BAL) in patients with IgG4-related lung disease exhibits lymphocytosis with a relatively normal $CD4^+/CD8^+$ lymphocyte ratio.[2,27,37,44] IgG4 level in the BAL has been found to be elevated in patients with IgG4-related lung disease and seems to correlate with the serum IgG4 level.[37] However, BAL data regarding IgG4-related lung disease are sparse and the role of BAL in the evaluation and management of these patients remains to be clarified.

TREATMENT

The goal for the treatment of IgG4-RD, in general, is the prevention of irreversible fibrosis and organ damage.[3,4,68] Corticosteroids are generally considered the first-line therapy for IgG4-RD. Intrathoracic manifestations of IgG4-RD respond well to corticosteroid therapy, similar to extrathoracic lesions.[2–4,19,23,24,27,31,35,52,68–70] However, it should be noted that there have been no randomized clinical trials conducted to investigate the efficacy of treatment for IgG4-RD.

Corticosteroids

The optimal dose of corticosteroid therapy in the treatment of IgG4-RD has not been determined, but most authors recommend oral prednisone or the equivalent at an initial dosage of 30 to 40 mg/d.[3,68,71] This initial dose is maintained for 2 to 4 weeks with favorable response typically seen by 2 weeks on treatment. Subsequently, the corticosteroid dose is gradually tapered over the following weeks to months while monitoring for possible recurrence or reactivation of disease.

It is recommended that all patients with symptomatic, active IgG4-RD be treated.[3,4,68] However, some patients with asymptomatic disease may not require pharmacologic therapy. For example, a patient who has a solitary lung mass resected that proves to be IgG4-related lung disease may be monitored without additional treatment. Similarly, asymptomatic intrathoracic lymphadenopathy by itself would not be an indication for treatment.

The duration of corticosteroid therapy is typically 3 to 6 months. Although most patients respond well to initial therapy, the durability of response is variable and relapses have been observed commonly. A recent study of 125 patients with IgG4-RD noted a relapse rate of 77% after remission induction with corticosteroid therapy.[8] Thus, some authors have advocated the use of a low-dose maintenance therapy, for example, prednisone 5 mg/d, for a longer period to reduce the risk of such relapse.[68,72–75]

Steroid-Sparing Immunosuppressive Agents

Various steroid-sparing immunosuppressive agents have been used in the treatment of IgG4-RD, but the evidence supporting their use is limited.[3,4,8,26,68] These agents have included azathioprine, mycophenolate mofetil, methotrexate, cyclophosphamide, 6-mercaptopurine, and tacrolimus.[2,3,8,9,26,68,76,77] The use of such agents should be considered in the initial treatment of IgG4-RD in patients at increased risk of serious adverse effects from corticosteroid administration. In addition, steroid-sparing immunosuppressive agents are used when adverse effects from corticosteroid therapy have occurred or the dose of corticosteroids cannot be reduced owing to persistent disease activity.

B-Cell Depletion Therapy

A relatively new concept in the treatment of IgG4-RD is B-cell depletion therapy. Several reports in recent years have described successful use of rituximab therapy, even in patients who failed to achieve a durable remission with steroid-sparing immunosuppressive agents.[37,78–85] Recently, Carruthers and colleagues[82] reported the treatment of 30 IgG4-RD patients with 2 doses of rituximab (1000-mg doses administered approximately 15 days apart) in an open-label pilot trial resulting in favorable disease responses in 97% of the participants. The majority of these patients had been treated previously with corticosteroids and steroid-sparing immunosuppressive agents that did not prevent relapse. At 12 months after rituximab therapy, 40% of the participants remained in complete remission.

PROGNOSIS

Prompt recognition and effective treatment prevents irreversible organ damage from the fibrotic changes that can result from persistently active IgG4-RD.[23,71,75,86] Although relapses are common, corticosteroid therapy is usually effective in reinducing remission. Deaths directly attributable to IgG4-RD are rare and have resulted from cardiac or aortic involvement.[8,9,26,87,88]

SUMMARY

IgG4-RD is an immune-mediated fibroinflammatory disorder that can affect virtually any organ or tissue in the human body. Any compartment in the thorax can be involved in IgG4-RD with or without associated extrathoracic manifestations.

In patients presenting with fibroinflammatory disease of obscure cause, the possibility of IgG4-RD should be considered. Although the etiology of IgG4-RD remains unclear, early diagnosis and treatment can manage most patients effectively with this corticosteroid-responsive disorder.

REFERENCES

1. Stone JH, Khosroshahi A, Deshpande V, et al. Recommendations for the nomenclature of IgG4-related disease and its individual organ system manifestations. Arthritis Rheum 2012;64(10):3061–7.
2. Ryu JH, Sekiguchi H, Yi ES. Pulmonary manifestations of immunoglobulin G4-related sclerosing disease. Eur Respir J 2012;39(1):180–6.
3. Kamisawa T, Zen Y, Pillai S, et al. IgG4-related disease. Lancet 2015;385(9976):1460–71.
4. Stone JH, Zen Y, Deshpande V. IgG4-related disease. N Engl J Med 2012;366(6):539–51.
5. Hamano H, Kawa S, Horiuchi A, et al. High serum IgG4 concentrations in patients with sclerosing pancreatitis [comment]. N Engl J Med 2001; 344(10):732–8.
6. Umehara H, Okazaki K, Masaki Y, et al. Comprehensive diagnostic criteria for IgG4-related disease (IgG4-RD), 2011. Mod Rheumatol 2012;22(1):21–30.
7. Zen Y, Nakanuma Y. IgG4-related disease: a cross-sectional study of 114 cases. Am J Surg Pathol 2010;34(12):1812–9.
8. Wallace ZS, Deshpande V, Mattoo H, et al. IgG4-related disease: clinical and laboratory features in one hundred twenty-five patients. Arthritis Rheumatol 2015;67(9):2466–75.
9. Fernandez-Codina A, Martinez-Valle F, Pinilla B, et al. IgG4-related disease: results from a multicenter Spanish registry. Medicine 2015;94(32): e1275.
10. Ebbo M, Daniel L, Pavic M, et al. IgG4-related systemic disease: features and treatment response in a French cohort: results of a multicenter registry. Medicine 2012;91(1):49–56.
11. Umehara H, Okazaki K, Masaki Y, et al. A novel clinical entity, IgG4-related disease (IgG4RD): general concept and details. Mod Rheumatol 2012;22(1):1–14.
12. Khosroshahi A, Stone JH. A clinical overview of IgG4-related systemic disease. Curr Opin Rheumatol 2011;23(1):57–66.
13. Yamamoto M, Takahashi H, Shinomura Y. Mechanisms and assessment of IgG4-related disease: lessons for the rheumatologist. Nat Rev Rheumatol 2014;10(3):148–59.
14. Mahajan VS, Mattoo H, Deshpande V, et al. IgG4-Related disease. Annu Rev Pathol 2014;9:315–47.
15. Takahashi H, Yamamoto M, Tabeya T, et al. The immunobiology and clinical characteristics of IgG4 related diseases. J Autoimmun 2012;39(1–2):93–6.

16. Wallace ZS, Mattoo H, Carruthers M, et al. Plasmablasts as a biomarker for IgG4-related disease, independent of serum IgG4 concentrations. Ann Rheum Dis 2015;74(1):190–5.

17. Zen Y, Nakanuma Y. Pathogenesis of IgG4-related disease. Curr Opin Rheumatol 2011;23(1):114–8.

18. Yi ES, Sekiguchi H, Peikert T, et al. Pathologic manifestations of Immunoglobulin(Ig)G4-related lung disease. Semin Diagn Pathol 2012;29(4):219–25.

19. Shrestha B, Sekiguchi H, Colby TV, et al. Distinctive pulmonary histopathology with increased IgG4-positive plasma cells in patients with autoimmune pancreatitis: report of 6 and 12 cases with similar histopathology. Am J Surg Pathol 2009;33(10):1450–62.

20. Deshpande V, Zen Y, Chan JK, et al. Consensus statement on the pathology of IgG4-related disease. Mod Pathol 2012;25(9):1181–92.

21. Stone JH, Brito-Zeron P, Bosch X, et al. Diagnostic approach to the complexity of IgG4-related disease. Mayo Clin Proc 2015;90(7):927–39.

22. Brito-Zeron P, Ramos-Casals M, Bosch X, et al. The clinical spectrum of IgG4-related disease. Autoimmun Rev 2014;13(12):1203–10.

23. Zen Y, Inoue D, Kitao A, et al. IgG4-related lung and pleural disease: a clinicopathologic study of 21 cases. Am J Surg Pathol 2009;33(12):1886–93.

24. Inoue D, Zen Y, Abo H, et al. Immunoglobulin G4-related lung disease: CT findings with pathologic correlations. Radiology 2009;251(1):260–70.

25. Shigemitsu H, Koss MN. IgG4-related interstitial lung disease: a new and evolving concept. Curr Opin Pulm Med 2009;15(5):513–6.

26. Inoue D, Yoshida K, Yoneda N, et al. IgG4-related disease: dataset of 235 consecutive patients. Medicine 2015;94(15):e680.

27. Matsui S, Hebisawa A, Sakai F, et al. Immunoglobulin G4-related lung disease: clinicoradiological and pathological features. Respirology 2013;18(3):480–7.

28. Raj R. IgG4-related lung disease. Am J Respir Crit Care Med 2013;188(5):527–9.

29. Zhang J, Chen H, Ma Y, et al. Characterizing IgG4-related disease with (18)F-FDG PET/CT: a prospective cohort study. Eur J Nucl Med Mol Imaging 2014;41(8):1624–34.

30. Zen Y, Kitagawa S, Minato H, et al. IgG4-positive plasma cells in inflammatory pseudotumor (plasma cell granuloma) of the lung. Hum Pathol 2005;36(7):710–7.

31. Taniguchi T, Ko M, Seko S, et al. Interstitial pneumonia associated with autoimmune pancreatitis [comment]. Gut 2004;53(5):770 [author reply: 770–1].

32. Yamashita K, Haga H, Kobashi Y, et al. Lung involvement in IgG4-related lymphoplasmacytic vasculitis and interstitial fibrosis: report of 3 cases and review

of the literature. Am J Surg Pathol 2008;32(11):1620–6.

33. Tanaka K, Nagata K, Tomii K, et al. A case of isolated IgG4-related interstitial pneumonia: a new consideration for the cause of idiopathic nonspecific interstitial pneumonia. Chest 2012;142(1):228–30.

34. Umeda M, Fujikawa K, Origuchi T, et al. A case of IgG4-related pulmonary disease with rapid improvement. Mod Rheumatol 2012;22(6):919–23.

35. Duvic C, Desrame J, Lévêque C, et al. Retroperitoneal fibrosis, sclerosing pancreatitis and bronchiolitis obliterans with organizing pneumonia. Nephrol Dial Transplant 2004;19(9):2397–9.

36. Tian X, Yi ES, Ryu JH. Lymphocytic interstitial pneumonia and other benign lymphoid disorders. Semin Respir Crit Care Med 2012;33(5):450–61.

37. Tsushima K, Tanabe T, Yamamoto H, et al. Pulmonary involvement of autoimmune pancreatitis. Eur J Clin Invest 2009;39(8):714–22.

38. Fujinaga Y, Kadoya M, Kawa S, et al. Characteristic findings in images of extra-pancreatic lesions associated with autoimmune pancreatitis. Eur J Radiol 2010;76(2):228–38.

39. Matsui S, Taki H, Shinoda K, et al. Respiratory involvement in IgG4-related Mikulicz's disease. Mod Rheumatol 2012;22(1):31–9.

40. Ito S, Ko SBH, Morioka M, et al. Three cases of bronchial asthma preceding IgG4-related autoimmune pancreatitis. Allergol Int 2012;61(1):171–4.

41. Virk JS, Stamatoglou C, Kwame I, et al. IgG4-sclerosing pseudotumor of the trachea: a case report and review of the literature. Arch Otolaryngol Head Neck Surg 2012;138(9):864–6.

42. Sekiguchi H, Horie R, Aksamit TR, et al. Immunoglobulin G4-related disease mimicking asthma. Can Respir J 2013;20(2):87–9.

43. Kobraei EM, Song TH, Mathisen DJ, et al. Immunoglobulin g4-related disease presenting as an obstructing tracheal mass: consideration of surgical indications. Ann Thorac Surg 2013;96(4):e91–3.

44. Ito M, Yasuo M, Yamamoto H, et al. Central airway stenosis in a patient with autoimmune pancreatitis. Eur Respir J 2009;33(3):680–3.

45. Shirai Y, Tamura Y, Yasuoka H, et al. IgG4-related disease in pulmonary arterial hypertension on long-term epoprostenol treatment. Eur Respir J 2014;43(5):1516–9.

46. Ishida M, Miyamura T, Sato S, et al. Pulmonary arterial hypertension associated with IgG4-related disease. Intern Med 2014;53(5):493–7.

47. Inoue M, Nose N, Nishikawa H, et al. Successful treatment of sclerosing mediastinitis with a high serum IgG4 level. Gen Thorac Cardiovasc Surg 2007;55(10):431–3.

48. Ikeda K, Nomori H, Mori T, et al. Successful steroid treatment for fibrosing mediastinitis and sclerosing cervicitis. Ann Thorac Surg 2007;83(3):1199–201.

49. Noh D, Park C-K, Kwon S-Y. Immunoglobulin G4-related sclerosing disease invading the trachea and superior vena cava in mediastinum. Eur J Cardiothorac Surg 2014;45(3):573–5.

50. Peikert T, Shrestha B, Aubry MC, et al. Histopathologic overlap between fibrosing mediastinitis and IgG4-related disease. Int J Rheumatol 2012;2012: 207056.

51. Naitoh I, Nakazawa T, Ohara H, et al. Clinical significance of extrapancreatic lesions in autoimmune pancreatitis. Pancreas 2010;39(1):e1–5.

52. Cheuk W, Yuen HKL, Chu SYY, et al. Lymphadenopathy of IgG4-related sclerosing disease. Am J Surg Pathol 2008;32(5):671–81.

53. Sekiguchi H, Horie R, Utz JP, et al. IgG4-related systemic disease presenting with lung entrapment and constrictive pericarditis. Chest 2012;142(3):781–3.

54. Choi IH, Jang S-H, Lee S, et al. A case report of IgG4-related disease clinically mimicking pleural mesothelioma. Tuberc Respir Dis 2014;76(1):42–5.

55. Ryu JH, Hu X, Yi ES. IgG4-related pleural disease. Curr Pulmonology Rep 2015;4(1):22–7.

56. Ishida A, Furuya N, Nishisaka T, et al. IgG4-related pleural disease presenting as a massive bilateral effusion. J Bronchology Interv Pulmonol 2014; 21(3):237–41.

57. Kojima M, Nakazato Y, Kaneko Y, et al. Cytological findings of IgG4-related pleural effusion: a case report. Cytopathology 2013;24(5):338–40.

58. Yamamoto H, Suzuki T, Yasuo M, et al. IgG4-related pleural disease diagnosed by a re-evaluation of chronic bilateral pleuritis in a patient who experienced occasional acute left bacterial pleuritis. Intern Med 2011;50(8):893–7.

59. Strehl JD, Hartmann A, Agaimy A. Numerous IgG4-positive plasma cells are ubiquitous in diverse localised non-specific chronic inflammatory conditions and need to be distinguished from IgG4-related systemic disorders. J Clin Pathol 2011; 64(3):237–43.

60. Chang SY, Keogh KA, Lewis JE, et al. IgG4-positive plasma cells in granulomatosis with polyangiitis (Wegener's): a clinicopathologic and immunohistochemical study on 43 granulomatosis with polyangiitis and 20 control cases. Hum Pathol 2013;44(11): 2432–7.

61. Sah RP, Chari ST. Serologic issues in IgG4-related systemic disease and autoimmune pancreatitis. Curr Opin Rheumatol 2011;23(1):108–13.

62. Ryu JH, Horie R, Sekiguchi H, et al. Spectrum of disorders associated with elevated serum IgG4 Levels encountered in clinical practice. Int J Rheumatol 2012;2012:232960.

63. Carruthers MN, Khosroshahi A, Augustin T, et al. The diagnostic utility of serum IgG4 concentrations in IgG4-related disease. Ann Rheum Dis 2015;74(1): 14–8.

64. Yu K-H, Chan T-M, Tsai P-H, et al. Diagnostic performance of serum IgG4 levels in patients with IgG4-related disease. Medicine 2015;94(41):e1707.

65. Ebbo M, Grados A, Bernit E, et al. Pathologies associated with serum IgG4 elevation. Int J Rheumatol 2012;2012:602809.

66. Ngwa TN, Law R, Murray D, et al. Serum immunoglobulin g4 level is a poor predictor of immunoglobulin g4-related disease. Pancreas 2014; 43(5):704–7.

67. Fox RI, Fox CM. IgG4 levels and plasmablasts as a marker for IgG4-related disease (IgG4-RD). Ann Rheum Dis 2015;74(1):1–3.

68. Khosroshahi A, Wallace ZS, Crowe JL, et al. International consensus guidance statement on the management and treatment of IgG4-related disease. Arthritis Rheumatol 2015;67(7):1688–99.

69. Hamano H, Arakura N, Muraki T, et al. Prevalence and distribution of extrapancreatic lesions complicating autoimmune pancreatitis. J Gastroenterol 2006;41(12):1197–205.

70. Campbell SN, Rubio E, Loschner AL. Clinical review of pulmonary manifestations of IgG4-related disease. Ann Am Thorac Soc 2014;11(9):1466–75.

71. Kamisawa T, Okazaki K, Kawa S, et al. Amendment of the Japanese consensus guidelines for autoimmune pancreatitis, 2013 III. Treatment and prognosis of autoimmune pancreatitis. J Gastroenterol 2014;49(6):961–70.

72. Ghazale A, Chari ST, Zhang L, et al. Immunoglobulin G4-associated cholangitis: clinical profile and response to therapy. Gastroenterology 2008; 134(3):706–15.

73. Raina A, Yadav D, Krasinskas AM, et al. Evaluation and management of autoimmune pancreatitis: experience at a large US center. Am J Gastroenterol 2009;104(9):2295–306.

74. Masaki Y, Shimizu H, Sato Nakamura T, et al. IgG4-related disease: diagnostic methods and therapeutic strategies in Japan. J Clin Exp Hematop 2014; 54(2):95–101.

75. Khosroshahi A, Stone JH. Treatment approaches to IgG4-related systemic disease. Curr Opin Rheumatol 2011;23(1):67–71.

76. Sodikoff JB, Keilin SA, Cai Q, et al. Mycophenolate mofetil for maintenance of remission in steroid-dependent autoimmune pancreatitis. World J Gastroenterol 2012;18(18):2287–90.

77. Hart PA, Kamisawa T, Brugge WR, et al. Long-term outcomes of autoimmune pancreatitis: a multicentre, international analysis. Gut 2013;62(12):1771–6.

78. Witzig TE, Inwards DJ, Habermann TM, et al. Treatment of benign orbital pseudolymphomas with the monoclonal anti-CD20 antibody rituximab. Mayo Clin Proc 2007;82(6):692–9.

79. Plaza JA, Garrity JA, Dogan A, et al. Orbital inflammation with IgG4-positive plasma cells: manifestation of

IgG4 systemic disease. Arch Ophthalmol 2011;129(4): 421–8.

80. Khosroshahi A, Bloch DB, Deshpande V, et al. Rituximab therapy leads to rapid decline of serum IgG4 levels and prompt clinical improvement in IgG4-related systemic disease. Arthritis Rheum 2010; 62(6):1755–62.

81. Topazian M, Witzig TE, Smyrk TC, et al. Rituximab therapy for refractory biliary strictures in immunoglobulin G4-associated cholangitis. Clin Gastroenterol Hepatol 2008;6(3):364–6.

82. Carruthers MN, Topazian MD, Khosroshahi A, et al. Rituximab for IgG4-related disease: a prospective, open-label trial. Ann Rheum Dis 2015;74(6):1171–7.

83. Della-Torre E, Feeney E, Deshpande V, et al. B-cell depletion attenuates serological biomarkers of fibrosis and myofibroblast activation in IgG4-related disease. Ann Rheum Dis 2015;74(12): 2236–43.

84. Khosroshahi A, Carruthers MN, Deshpande V, et al. Rituximab for the treatment of IgG4-related disease: lessons from 10 consecutive patients. Medicine 2012;91(1):57–66.

85. Murakami J, Matsui S, Ishizawa S, et al. Recurrence of IgG4-related disease following treatment with rituximab. Mod Rheumatol 2013;23(6):1226–30.

86. Hirano K, Tada M, Isayama H, et al. Long-term prognosis of autoimmune pancreatitis with and without corticosteroid treatment. Gut 2007;56(12):1719–24.

87. Patel NR, Anzalone ML, Buja LM, et al. Sudden cardiac death due to coronary artery involvement by IgG4-related disease: a rare, serious complication of a rare disease. Arch Pathol Lab Med 2014; 138(6):833–6.

88. Holmes BJ, Delev NG, Pasternack GR, et al. Novel cause of sudden cardiac death: IgG4-related disease. Circulation 2012;125(23):2956–7.

Diffuse Idiopathic Pulmonary Neuroendocrine Cell Hyperplasia and Neuroendocrine Hyperplasia of Infancy

Laurie L. Carr, MD[a],*, Jeffrey A. Kern, MD[a],
Gail H. Deutsch, MD[b]

KEYWORDS

- Diffuse idiopathic neuroendocrine cell hyperplasia • Neuroendocrine hyperplasia of infancy
- Pulmonary neuroendocrine cells

KEY POINTS

- Diffuse idiopathic neuroendocrine cell hyperplasia (DIPNECH) in adults and neuroendocrine hyperplasia of infancy (NEHI) in children are rare lung diseases characterized by marked increases in neuroendocrine cells.
- DIPNECH is a progressive disease found in middle-aged women who present with chronic cough and dyspnea. Imaging reveals air trapping, pulmonary nodules, and bronchial carcinoids or tumorlets.
- DIPNECH is associated with obstructive lung disease, thought to be owing to the secretion of neuropeptides that drive tissue remodeling in small airways.
- NEHI presents in otherwise well infants with chronic tachypnea, retractions, crackles and hypoxemia. Chest computed tomography demonstrates hyperinflation and ground glass opacities in a characteristic distribution.
- Lung biopsies show minimal alterations with neuroendocrine cell hyperplasia in distal airways. Pulmonary symptoms tend to improve with age in patients with NEHI.

INTRODUCTION

Pulmonary neuroendocrine cells (PNEC) are located anatomically throughout the respiratory tract from the trachea to the terminal airways. They are among the first specialized cell types to differentiate within the primitive airway epithelium, originating from the foregut endoderm early in development.[1] These cells are distinguished histologically by their bottle shape and ultrastructurally by the presence of dense core vesicles containing bioactive mediators including calcitonin, chromogranin A, gastrin releasing peptide/bombesin,

Disclosure Statement: Dr J.A. Kern is a consultant to Gensignia Life Sciences, Inc, and serves on the scientific advisory boards of Strand Life Sciences, and Uptake Medical, Inc.
[a] Division of Oncology, National Jewish Health, 1400 Jackson Street, Denver, CO 80206, USA; [b] Department of Pathology, Seattle Children's Hospital, University of Washington, 4800 Sand Point Way Northeast, Seattle, WA 98105, USA
* Corresponding author.
E-mail address: carrl@njhealth.org

Clin Chest Med 37 (2016) 579–587
http://dx.doi.org/10.1016/j.ccm.2016.04.018

and serotonin. PNEC are present within the pulmonary epithelium as individual cells, or organized in extensively innervated groups, termed neuroepithelial bodies. These cells are thought to function as airway receptors controlling bronchomotor and vasomotor tone in response to alterations in airway gas composition, especially oxygen.[2] However, their exact function remains unknown. There are far more identifiable PNECs in the fetus and newborn than in the adult.[3] Although increased PNEC cells within the pulmonary epithelium can be seen in multiple chronic lung diseases, their significance and impact on disease manifestations is not known. In contrast, pulmonary disorders in which neuroendocrine cell hyperplasia is the primary finding are extremely rare, and associated with significant symptoms. Increased PNEC defines diffuse idiopathic neuroendocrine epithelial cell hyperplasia (DIPNECH) in adults and neuroendocrine hyperplasia of infancy (NEHI) in infants. This review focuses on these 2 distinct and rare lung diseases.

DIFFUSE IDIOPATHIC NEUROENDOCRINE EPITHELIAL CELL HYPERPLASIA

The prevalence of DIPNECH in the adult population is not known and a lack of specific diagnostic criteria has led to a confusing literature composed of a heterogeneous patient population. Although rare, this disease is becoming more commonly recognized. In 1976, Churg and Warnock[4] reported the finding of pulmonary carcinoid tumorlets in a review of indexed autopsy and surgical pathology cases. Seven cases of multiple pulmonary carcinoid tumorlets, a nodular proliferation of neuroendocrine cells less than 5 mm in size, were identified, all in women. These changes were accompanied by periarterial and peribronchial fibrosis, in which "the bronchus or bronchiole was completely obliterated by scar tissue or tumor and only the periarterial location indicated that an air passage had previously existed." This early description of multiple carcinoid tumorlets associated with an obliterative bronchiolitis (OB) is consistent with DIPNECH and may have been the first report of the disease. Aguayo and colleagues[5] in a series of case reports, later proposed that PNEC hyperplasia be considered a distinct clinical entity causing airway disease with airway wall thickening and fibrosis, radiographic abnormalities, irreversible airway obstruction and long standing symptoms of cough and exertional dyspnea. They labeled the syndrome as DIPNECH.

DIPNECH presents as chronic, persistent cough and dyspnea in middle-aged women. However, it has also been identified as an incidental finding on chest imaging of asymptomatic patients.[6,7] In those who present with cough or dyspnea, the symptoms have often been present for years, even decades, commonly misdiagnosed as asthma or another obstructive lung disease. The cough is frequently described as a persistent daily cough without sputum production. It is exacerbated by prolonged speaking, such as during long telephone conversations, but seldom interferes with sleep. Patients and their families frequently describe "coughing fits" that lead to decreased social interactions. Dyspnea can be more subtle, but tends to progress slowly over time. DIPNECH has a striking yet unexplained gender bias toward women.

Imaging

The appearance of DIPNECH on computed tomography (CT) imaging is distinctive and often provides the first indication of the disease in those undergoing evaluation for chronic cough or dyspnea (**Fig. 1**). With 1 reported exception, the imaging findings are bilateral and diffuse in nature.[8] Consistent findings involve a combination of airway abnormalities and pulmonary nodules. Of note, there have been reports of normal CT imaging on patients found to have DIPNECH on subsequent lung biopsy.

Airway abnormalities

The finding of mosaic attenuation with air trapping on expiratory, high-resolution CT (HRCT) is a consistent feature of DIPNECH and limits the differential diagnosis to pulmonary disease affecting the small airways, essentially to follicular or constrictive bronchiolitis. Mosaic perfusion is presumably caused by hypoventilation of the alveoli distal to the bronchiolar obstruction, leading to secondary vasoconstriction. At our institution, in a review of 18 DIPNECH patients with HRCT including expiratory images, all had a significant degree of air trapping, and most subjects (12/18) had 51% to 100% of lung parenchymal involvement.[6] Lee and colleagues[9] reported 5 patients with a mosaic pattern of air trapping, accentuated on expiratory CT, that was the predominant finding in all patients. Often the degree of air trapping is significant enough to detect mosaic attenuation even on inspiratory images.[6,10]

Diffuse bronchial wall thickening is another commonly detected CT abnormality. First reported by Aguayo and colleagues[5] in their original case series, subsequent case reviews have confirmed this feature.[9] In our review, bronchial wall thickening occurred in 80% of subjects (21/26).[6] Additional, but less common airway changes include mucoid impaction and mild bronchiectasis.

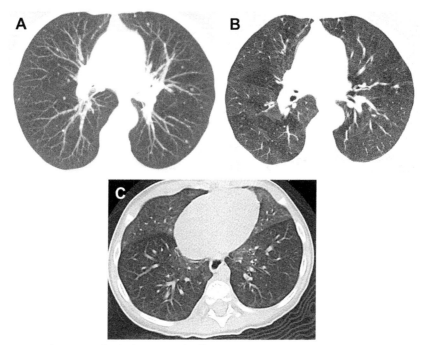

Fig. 1. Chest computed tomography (CT) images of diffuse idiopathic pulmonary neuroendocrine cell hyperplasia (DIPNECH) and neuroendocrine hyperplasia of infancy (NEHI). (*A*) DIPNECH: Axial image from chest CT in an adult female with multiple scattered pulmonary nodules present on inspiratory CT. (*B*) Expiratory phase CT of a similar patient shows extensive areas of air trapping. (*C*) NEHI: High-resolution CT scan demonstrating ground glass attenuation in the right middle lobe and lingula.

Pulmonary nodules

The presence of pulmonary nodules on the background of mosaic attenuation comprise the defining features of DIPNECH. Owing to concerns for metastatic cancer, this finding often leads to further evaluation.[6,10] DIPNECH nodules are typically noncalcified, rounded, and well-defined. The majority are 6 to 10 mm in size, although it is not uncommon to have a nodule reach 40 mm. Although diffusely distributed, they are often most prominent in lower or midlung fields. The majority of subjects in our series had more than 20 pulmonary nodules, with 35% (9/26) demonstrating more than 50 pulmonary nodules. The nodules have an indolent growth pattern. In our cohort of 21 patients who had longitudinal imaging with an average length of follow-up 1054 days (±883 days), the number of nodules was stable in most subjects (90%), but 52% showed slight growth in the size of nodules over time. Upon resection, the nodules are classified histologically as typical carcinoid tumors or carcinoid tumorlets based on their size.

Biochemical Testing

Serotonin is not generally produced in cells of foregut origin, owing to a lack of the enzyme aromatic amino acid decarboxylase. Carcinoid syndrome is therefore rarely seen in bronchial carcinoids or DIPNECH, because the neuroendocrine cells in these disorders arise from the foregut endoderm. Biochemical testing for serum chromogranin A and 24-hour urine collection for 5-hydroxyindole-acetic acid can be performed in DIPNECH patients and an elevation in serum chromogranin A has been reported. Sandostatin analog therapy can reduce serum chromogranin A levels, indicating a targeted response from a surrogate biomarker.[6,7] However, urine 5-hydroxyindoleacetic acid levels are usually normal.[6–8]

Physiology

Lung physiology in DIPNECH patients is typically similar to that seen with other forms of obstructive bronchiolitis, although some patients may present with normal lung function. Spirometry characteristically reveals airway obstruction with a reduced forced expiratory volume in 1 second and a reduced forced expiratory volume in 1 second/forced vital capacity (FVC) ratio without a significant response to bronchodilators. Air trapping is common, leading to increased residual volume. The combination of airway obstruction owing to bronchiolitis obliterans and reduced FVC owing to residual volume expansion can lead to a mixed obstructive/restrictive pattern on pulmonary function tests (PFT). The diffusing capacity for carbon monoxide is usually normal because the alveoli are not involved and gas transfer surface area is normal. Patients generally have a prolonged course of airway obstruction with long periods of stability, although there is some heterogeneity in the progression of their obstructive disease. In our series, 8 of 27 subjects with multiple PFTs available for analysis had episodes in which the forced expiratory volume in 1 second declined by more than 10% within a 2-year interval. The morbidity and mortality associated with this disease is driven by the bronchiolitis.

Pathology

Formal diagnostic criteria for a pathologic diagnosis of DIPNECH are evolving. The World Health Organization defines pulmonary neuroendocrine hyperplasia as "proliferating PNCs confined to the mucosa as small groups or as a monolayer ... or aggregates that protrude into the lumen as nodular or papillary growths."[11] Carcinoid tumorlets are formed when PNECs become invasive across the basal lamina to form nodules less than 5 mm in diameter, with irregular margins and a fibrotic stroma (**Fig. 2**). When these nodules are greater than 5 mm in size, they are classified as bronchial carcinoid tumors. The degree of PNEC hyperplasia required to establish a diagnosis of DIPNECH has not been formalized. Marchevsky and Walts[12] proposed more definitive criteria for pathologic diagnosis based on review of surgical lung resections, namely, multifocal neuroendocrine cell hyperplasia, defined by the presence of 5 or more PNEC in at least 3 separate small airways combined with 3 or more carcinoid tumorlets. Because PNEC hyperplasia occurs in the setting of chronic lung disease, it is important to exclude secondary hyperplasia before making a DIPNECH diagnosis.

In the setting of high clinical suspicion, confirmation with a pathologic diagnosis is not always necessary, especially given that there is no specific therapeutic intervention that has been shown to change the course of this disease. In addition, the optimal approach to obtaining tissue is debated. The pathologic criteria proposed by

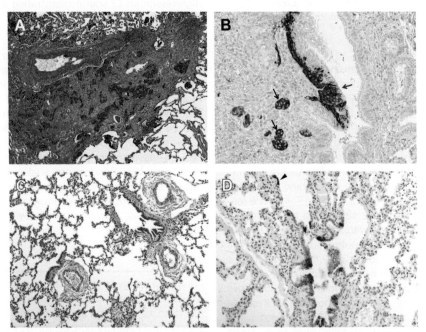

Fig. 2. (*A*) Diffuse idiopathic pulmonary neuroendocrine cell hyperplasia (DIPNECH): Small airway constrictive changes: airway replacement by pulmonary neuroendocrine cell hyperplasia and scarring (hematoxylin and eosin; original magnification ×40). (*B*) DIPENCH: Proliferation of neuroendocrine cells confined to the bronchiolar epithelium (*blue arrow*) and carcinoid tumorlets (*black arrows*). Immunoperoxidase (synaptophysin; original magnification ×60). (*C*) Neuroendocrine hyperplasia of infancy (NEHI). Near-normal airway and alveolar architecture with mildly increased bronchiolar smooth muscle and increased alveolar macrophages (hematoxylin and eosin; original magnification ×40). (*D*) NEHI: An increased number of neuroendocrine cells in the bronchiolar epithelium and as clusters (neuroendocrine body) in the alveolar duct (*arrowhead*). Immunoperoxidase (bombesin; original magnification ×200).

Marchevsky and Walts[12] was based on review of surgical lung biopsies; however, it may be feasible to use a less invasive strategy to diagnosis DIPNECH. The combination of compatible clinical criteria including presenting symptoms, patient demographics, pulmonary function and imaging, and confirmation of PNEC hyperplasia on transbronchial biopsy may suffice (**Table 1**). At our institution, 10 patients with clinical findings consistent with DIPNECH underwent transbronchial biopsy. Of these, 6 patients had confirmation of neuroendocrine cell hyperplasia upon histologic review. Transbronchial biopsies in the remaining 4 patients were nondiagnostic.

DIPNECH has been categorized by World Health Organization as a preinvasive lesion based on consistent findings of typical carcinoid tumors arising within DIPNECH. There have also been reports of atypical carcinoids arising in DIPNECH with lymph node involvement.[7,8,13] To date, no cases of more aggressive neuroendocrine cell cancers, such as small cell carcinoma or large cell neuroendocrine tumors, have been reported. The characterization of DIPNECH as a premalignant condition suggests a program for surveillance with imaging and biopsy that is a poor fits for the natural history of DIPNECH as we currently understand it. For example, the National Comprehensive Cancer Network recommends mediastinal lymph node sampling and follow-up for 10 years with annual CT of the chest for bronchial carcinoids.[14] It is difficult to reconcile these aggressive recommendations for bronchial carcinoid management with the management of DIPNECH because multiple carcinoids may arise over the course of the disease.

Neuroendocrine hyperplasia is known to be associated with OB. The relationship between DIPNECH and OB is not well-understood, and the prevalence of this associated condition is variable in reported case series. PNEC secretory products, such as the bombesinlike gastrin-releasing peptide, have biologic effects on airway epithelial cell and fibroblast proliferation.[2] Additional PNEC secretory products, such as serotonin, are known to cause potent pulmonary vasoconstriction and bronchoconstriction.[15] Inappropriate and excessive production of these secretory products may lead to the constrictive fibrotic lesions often seen in bronchioles of DIPNECH patients. The variability in reporting OB with DIPNECH in case series may be owing to a

Table 1
Diagnostic findings in DIPNECH and NEHI

	DIPNECH	NEHI
Demographics	Women age 45–70	Infancy with most in first year of life
Symptoms	Chronic cough and dyspnea, for >5–10 y	Tachypnea, retractions, crackles, and hypoxemia
Imaging/HRCT	Diffuse pulmonary nodules 4–10 mm Mosaic attenuation or air trapping Bronchial wall thickening	Ground glass opacities centrally, right middle lobe and lingula Air trapping
Pulmonary function testing	Fixed obstruction, or mixed obstructive/ restrictive lung disease Increased RV, TLC Low DLCO that corrects with VA	Mixed obstructive/restrictive pattern with profound air trapping Marked increase in FRC, RV and RV/TLC Proportionate reduction in FEV and FVC
Histology	Proliferation of neuroendocrine cells per WHO, "proliferating PNCs confined to the mucosa as small groups or as a monolayer … or aggregates that protrude into the lumen as nodular or papillary growths" Presence of constrictive bronchiolitis Absence of underlying chronic lung disease or primary malignancy to exclude reactive PNECH	Near normal histology with absence of underlying chronic lung disease Bombesin immunopositive cells in the majority of distal airways Prominent neuroepithelial bodies in alveolar ducts
Laboratory tests	Elevated serum chromogranin A level	None to date

Abbreviations: DIPNECH, diffuse idiopathic pulmonary neuroendocrine cell hyperplasia; DLCO, diffusion capacity; FEV, forced expiratory volume; FRC, functional residual capacity; FVC, forced vital capacity; HRCT, high-resolution computed topography; NEHI, neuroendocrine hyperplasia of infancy; PNC, pulmonary neuroendocrine cell; PNECH, pulmonary neuroendocrine cell hyperplasia; RV, residual volume; TLC, total lung capacity; VA, alveolar volume; WHO, World Health Organization.

lack of formal diagnostic criteria for this disease. Variability in reporting may also be owing to the limited amount of tissue available for histologic review. Because OB can be focal or patchy, findings can be missed with small tissue samples, such as transbronchial biopsies. In our cohort, of 12 surgical lung biopsy samples available for histologic review, 7 had constrictive bronchiolitis.

Management and Treatment

To date, there have been no clinical trials in DIP-NECH patients to inform treatment decisions. Although inhaled or oral steroids are often prescribed, there are no data to suggest that pulmonary function improves with their use. Owing to the indolent nature of the disease, conservative management is often used to prevent the adverse effects of overtreatment with glucocorticoids and/ or surgical resection. However, a subset of DIP-NECH patients who experience an accelerated rate of lung function decline, as well as some of those with a long course of the more typical slow progression, develop debilitating and even life-threatening disease. Sandostatin analogs have been shown to palliate the debilitating cough associated with DIPNECH.[6] The effect of sandostatin analogs on pulmonary function is less clear and is difficult to study owing to slow progression, small patient numbers, and variability inherent in spirometric measurements. If the neuropeptides being released by the PNECs play a role in the pathogenesis of bronchiolitis, perhaps early treatment with sandostatin, to reduce the offending agent, should be considered.

Early translational studies have demonstrated activation of the mammalian target of rapamycin (mTOR) pathway in DIPNECH.[16] In addition, recent clinical trials using everolimus in the setting of bronchial carcinoids have demonstrated tumor response and improvement in progression-free survival.[17] There is reason to believe mTOR inhibition may also be an effective therapy for DIP-NECH. Although mTOR inhibition has been shown to reduce bronchial carcinoid growth, the effect on the bronchiolitis associated with DIP-NECH, which is the source of the morbidity and mortality of this disease, is not known. In addition, oral mTOR inhibitors have significant adverse effects that may make patient compliance in the treatment of a life-long disease difficult.

Finally, single lung transplantation has been performed in the setting of DIPNECH with severe OB.[18] A follow-up report 2 years after transplant described no progression of the remaining nodules in the native lung while on immunosuppression and no new nodules developed in the transplanted lung. Although immunosuppression did not seem to exacerbate disease progression, this is a short interval to detect changes in this indolent disease.

NEUROENDOCRINE HYPERPLASIA OF INFANCY

Neuroendocrine cell hyperplasia of infancy (NEHI), previously termed "persistent tachypnea of infancy," is a rare form of childhood interstitial lung disease that has characteristic clinical, radiographic, and histologic features.[19,20] NEHI typically presents in otherwise healthy infants with chronic tachypnea and intercostal retractions in the first few months to year of life. Most patients with NEHI are born at term after uncomplicated pregnancies, but cases occurring in late preterm infants have been reported.[19,21] Many patients come to attention with persistent symptoms after a presumed viral infection, although further history usually reveals respiratory symptoms that predate the acute illness. Tachypnea is the most common clinical feature at presentation, and is often associated with chronic subglottic, intercostal, and subcostal retractions.[19,22,23] Physical examination is notable for prominent crackles and frequent hypoxemia; wheezing is noted occasionally. Patients with NEHI frequently have failure to thrive and gastroesophageal reflux is common.[19,23,24] The presence of these symptoms is thought to be related to the pulmonary physiology, but it is unknown whether gastrointestinal abnormalities might also occur in NEHI. The incidence and prevalence of NEHI has not yet been established, although cases have been identified at many different institutions around the world. In a large case series from 11 centers in North America reported by the Children's Interstitial Lung Disease Research Network (CHILDRN), NEHI represented 10% of all lung biopsies from children less than 2 years of age.[22] Based on recent recognition of the disorder and retrospective review revealing cases previously diagnosed with other nonspecific types of chronic lung disease, the prevalence of NEHI is likely greater than currently estimated.[25]

Imaging

Like DIPNECH, the HRCT imaging appearance in NEHI is frequently distinct enough to confirm the diagnosis in the appropriate clinical context, obviating the need for lung biopsy. Chest radiographs may be normal or show hyperexpansion.[19] By HRCT, there are ground glass opacities that are seen centrally, in the right middle lobe and lingula (see Fig. 1). Air trapping with a mosaic pattern is often demonstrated on expiratory images. No other airway or parenchymal abnormalities are usually seen. A study by Brody and colleagues,[26] in which 2 expert radiologists evaluated HRCT scans from 23 children with biopsy-proven NEHI and 6 children with other forms of interstitial lung disease, NEHI was identified correctly in all cases. However, the sensitivity was imperfect because the radiologists did not suggest the diagnosis of NEHI in up to 22% of cases.

Physiology

Infant PFTs in NEHI reveal a mixed physiologic pattern, including severe air trapping resulting in a low FVC. There are proportionate reductions in the forced expiratory volume in 0.5 seconds and FVC, with particularly reduced force expiratory volume at 75% and 85% of FVC. Functional residual capacity, residual volume, and residual volume/total lung capacity are markedly elevated.[21,23,27] Studies have suggested that infant PFT may correlate with number of bombesin-immunopositive neuroendocrine cells seen on lung biopsy as well as long-term pulmonary function and oxygen requirement.[21,27] The specificity of infant PFT findings in NEHI compared with other respiratory disorders, including bronchiolitis obliterans, has not been evaluated systematically.

Pathology

In contrast with the severity of clinical symptoms, lung biopsies in NEHI are near normal, with minimal nonspecific changes of airway obstruction including a mild increase in alveolar macrophages and smooth muscle hyperplasia in the bronchiolar wall (see **Fig. 2**). Patchy mild inflammation or fibrosis reflective of chronic bronchiolitis may be present, especially after a viral infection, but the degree of pathologic change is usually insufficient to provide a compelling explanation for the patient's often significant symptomatology. Pathologic confirmation of the diagnosis rests is based on documentation of an increased proportion of neuroendocrine cells within distal airways, best seen using immunostains against bombesin and serotonin.[19] Other neuroendocrine markers, including synaptophysin, chromogranin, neuron specific enolase, and PGP 9.5, have been shown to be less reliable in demonstrating this increase in neuroendocrine cell numbers. Immunohistochemical assessment requires an adequate biopsy with at least 10 airways present for evaluation. Currently, formal criteria for defining neuroendocrine cell excess in NEHI are lacking, and in the absence of a pathologist experienced with the disorder, morphometric quantification of bombesin staining may be useful for establishing the diagnosis. In general, bombesin immunopositive cells in NEHI are prominent in the distal respiratory bronchioles and as clusters (neuroepithelial bodies) in the alveolar ducts. Two individual airways with more than 10% bombesin-immunopositive area or cell number of the airway epithelium, is suggestive of the diagnosis. Correlation of the histology with the clinical presentation and radiographic findings in all cases is essential, because increased neuroendocrine cells have been reported in other pediatric lung disorders, including chronic neonatal lung disease of prematurity, sudden infant death syndrome, pulmonary hypertension, and cystic fibrosis. Likewise, failure to demonstrate an increase in bombesin immunopositive cells does not exclude the diagnosis because wide intrasubject and intersubject variability in neuroendocrine cell number has been reported, which does not relate to imaging appearance of the region biopsied.[21] More than 1 biopsy site is recommended to enhance sensitivity.

Management and Treatment

There have been no controlled trials and there is no known definitive therapy for NEHI. Management of the disorder largely consists of supportive and preventive care. Most children require supplemental oxygen for months, and many require nutritional support and treatment of gastroesophageal reflux. Glucocorticoids are not helpful in most cases.[19,23] Although the clinical condition tends to gradually improve over time, patients may remain symptomatic for many years with respiratory illnesses or exercise.[23,24,27] In 1 series, several patients developed a phenotype of nonatopic asthma.[23] HRCT abnormalities may persist for years.[24,28] No deaths have been reported in the setting of NEHI and no patients have progressed to respiratory failure or required lung transplantation. Of interest, there have been no reports of DIPNECH occurring in a patient or a family member with NEHI.

Pathogenesis

The etiology of NEHI is unknown, but based on the report of several families with multiple siblings affected, genetic mechanisms may play a role.[29] In a single family, a heterozygous mutation in *NKX2.1* was identified in an individual with biopsy-proven NEHI and 4 adult family members with a history of lung disease in childhood.[28] *NKX2.1* mutations have not been identified in other unrelated subjects with NEHI.

Although the name NEHI was coined based on the increased neuroendocrine cells seen on lung biopsy, it is unknown whether these cells are involved in the pathogenesis of the disorder or are simply a marker. A relationship of increased neuroendocrine cells to airway injury or neuroendocrine cell proliferation has not been demonstrated and neuroendocrine cell number and distribution seems to be distinct from other pediatric disorders in which increased neuroendocrine cells are observed.[21] Of interest, while NEHI presents clinically with small airway obstruction; there is no evidence of airway occlusion on lung biopsy. Neuroendocrine cells are airway chemoreceptors and release potent bronchoconstrictive and vasoactive peptides, including bombesin and serotonin, in response to hypoxia and other stimuli, which may result in hyperresponsiveness of small airways.[30] There is an association between density of airway neuroendocrine cells and airway obstruction on infant PFTs in patients with NEHI.[21]

SUMMARY AND DISCUSSION

The presence of neuroendocrine cell hyperplasia in small airways is the defining feature of DIPNECH in adults and NEHI in young children. The underlying etiology of NEC hyperplasia is unknown in either of these rare lung diseases. Although both disorders manifest with dyspnea, obstruction and severe air trapping, symptoms in NEHI typically improve over time, whereas DIPNECH is progressive in nature. In addition, DIPNECH has a gender bias toward women, whereas NEHI is found in both genders equally. The similarities in physiologic manifestations are presumably owing to the effect of the secretory products of the PNECs on the small airways. The differences may represent different etiologies or different host response to similar inciting events. Both DIPNECH and NEHI are relatively new syndromes only recently recognized in pulmonary pathology. Importantly, both are rare. To achieve advances in the diagnosis and management of these disorders, we recommend that patients be referred to experienced centers for care and the generation of cohorts of sufficient size to advance our understanding of these syndromes.

REFERENCES

1. Song H, Yao E, Lin C, et al. Functional characterization of pulmonary neuroendocrine cells in lung development, injury, and tumorigenesis. Proc Natl Acad Sci U S A 2012;109(43):17531–6.
2. Pulmonary Neuroendocrine Cells. Their secretory products and their potential roles in health and chronic lung disease in infancy. Am Rev Respir Dis 1989;140(6):1807–12.
3. Cutz E, Gillan JE, Track NS. Pulmonary endocrine cells in the developing human lung and during neonatal adaptation. The endocrine lung in health and disease. Philadelphia: Saunders; 1984.
4. Churg A, Warnock ML. Pulmonary tumorlet. A form of peripheral carcinoid. Cancer 1976;37(3):1469–77.
5. Aguayo SM, Miller YE, Waldron JA Jr. Idiopathic diffuse hyperplasia of pulmonary neuroendocrine cells and airways disease. N Engl J Med 1992;327(18):1285.
6. Carr LL, Chung JH, Achcar RD, et al. The clinical course of diffuse idiopathic pulmonary neuroendocrine cell hyperplasia. Chest 2015;147(2):415.
7. Gorshtein A, Gross DJ, Barak D, et al. Diffuse idiopathic pulmonary neuroendocrine cell hyperplasia and the associated lung neuroendocrine tumors. Cancer 2011;118(3):612.
8. Irshad S, McLean E, Rankin S, et al. Unilateral diffuse idiopathic pulmonary neuroendocrine cell hyperplasia and multiple carcinoids treated with surgical resection. J Thorac Oncol 2010;5(6):921.
9. Lee JS, Brown KK, Cool C. Diffuse pulmonary neuroendocrine cell hyperplasia: radiologic and clinical features. J Comput Assist Tomogr 2002;26(2):10.
10. Davies SJ, Gosney JR, Hansell DM, et al. Diffuse idiopathic pulmonary neuroendocrine cell hyperplasia: an under-recognized spectrum of disease. Thorax 2007;62:248.
11. Travis WD, World Health Organization. International Association for the Study of Lung Cancer, International Academy of Pathology. Pathology and Genetics of Tumours of the Lung, Pleura, Thymus and Heart. Thymus 2004. p. 78–9.
12. Marchevsky AM, Walts AE. Diffuse idiopathic pulmonary neuroendocrine cell hyperplasia (DIPNECH). Semin Diagn Pathol 2015;32(6):438–44.
13. Aubry M-C. Significance of multiple carcinoid tumors and tumorlets in surgical lung specimens. Chest 2007;131(6):1635.
14. National Comprehensive Cancer Network (NCCN). NCCN Clinical Practice Guidelines in Oncology: Small Cell Lung Cancer. Version 2.2014. 2013.
15. Johnson DE, Wobken JD, Landrum BG. Changes in bombesin, calcitonin, and serotonin immunoreactive pulmonary neuroendocrine cells in cystic fibrosis and after prolonged mechanical ventilation. Am Rev Respir Dis 2012;137(1):123–31.
16. Rossi G, Cavazza A, Graziano P, et al. mTOR/p70S6K in diffuse idiopathic pulmonary neuroendocrine cell hyperplasia. Am J Respir Crit Care Med 2012;185(3):341.
17. Yao JC, Fazio N, Singh S, et al. Everolimus for the treatment of advanced, non-functional neuroendocrine tumours of the lung or gastrointestinal tract (RADIANT-4): a randomized, placebo-controlled, phase 3 study. Lancet 2016;387(10022):968–77.

18. Sheerin N, Harrison NK, Sheppard MN, et al. Obliter-ative bronchiolitis caused by multiple tumourlets and microcarcinoids successfully treated by single lung transplantation. Thorax 1995;50(2):207–9.

19. Deterding RR, Pye C, Fan LL, et al. Persistent ta-chypnea of infancy is associated with neuroendo-crine cell hyperplasia. Pediatr Pulmonol 2005; 40(2):157–65.

20. Deterding RR, Fan LL, Morton R, et al. Persistent ta-chypnea of infancy (PTI)–a new entity. Pediatr Pul-monol 2001;(Suppl 23):72–3.

21. Young LR, Brody AS, Inge TH, et al. Neuroendocrine cell distribution and frequency distinguish neuroen-docrine cell hyperplasia of infancy from other pulmo-nary disorders. Chest 2011;139(5):1060–71.

22. Deutsch GH, Young LR, Deterding RR, et al. Diffuse lung disease in young children. Am J Respir Crit Care Med 2012;176(11):1120–8.

23. Lukkarinen H, Pelkonen A, Lohi J, et al. Neuroendo-crine cell hyperplasia of infancy: a prospective follow-up of nine children. Arch Dis Child 2013; 98(2):141–4.

24. Gomes VCC, Silva MCC, Maia Filho JH, et al. Diag-nostic criteria and follow-up in neuroendocrine cell hyperplasia of infancy: a case series. J Bras Pneu-mol 2013;39(5):569–78.

25. Soares JJ, Deutsch GH, Moore PE, et al. Childhood interstitial lung diseases: an 18-year retrospective analysis. Pediatrics 2013;132(4):684–91.

26. Brody AS, Guillerman RP, Hay TC, et al. Neuroendo-crine cell hyperplasia of infancy: diagnosis with high-resolution CT. AJR Am J Roentgenol 2010; 194(1):238–44.

27. Kerby GS, Wagner BD, Popler J, et al. Abnormal in-fant pulmonary function in young children with neuroendocrine cell hyperplasia of infancy. Pediatr Pulmonol 2013;48(10):1008–15.

28. Young LR, Deutsch GH, Bokulic RE, et al. A mutation in TTF1/NKX2.1 is associated with familial neuroen-docrine cell hyperplasia of infancy. Chest 2013; 144(4):1199–206.

29. Popler J, Gower WA, Mogayzel PJ, et al. Familial neuroendocrine cell hyperplasia of infancy. Pediatr Pulmonol 2010;45(8):749–55.

30. Cutz E, Yeger H, Pan J. Pulmonary neuroendo-crine cell system in pediatric lung disease-recent advances. Pediatr Dev Pathol 2007;10(6): 419–35.

Benign Metastasizing Leiomyoma

Gustavo Pacheco-Rodriguez, PhD[a], Angelo M. Taveira-DaSilva, MD, PhD[b],
Joel Moss, MD, PhD[b],*

KEYWORDS

- Leiomyomas • Metastasis • Estrogen • Rare lung disease • Smooth muscle cells

KEY POINTS

- Benign metastasizing leiomyoma (BML) is predominantly a disease of premenopausal women, which is strongly associated with uterine leiomyomas and involvement of the lung, but may also involve the heart, lymph nodes, and vertebral spine.
- BML has also been diagnosed in men and children.
- Lung BML nodules may be solitary or multiple, and unilateral or bilateral.
- Currently available treatments for BML involve reduction of estrogen and progesterone by pharmacologic or surgical intervention; but asymptomatic patients do not necessarily require treatment.
- BML should be considered in premenopausal women who have a history of uterine leiomyoma and prior uterine surgery and present with lung-related symptoms.

INTRODUCTION

Benign metastasizing leiomyoma (BML) is a rare disease characterized by the presence of multiple, bilateral lung nodules of different sizes[1] that may be mistaken for metastatic cancer. BML is most commonly found in premenopausal women who have undergone myomectomy or hysterectomy for treatment of uterine leiomyomas[2]; however, the disease also occurs in the absence of these surgical procedures.[3] BML is characterized by the proliferation of pathologically benign smooth muscle cells that form tumors in different sites, including lung, lymph nodes, heart, skeletal muscle, and pelvic cavity. Occasionally, BML tumors may be found in multiple organs, including the lungs, liver, muscles, heart, and pelvic cavity.[4] BML has been misclassified as a low-grade leiomyosarcoma.[5] Although lungs and lymph nodes are the most common sites in which BML cells are found, they also can be present in the mediastinum, retroperitoneum, vascular channels, bone, spine, and soft tissues.[6–8] In a series of 10 patients with spine involvement, 50% presented with lung lesions.[8] BML also has been reported in men and children. Although uterine leiomyoma are more prevalent in the African American population,[9] BML does not show an ethnic predisposition. A definitive diagnosis requires a medical history, imaging studies, for example, a computed tomography (CT) of the thorax and abdomen, and pathologic examination of tissues obtained by biopsy or surgical resection of the tumors. The molecular mechanisms and genetic factors that contribute to the pathogenesis of this disease have not been elucidated. BML typically responds to antiestrogen therapies and the respiratory

The authors report no conflict of interest. This work was supported by the Intramural Research Program of the National Institutes of Health, National Heart, Lung, and Blood Institute.
[a] Cardiovascular and Pulmonary Branch, National Heart, Lung, and Blood Institute, National Institutes of Health, Building 10, Room 5N307, 9000 Rockville Pike, Bethesda, MD 20892-1434, USA; [b] Cardiovascular and Pulmonary Branch, National Heart, Lung, and Blood Institute, National Institutes of Health, Building 10, Room 6D05, MSC-1590, 9000 Rockville Pike, Bethesda, MD 20892-1590, USA
* Corresponding author.
E-mail address: mossj@nhlbi.nih.gov

Clin Chest Med 37 (2016) 589–595
http://dx.doi.org/10.1016/j.ccm.2016.04.019
0272-5231/16/$ – see front matter © 2016 Elsevier Inc. All rights reserved.

symptoms, such as dyspnea, have also been re-ported to treatment.[10,11]

CLINICAL PRESENTATION

The symptoms of BML vary depending on the or-gan or organs affected.[11–13] From the respiratory standpoint, patients may be asymptomatic or they may present with mild pulmonary manifesta-tions, including shortness of breath, cough, wheezing, and pleuritic chest pain. In patients with BML involving the spine, leg pain and pares-thesias have been reported.[8] The posterior verte-bral body is commonly involved. Because pneumothoraces and cysts occur in patients with BML, the disease may be confused with lymphan-gioleiomyomatosis (LAM), a multisystem disease characterized by lung cysts and recurrent pneumothoraces, caused by proliferation of abnormal-appearing smooth muscle cells.[14] BML in other sites, such as uterus, heart, and lymph nodes, is usually asymptomatic. The symptoms of uterine fibroids, which are highly associated with pulmonary BML, may include abnormal uter-ine bleeding, pelvic pressure/pain, and reproduc-tive dysfunction. Although most cases of BML have been reported in patients following myomec-tomies and/or hysterectomies, some cases of BML are not associated with prior surgical proce-dures.[2] BML mainly presents in premenopausal women, and respiratory symptoms may be pre-sent in up to 30% of the cases.[15]

IMAGING STUDIES

On imaging studies, such as CT scans of the lungs, BML presents as well-circumscribed nodules scattered throughout the lungs (**Fig. 1**).[3] The nod-ules can be large or small (see **Fig. 1**C, D). Bilateral pulmonary nodules are more common than multi-ple unilateral lesions or solitary nodules.[15,16] The nodules in BML can cavitate,[17] leading to forma-tion of thin-walled or thick-walled cysts. BML nod-ules have been identified by chest radiograph, CT scan, 18F-fluorodeoxyglucose (FDG)-PET posi-tron emission tomography, and MRI. BML tumors have a low metabolic rate, similar to other low-grade neoplasms (eg, adenomas, bronchoalveolar carcinomas, carcinoid tumors, and lymphomas). 18F-FDG-PET, however, has helped to distinguish BML from leiomyosarcoma, which is a more glyco-lytically active tumor.

PATHOLOGY

The World Health Organization classification of lung tumors does not include BML but includes LAM, which may be confused with BML.[18] The pri-mary disorders in the differential diagnosis of nodular smooth muscle lung lesions are metasta-tic malignancies, lung cancer, hamartomas, peri-vascular epithelioid cell tumors (PEComa), leiomyosarcomas, and inflammatory or infectious processes. PEComas are tumors composed of cells with melanocytic and smooth muscle

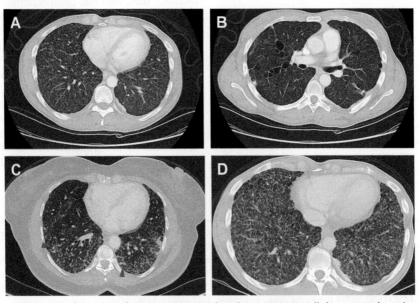

Fig. 1. High-resolution CT of the chest from 3 patients with pulmonary BML. All these cases have been confirmed with a biopsy. (*A*) Multiple nodules (*arrowheads*) with a diffuse distribution in both lungs. (*B*) Presence of cysts (*arrowheads*) in the same patient. (*C*) An example of relatively large lung nodules (*arrowhead*). (*D*) Numerous small miliary nodules scattered throughout both lungs.

properties, which have been associated recently with mutations in the tuberous sclerosis complex genes.[19] Some of the characteristic PEComas are angiomyolipomas, pulmonary lymphangioleiomyomatosis, and clear-cell (sugar) tumors.[19] Leiomyomas or fibroids are common benign and clonal smooth muscle tumors characterized by the presence of estrogen and progesterone receptors.[20] Uterine leiomyomas are the most frequent indication for surgeries and manipulation of the reproductive tract.[21,22] BML nodules are not generally cavitary and show low cellularity. Lung nodules are composed of proliferative smooth muscle cells arranged in intersecting fascicles (**Fig. 2**), which express smooth muscle proteins such as smooth muscle actin, desmin, and caldesmon.[23] BML cells have a low mitotic index, without nuclear atypia, and do not invade the surrounding tissue. The growth of the BML tumors is slow, with the size of the nodules frequently reported as unchanged over long periods of time. Similar to the cells of uterine leiomyomas, lung BML cells are reactive to antibodies against estrogen and progesterone

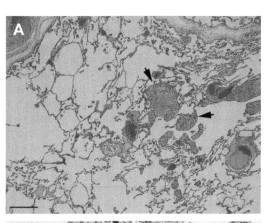

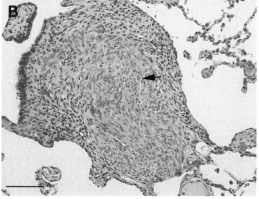

Fig. 2. (*A*) Proliferative smooth muscle cells in the lung (*arrows*) of a patient with BML (H&E, original magnification ×50, bar = 250 μm). (*B*) Well-differentiated smooth muscle cells growing in fascicles (*arrow*) (H&E, original magnification ×200, bar = 100 μm).

receptors.[2] Some BML lung lesions show vascular structures, with nodules at the periphery of the vessels. BML lesions express high levels of the tumor suppressor gene p53, but its role in pathogenesis has not been defined. BML lung lesions also show immunoreactivity with antibodies against proliferating antigen Ki-67.[23] BML is a disease considered in the differential diagnosis of multiple pulmonary leiomyomatous hamartomas (MPLH)[24] or leiomyomatous hamartoma, a rare disease of men and women characterized by lesions composed of smooth muscle cells with eosinophilic fibrillary cytoplasm.[24] Although most of the BML lesions have been reported as nonreactive to the antibody HMB-45,[23] which recognizes Pmel17, a melanosomal protein expressed in lung hamartomas, PEComas, and LAM,[25,26] BML lesions may show low reactivity.[3]

There have been many attempts to characterize BML nodules immunologically. BML smooth muscle cells are not reactive to common markers (eg, EMA, CD10, CD117, TTF-1, BCL-2, GPAP, calretinin, cytokeratin, chromogranin) tested routinely in clinical laboratories. An antigen that may be promising for distinguishing BML from other smooth muscle tumors is S-100, which appears to be expressed at low levels in BML. These findings contrast with pulmonary metastases of uterine PEComas, which despite exhibiting a similar presentation to BML, are composed of proliferating smooth muscle cells that are reactive to the antibody HMB-45.[27] Thus, BML lung nodules have some distinct histopathological characteristics that can be used to differentiate them from other diseases associated with smooth muscle nodules.

Cytogenetic studies of cells from BML lung tissue specimens have shown that the cells have chromosomal abnormalities.[28] In 5 cases, 19q and 22q terminal deletions were observed. These chromosomal abnormalities differ from those reported more frequently in uterine leiomyomas, which often involve translocations of chromosomes 12q14-15 and deletions of chromosome 7.[29] Interestingly, a case of BML showed different chromosomal deletions in cells isolated from different metastatic sites.[30] In a few cases, BML cells lacked estrogen or progesterone receptors, suggesting that the site of origin was not the uterus; however, it is also possible that the receptors had been downregulated.[31] Interestingly, there are genetic studies that suggest that BML is clonal in origin.[32]

PATHOGENESIS

Benign lung tumors can be of either epithelial or mesenchymal origin. BML has been classified as benign tumors of mesenchymal origin, which also include smooth muscle tumors of the uterus.[33] The sources of the cells that form these lung nodular structures remain unknown but due to the strong association with uterine leiomyomas (fibroids), it is believed that they arise from the uterus. Estrogens appear to play an important role in the origin of BML. Estrogen metabolites may promote mutagenesis giving rise to BML.[34] It has been postulated that BML cells originate from a single site.[32] Although among uterine tumors BML has been mainly associated with leiomyomas,[2] the type of leiomyomas is unclear (eg, mitotically active, cellular, hemorrhagic cellular, atypical, epithelioid, myxoid, vascular, lipoleiomyomas). Other types of smooth muscle tumors of the uterus that could be associated with BML are smooth muscle tumors of uncertain malignant potential, leiomyosarcomas, and endometrial stromal tumors.[33,35,36] BML has been considered by some as a low-grade endometrial stromal sarcoma[37] and malignant uterine leiomyoma,[38] but the evidence supporting these concepts is not very strong.

The most accepted hypothesis regarding the etiology of BML is that cells of pulmonary BML nodules are derived from uterine cells dislodged from the uterus at the time of myomectomy and hysterectomy performed for treatment of fibroids. Alternatively, it is also possible that BML could originate from lung smooth muscle cells or other sites containing smooth muscle cells.

DIAGNOSIS

This unusual diagnosis is most frequently made by the accidental detection of lung nodules by imaging procedures done for other reasons in women with a history of prior hysterectomy or myomectomy. In cases of BML presenting with symptoms of cough, wheezing, and chest pain, subsequent radiographs or chest CT scans may reveal the presence of lung nodules. BML lung nodules have been detected in premenopausal women from just after a few months to more than 30 years following myomectomy or hysterectomy. Currently, there is no straightforward and simple way to diagnose BML based on clinical criteria (**Fig. 3**). The main feature of this disease is the finding of single or multiple lung nodules that are well-circumscribed and range in size from a few millimeters to several centimeters. The presence of cysts has resulted in a misdiagnosis of LAM in some cases of BML[3,39]; however, in contrast to LAM,[14] lymphatic involvement has not been reported in BML.[14] As mentioned previously, lung BML is usually asymptomatic. A special case in which nonpulmonary symptoms could lead to a diagnosis of BML is intravenous leiomyomatosis associated with uterine leiomyomas.[40] Intravenous leiomyomatosis is a rare form of leiomyoma originating from the uterus that is characterized by intravascular tumor invasion through the uterine veins, reaching into the inferior vena cava, the right heart chambers, and pulmonary artery.[40,41,42] Leiomyomatosis peritonealis is a rare condition characterized by the presence of multiple subperitoneal or peritoneal smooth muscle nodules throughout the peritoneal surface, and should be considered in patients presenting with peritoneal lesions.[43] According to guidelines for treatment and follow-up of lung nodules smaller than 8 mm diameter, it is important to determine the distribution of the nodules, and risk factors to help establish a diagnosis and follow-up plan.[44,45] Lung

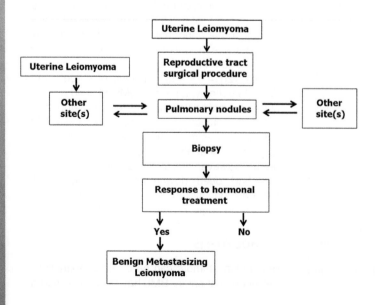

Fig. 3. Considerations in the diagnosis and management of BML.

biopsies have been more frequently used to establish a diagnosis of BML and rule out the presence of a malignant tumor.

In most cases, patients with BML present with multiple lung nodules that develop some time after a myomectomy or hysterectomy for treatment of uterine fibroids.[3] The differential diagnosis of BML includes a large number of lung diseases that present as diffuse pulmonary nodules with or without cystic lesions. Among these are sarcoidosis, silicosis, and hematogenous malignancies, such as thyroid carcinoma, choriocarcinoma, seminoma, squamous cell carcinoma, adenocarcinoma, lymphoma, bronchoalveolar carcinoma, and Kaposi sarcoma.[45] Several pulmonary infections may present with pulmonary nodules, namely, septic emboli caused by endocarditis, tuberculosis, fungal infections, paragonimiasis and parasitic diseases. Several nodular and cystic diseases, including LAM, Langerhans cell histiocytosis, lymphocytic interstitial pneumonia, Birt-Hogg-Dubé syndrome, and light chain deposition disease, must be considered in the differential diagnosis.[46–48] A careful history and physical examination can quickly rule out many of the listed conditions. Lack of systemic symptoms or any symptoms at all, along with a history of uterine fibroids and prior uterine surgery is highly suggestive of BML. CT imaging of the chest and abdomen may detect the presence of a malignancy or infection. Ultimately, tissue diagnosis may be required to rule out some of those diagnoses and establish the diagnosis of BML. This may consist of a transbronchial biopsy or an open lung biopsy (see **Fig. 3**).

Because there are no reports of large cohorts of patients with BML, it has not been possible to identify circulating factors or cell markers that may assist in the diagnosis of BML. Similarly, no hematological abnormalities have been detected in patients with BML.

TREATMENT

There is no standard treatment for patients with BML. In the case of an asymptomatic premenopausal woman found to have developed lung nodules sometime after having had a uterine procedure to resect fibroids, a conservative approach may be undertaken. The slow-growing behavior of BML suggests that they may be left untreated unless there are symptoms. Frequently, treatment of patients with pulmonary BML has involved uterine fibroid resection and manipulation of hormonal status. Changes in BML lung tumor size associated with menopause or during pregnancy have provided evidence for a role of hormonal changes in the development progression of BML.[49–51] Because BML is highly associated with uterine leiomyomas, treatments for uterine fibroids, which reduce estrogen action, are often considered for patients with BML.[3,52,53] Because progestins and estrogens seem to increase the growth of BML lung nodules, treatments that include GnRH (gonadotropin-releasing hormone) analogs, selective estrogen receptor modulators, selective progesterone receptor modulators, and aromatase inhibitors have been used.[52,53] In cases of BML that are refractory to anti-estrogen therapy, such as aromatase inhibitors, surgical treatment can be considered.[52]

Surgical procedures used to treat uterine leiomyomas include minimally invasive techniques and hysteroscopic myomectomy, dilation of the cervix, curettage, laparoscopic myomectomy, abdominal myomectomy, and hysterectomy.[36,53]

Different combinations of drugs have been used. Patients with BML have been treated with leuprolide acetate, letrozole, leuprolide acetate, aromatase inhibitor, and antiprogestin (CDB-2914). Changes in bone mineral density may occur due to the antiestrogenic therapy. Although bilateral oophorectomy has been the most used method, unilateral oophorectomy has been shown to be sufficient to cause resolution of lung BML tumors. For patients with pulmonary involvement, hysterectomy, salpingo-oophorectomy, or antiestrogen therapy is recommended if lung symptoms are present. However, lung function should be monitored. Surgery should be considered for patients with spine-related symptoms.[30]

PROGNOSIS

The prognosis of patients with BML is favorable. The lung lesions are usually identified many years (months to more than 30 years) after hysterectomy or myomectomy and the growth rate of these tumors is slow. Because uterine fibroid and leiomyomas appear more prevalent in individuals of African descent,[9,54] it has been suggested that vigilance for subsequent BML should be more intensive in this demographic. Involvement of other sites (eg, heart, veins, spine) could influence the prognosis of patients with BML.

SUMMARY

BML is characterized by the presence of a single nodule or multiple nodules scattered throughout the lungs. Pulmonary BML has been mainly associated with uterine leiomyomas. Pathologically, BML resembles lung hamartomas (the most common benign lung tumor), low-grade leiomyosarcomas, and diseases characterized by smooth muscle cell proliferation (eg, LAM). Patients with pulmonary BML are usually asymptomatic but may present with respiratory symptoms or manifestations, including shortness of breath or pneumothorax. In most cases, patients present with multiple pulmonary tumors, which develop after myomectomy and hysterectomy, although less frequently, lung nodules may develop before hysterectomy.[3] Other diseases that may mimic BML include primary leiomyoma, primary leiomyosarcoma, metastatic leiomyosarcoma, pulmonary hamartoma, leiomyomatous hyperplasia, infectious processes including tuberculosis, and LAM. Transbronchial and open lung biopsy have been used to diagnose BML. Pharmacologic or surgical interventions to decrease estrogen burden in patients with BML can result in regression. Because some cases show recurrent nodules, continued monitoring is important.

REFERENCES

1. Cohen JD, Robins HI. Response of "benign" metastasizing leiomyoma to progestin withdrawal. Case report. Eur J Gynaecol Oncol 1993;14(1):44–5.
2. Pitts S, Oberstein EM, Glassberg MK. Benign metastasizing leiomyoma and lymphangioleiomyomatosis: sex-specific diseases? Clin Chest Med 2004;25(2):343–60.
3. Taveira-DaSilva AM, Alford CE, Levens ED, et al. Favorable response to antigonadal therapy for a benign metastasizing leiomyoma. Obstet Gynecol 2012;119(2 Pt 2):438–42.
4. Cai A, Li L, Tan H, et al. Benign metastasizing leiomyoma. Case report and review of the literature. Herz 2014;39(7):867–70.
5. Motegi M, Takayanagi N, Sando Y, et al. [A case of so-called benign metastasizing leiomyoma responsive to progesterone]. Nihon Kyobu Shikkan Gakkai Zasshi 1993;31(7):890–5.
6. Kang MW, Kang SK, Yu JH, et al. Benign metastasizing leiomyoma: metastasis to rib and vertebra. Ann Thorac Surg 2011;91(3):924–6.
7. Jo JH, Lee JH, Kim DC, et al. A case of benign metastasizing leiomyoma with multiple metastasis to the soft tissue, skeletal muscle, lung and breast. Korean J Intern Med 2006;21(3):199–201.
8. Hur JW, Lee S, Lee J-B, et al. What are MRI findings of spine benign metastasizing leiomyoma? Case report with literature review. Eur Spine J 2015;24(Suppl 4):S600–5.
9. Blake RE. Leiomyomata uteri: hormonal and molecular determinants of growth. J Natl Med Assoc 2007;99(10):1170–84.
10. Wentling GK, Sevin BU, Geiger XJ, et al. Benign metastasizing leiomyoma responsive to megestrol: case report and review of the literature. Int J Gynecol Cancer 2005;15(6):1213–7.
11. Ki EY, Hwang SJ, Lee KH, et al. Benign metastasizing leiomyoma of the lung. World J Surg Oncol 2013;11:279.
12. Gatti JM, Morvan G, Henin D, et al. Leiomyomatosis metastasizing to the spine. A case report. J Bone Joint Surg Am 1983;65(8):1163–5.
13. Paley D, Fornasier VL. Leiomyomatosis metastasizing to the spine. J Bone Joint Surg Am 1984;66(4):630.
14. Taveira-DaSilva AM, Pacheco-Rodriguez G, Moss J. The natural history of lymphangioleiomyomatosis: markers of severity, rate of progression and prognosis. Lymphat Res Biol 2010;8(1):9–19.
15. Miller J, Shoni M, Siegert C, et al. Benign metastasizing leiomyomas to the lungs: an institutional case series and a review of the recent literature. Ann Thorac Surg 2016;101(1):253–8.
16. Orejola WC, Vaidya AP, Elmann EM. Benign metastasizing leiomyomatosis of the lungs presenting a miliary pattern. Ann Thorac Surg 2014;98(5):e113–4.
17. Loukeri AA, Pantazopoulos IN, Tringidou R, et al. Benign metastasizing leiomyoma presenting as cavitating lung nodules. Respir Care 2014;59(7):e94–7.
18. Travis WD, Brambilla E, Nicholson AG, et al. The 2015 World Health Organization classification of lung tumors: impact of genetic, clinical and radiologic advances since the 2004 classification. J Thorac Oncol 2015;10(9):1243–60.
19. Thway K, Fisher C. PEComa: morphology and genetics of a complex tumor family. Ann Diagn Pathol 2015;19(5):359–68.
20. Commandeur AE, Styer AK, Teixeira JM. Epidemiological and genetic clues for molecular mechanisms involved in uterine leiomyoma development and growth. Hum Reprod Update 2015;21(5):593–615.
21. Farquhar CM, Steiner CA. Hysterectomy rates in the United States 1990-1997. Obstet Gynecol 2002;99(2):229–34.
22. Wu JM, Wechter ME, Geller EJ, et al. Hysterectomy rates in the United States, 2003. Obstet Gynecol 2007;110(5):1091–5.
23. Kayser K, Zink S, Schneider T, et al. Benign metastasizing leiomyoma of the uterus: documentation of clinical, immunohistochemical and lectin-histochemical data of ten cases. Virchows Arch 2000;437(3):284–92.
24. Nistal M, Hardisson D, Riestra ML. Multiple pulmonary leiomyomatous hamartomas associated with a bronchogenic cyst in a man. Arch Pathol Lab Med 2003;127(4):e194–6.
25. Folpe AL, Kwiatkowski DJ. Perivascular epithelioid cell neoplasms: pathology and pathogenesis. Hum Pathol 2010;41(1):1–15.

26. Matsumoto Y, Horiba K, Usuki J, et al. Markers of cell proliferation and expression of melanosomal antigen in lymphangioleiomyomatosis. Am J Respir Cell Mol Biol 1999;21(3):327–36.

27. Martignoni G, Pea M, Reghellin D, et al. PEComas: the past, the present and the future. Virchows Arch 2008;452(2):119–32.

28. Nucci MR, Drapkin R, Dal Cin P, et al. Distinctive cytogenetic profile in benign metastasizing leiomyoma: pathogenetic implications. Am J Surg Pathol 2007;31(5):737–43.

29. Markowski DN, Holzmann C, Bullerdiek J. Genetic alterations in uterine fibroids–a new direction for pharmacological intervention? Expert Opin Ther Targets 2015;19(11):1485–94.

30. Shariftabrizi A, Abdullah A, Jacob S, et al. Incidental finding of synchronous, benign, metastasizing leiomyoma with distinct cytogenetics in the lung and uterus. Conn Med 2015;79(1):37–9.

31. Thomas C, Gustafsson JA. The different roles of ER subtypes in cancer biology and therapy. Nat Rev Cancer 2011;11(8):597–608.

32. Patton KT, Cheng L, Papavero V, et al. Benign metastasizing leiomyoma: clonality, telomere length and clinicopathologic analysis. Mod Pathol 2006; 19(1):130–40.

33. Hendrickson MR, Tavassoli FA, Kempson RL, et al. Mesenchymal tumours and related lesions. In: Tavassoli FA, Devilee P, editors. World Health Organization classification of tumours: pathology and genetics of tumours of the breast and female genital organs. Lyon (France): IARC Press; 2003. p. 233–44.

34. Roy D, Liehr JG. Estrogen, DNA damage and mutations. Mutat Res 1999;424(1–2):107–15.

35. Kempson RL, Hendrickson MR. Smooth muscle, endometrial stromal, and mixed Mullerian tumors of the uterus. Mod Pathol 2000;13(3):328–42.

36. Chen S, Zhang Y, Zhang J, et al. Pulmonary benign metastasizing leiomyoma from uterine leiomyoma. World J Surg Oncol 2013;11:163.

37. Tatebe S, Oka K, Kuraoka S, et al. Benign metastasizing leiomyoma of the lung: potential role of low-grade malignancy. Thorac Cardiovasc Surg 2009; 57(3):180–3.

38. Ip PP, Tse KY, Tam KF. Uterine smooth muscle tumors other than the ordinary leiomyomas and leiomyosarcomas: a review of selected variants with emphasis on recent advances and unusual morphology that may cause concern for malignancy. Adv Anat Pathol 2010;17(2):91–112.

39. Banner AS, Carrington CB, Emory WB, et al. Efficacy of oophorectomy in lymphangioleiomyomatosis and benign metastasizing leiomyoma. N Engl J Med 1981;305(4):204–9.

40. Worley MJ Jr, Aelion A, Caputo TA, et al. Intravenous leiomyomatosis with intracardiac extension: a single-institution experience. Am J Obstet Gynecol 2009;201(6):574.e1–5.

41. Gui T, Qian Q, Cao D, et al. Computerized tomography angiography in preoperative assessment of intravenous leiomyomatosis extending to inferior vena cava and heart. BMC Cancer 2015;16(1):73.

42. Consamus EN, Reardon MJ, Ayala AG, et al. Metastasizing leiomyoma to heart. Methodist Debakey Cardiovasc J 2014;10(4):251–4.

43. Lim SY, Park JC, Bae JG, et al. Pulmonary and retroperitoneal benign metastasizing leiomyoma. Clin Exp Reprod Med 2011;38(3):174–7.

44. Gould MK, Donington J, Lynch WR, et al. Evaluation of individuals with pulmonary nodules: when is it lung cancer? Diagnosis and management of lung cancer, 3rd ed: American College of Chest Physicians evidence-based clinical practice guidelines. Chest 2013;143(Suppl 5):e93S–120S.

45. Boitsios G, Bankier AA, Eisenberg RL. Diffuse pulmonary nodules. AJR Am J Roentgenol 2010; 194(5):W354–66.

46. Richards JC, Lynch DA, Chung JH. Cystic and nodular lung disease. Clin Chest Med 2015;36(2): 299–312.

47. Gupta N, Vassallo R, Wikenheiser-Brokamp KA, et al. Diffuse cystic lung disease. Part I. Am J Respir Crit Care Med 2015;191(12):1354–66.

48. Gupta N, Vassallo R, Wikenheiser-Brokamp KA, et al. Diffuse cystic lung disease. Part II. Am J Respir Crit Care Med 2015;192(1):17–29.

49. Arai T, Yasuda Y, Takaya T, et al. Natural decrease of benign metastasizing leiomyoma. Chest 2000; 117(3):921–2.

50. Thomas EO, Gordon J, Smith-Thomas S, et al. Diffuse uterine leiomyomatosis with uterine rupture and benign metastatic lesions of the bone. Obstet Gynecol 2007;109(2 Pt2):528–30.

51. Horstmann JP, Pietra GG, Harman JA, et al. Spontaneous regression of pulmonary leiomyomas during pregnancy. Cancer 1977;39(1):314–21.

52. Lewis EI, Chason RJ, DeCherney AH, et al. Novel hormone treatment of benign metastasizing leiomyoma: an analysis of five cases and literature review. Fertil Steril 2013;99(7):2017–24.

53. Khan AT, Shehmar M, Gupta JK. Uterine fibroids: current perspectives. Int J Womens Health 2014;6: 95–114.

54. Baird DD, Dunson DB, Hill MC, et al. High cumulative incidence of uterine leiomyoma in black and white women: ultrasound evidence. Am J Obstet Gynecol 2003;188(1):100–7.

Index

Note: Page numbers of article titles are in **boldface** type.

chestmed.theclinics.com

Moving?

Make sure your subscription moves with you!

To notify us of your new address, find your **Clinics Account Number** (located on your mailing label above your name), and contact customer service at:

Email: journalscustomerservice-usa@elsevier.com

800-654-2452 (subscribers in the U.S. & Canada)
314-447-8871 (subscribers outside of the U.S. & Canada)

Fax number: 314-447-8029

Elsevier Health Sciences Division
Subscription Customer Service
3251 Riverport Lane
Maryland Heights, MO 63043

ELSEVIER

Printed and bound by CPI Group (UK) Ltd, Croydon, CR0 4YY

08/05/2025

01864686-0011